Seventh Edition

Pharmacy
Calculations
for Technicians

Skye A. McKennon

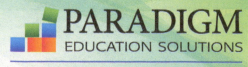

PARADIGM
EDUCATION SOLUTIONS

A DIVISION OF KENDALL HUNT

Minneapolis • Dubuque

VP of Content Strategy: Christine Hurney
Executive Acquiring Editor: Nancy Roberts
Development Editor: Nora Lambrecht
Director of Marketing: Keri Haas
Marketing and Communications Manager: Selena Hicks
Digital Project Manager: Tom Modl
Director of Publishing Services: Wendy S. Jochum
Publishing Specialist Supervisor: Carrie A. Maro
Supervisor of Prepress and Manufacturing: Cari M. Rieckens
Publishing Specialist: Nick Carolan

Care has been taken to verify the accuracy of information presented in this book. However, the authors, editors, and publisher cannot accept responsibility for web, email, newsgroup, or chat room subject matter or content, or for consequences from the application of the information in this book, and make no warranty, expressed or implied, with respect to its content.

Trademarks: Some of the product names and company names included in this book have been used for identification purposes only and may be trademarks or registered trade names of their respective manufacturers and sellers. The authors, editors, and publisher disclaim any affiliation, association, or connection with, or sponsorship or endorsement by, such owners.

Photo Credits: Following the index.

We have made every effort to trace the ownership of all copyrighted material and to secure permission from copyright holders. In the event of any question arising as to the use of any material, we will be pleased to make the necessary corrections in future printings. Thanks are due to the authors, publishers, and agents listed in the Photo Credits for permission to use the materials therein indicated.

Cover image © Shutterstock.com

© 2022, 2017, 2014 Paradigm Education Solutions, a division of Kendall Hunt
7900 Xerxes Avenue S STE 310
Minneapolis, MN 55431-1118
Email: CustomerService@ParadigmEducation.com
Website: ParadigmEducation.com

ISBN: 978-0-76389-303-3

Published in the United States of America

Brief Contents

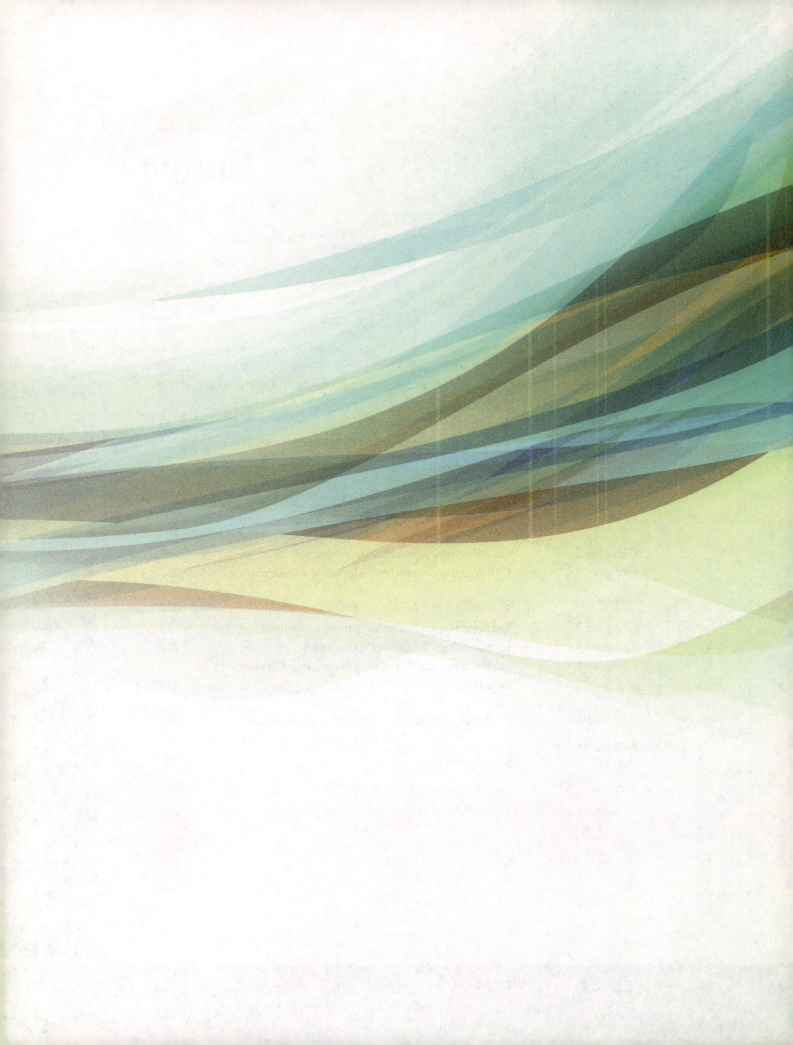

Contents

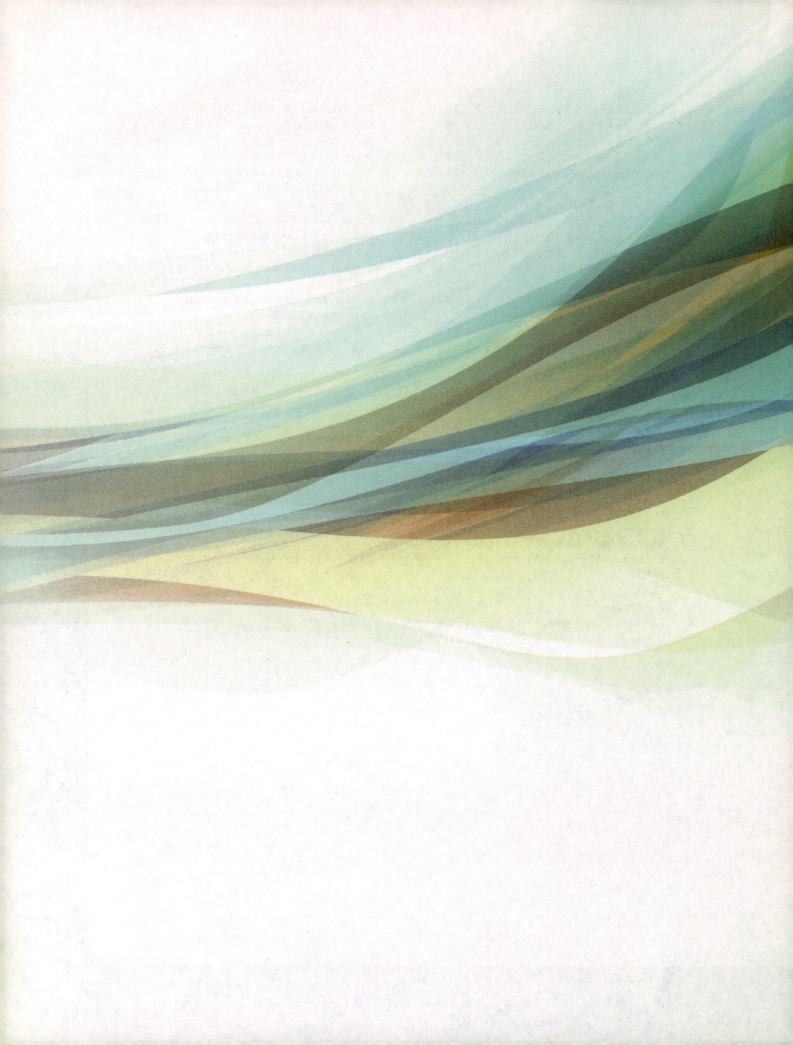

Pharmacy Calculations for Technicians: What Makes This New Edition Exciting?

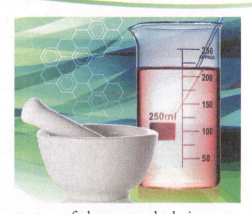

*P*harmacy Calculations for Technicians, Seventh Edition, provides entry-level and advanced-level mathematical concepts and calculation skills that pharmacy technicians need to prepare for the externship experience and certification exam and to achieve success in a career position at a community or an institutional pharmacy. Guided by clear, complete examples and practice problems, students review mathematical operations and concepts and learn different types of pharmacy calculation problems and the methods and formulas used to solve them.

The courseware program provides students with an understanding of measurement systems and conversions, an explanation of the elements of prescriptions and medication orders, and a proficiency in using the ratio-proportion and dimensional analysis calculation methods. In addition, the courseware offers plenty of practice in performing calculations for the preparation of medication doses, parenteral solutions, and compounded products. Finally, the courseware addresses calculations related to pharmacy operations, including inventory applications, purchasing needs, profit margins, and insurance reimbursements. With this comprehensive coverage of content, *Pharmacy Calculations for Technicians*, Seventh Edition, provides pharmacy technicians with the knowledge, skills, and confidence to provide safe and effective care for the patients they serve.

New Features in the Seventh Edition

The seventh edition offers several new features that benefit both students and instructors.

- **Cirrus™ Learning Environment:** This new and robust learning environment provides online access to course content, including an eBook, Watch & Learn videos, assessments, flash cards, handouts, and other activities.

- **Revised Contents:** The chapters have been reorganized to better align with the *ASHP/ACPE Accreditation Standards*. This stepped approach to learning allows students to master entry-level mathematical concepts and calculation skills before progressing to advanced-level skills in later chapters.

- **ASHP/ACPE Accreditation Standards:** The specific *ASHP/ACPE Accreditation Standards* that are covered in each chapter are listed in Appendix D.*

*Appendix D identifies the *ASHP/ACPE Accreditation Standards* associated with the chapter content. This list is meant for guidance purposes only and was created by the author of this text. Neither ASHP nor ACPE has participated in or had any role in creating the list of standards or any other content that is included in this book.

- **Targeted Learning Objectives:** The Learning Objectives for each chapter are correlated with specific, numbered sections of the chapter for easy student reference.
- **Chapter Introduction:** An introductory paragraph in each chapter provides students with a context for learning by relating the chapter content to real-world practice of a pharmacy technician.
- **Prescription and Medication Orders:** Literacy skills of *both* prescriptions and medication orders are addressed, including their applications, types, and elements.
- **Varied Problem-Solving Approaches:** Each chapter provides multiple approaches to solving pharmacy calculation problems to reinforce the concept that students should choose the method that they are most comfortable using and that ensures accuracy in their calculations.
- **Multiple Examples:** Each example problem follows a set format that introduces the problem, walks students through the problem-solving steps, and provides a clear, one-statement answer that repeats the wording of the initial question. This "bookend" format to solving word problems provides an effective approach for student learning.
- **Check Your Understanding Assessment:** An end-of-chapter section provides a quick, objective assessment of students' comprehension of key terms and mathematical concepts.

Consistency: Established Features

The seventh edition continues to offer tried-and-true features that complement the chapter content and contribute to student learning.

- Medication labels to promote student literacy and accurate interpretation
- Body system icons to accompany names of medications, providing a connection between specific drugs and the body systems they are used to treat
- Margin tips that reflect important chapter concepts and highlight safety alerts
- Figures and tables to illustrate and summarize mathematical concepts
- Key terms that are essential to understanding mathematical concepts and calculations
- End-of-chapter list of formulas that are introduced in the chapter
- Answer keys that reinforce self-study and promote student confidence in their problem-solving abilities
- An appendix that offers commonly used pharmacy abbreviations and acronyms for easy student reference

Study Assets: A Visual Walk-Through

Print and eBook Features
Learning Objectives

Each chapter begins with accreditation-targeted learning objectives establishing clear goals to focus each chapter.

Workplace Wisdom Boxes

Workplace Wisdom features identify important information related to the program and the art of pharmacy calculation.

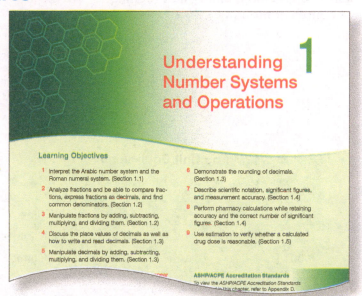

1

Understanding Number Systems and Operations

Learning Objectives

1 Interpret the Arabic number system and the Roman numeral system. (Section 1.1)

2 Analyze fractions and be able to compare fractions, express fractions as decimals, and find common denominators. (Section 1.2)

3 Manipulate fractions by adding, subtracting, multiplying, and dividing them. (Section 1.2)

4 Discuss the place values of decimals as well as how to write and read decimals. (Section 1.3)

5 Manipulate decimals by adding, subtracting, multiplying, and dividing them. (Section 1.3)

6 Demonstrate the rounding of decimals. (Section 1.3)

7 Describe scientific notation, significant figures, and measurement accuracy. (Section 1.4)

8 Perform pharmacy calculations while retaining accuracy and the correct number of significant figures. (Section 1.4)

9 Use estimation to verify whether a calculated drug dose is reasonable. (Section 1.5)

ASHP/ACPE Accreditation Standards
To view the ASHP/ACPE Accreditation Standards in this chapter, refer to Appendix D.

WORKPLACE WISDOM

In pharmacy practice, leading zeros are always used before a decimal point. For example, a one-half milligram should be written as 0.5 mg instead of .5 mg. The use of a leading zero helps to prevent medication errors. In fact, the US Food and Drug Administration has received reports of tenfold drug dosing errors due to prescriptions omitting a leading zero.

Examples

Examples provide realistic problem statements and show clear, step-by-step solutions. Many include authentic medication labels so students can gain confidence in reading and accurately interpreting labels.

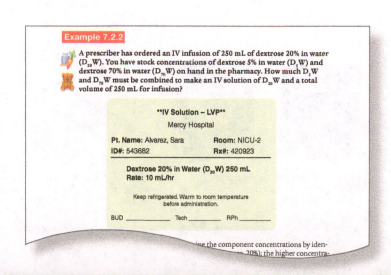

Example 7.2.2

A prescriber has ordered an IV infusion of 250 mL of dextrose 20% in water ($D_{20}W$). You have stock concentrations of dextrose 5% in water (D_5W) and dextrose 70% in water ($D_{70}W$) on hand in the pharmacy. How much D_5W and $D_{70}W$ must be combined to make an IV solution of $D_{20}W$ and a total volume of 250 mL for infusion?

IV Solution – LVP
Mercy Hospital

Pt. Name: Alvarez, Sara   Room: NICU-2
ID#: 543682   Rx#: 420923

Dextrose 20% in Water ($D_{20}W$) 250 mL
Rate: 10 mL/hr

Keep refrigerated. Warm to room temperature before administration.

BUD _____   Tech _____   RPh _____

...ine the component concentrations by identi-... 20%); the higher concentra-

Figures, Medication Labels, Tables, and Photographs

Engaging study tools enhance visual learning and aid memory and retention of course content.

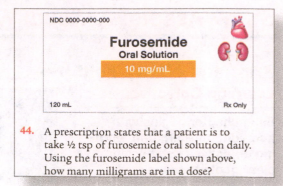

44. A prescription states that a patient is to take ½ tsp of furosemide oral solution daily. Using the furosemide label shown above, how many milligrams are in a dose?

TABLE 4.4 Metric Unit Equivalents

Kilo	Base	Milli	Micro
0.001 kg	1 g	1,000 mg	1,000,000 mcg
0.001 kL	1 L	1,000 mL	1,000,000 mcL
0.001 km	1 m	1,000 mm	1,000,000 mcm

FIGURE 4.1 Levothyroxine Tablet Strengths and Colors

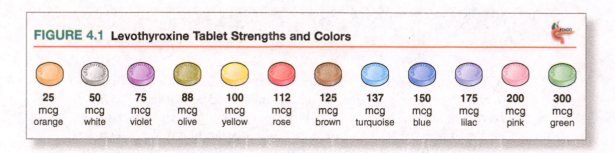

| 25 mcg orange | 50 mcg white | 75 mcg violet | 88 mcg olive | 100 mcg yellow | 112 mcg rose | 125 mcg brown | 137 mcg turquoise | 150 mcg blue | 175 mcg lilac | 200 mcg pink | 300 mcg green |

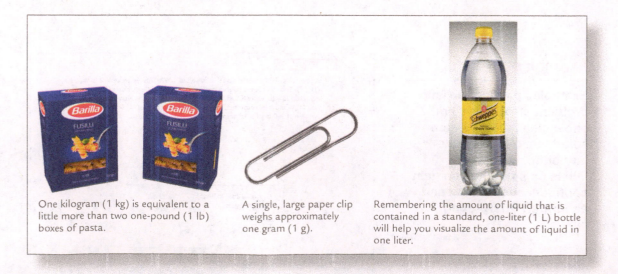

One kilogram (1 kg) is equivalent to a little more than two one-pound (1 lb) boxes of pasta.

A single, large paper clip weighs approximately one gram (1 g).

Remembering the amount of liquid that is contained in a standard, one-liter (1 L) bottle will help you visualize the amount of liquid in one liter.

Margin Features

Feature boxes spotlight important information.

 Put Down Roots

Offers word origins to make terms memorable.

 Work Wise

Gives advice on professional and soft skills.

 Safety Alert

Calls out warnings to avoid problems.

 Math Morsel

Supplies calculating hints.

 For Good Measure

Assists in accuracy with measuring.

 Name Exchange

Reminds about items with two names, such as brand and generic drugs.

 Quick Study

Suggests memory cues for common mathematical terms.

 Pharm Fact

Highlights interesting trivia and fun facts.

Body System Icons

Quick reference icons identify connections between drugs and the body systems they are prescribed to treat.

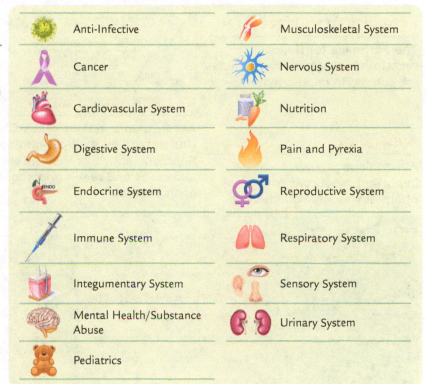

Anti-Infective	Musculoskeletal System
Cancer	Nervous System
Cardiovascular System	Nutrition
Digestive System	Pain and Pyrexia
Endocrine System	Reproductive System
Immune System	Respiratory System
Integumentary System	Sensory System
Mental Health/Substance Abuse	Urinary System
Pediatrics	

Problem Sets

Activities located at the end of each section of text reinforce chapter content and provide opportunities for students to practice their skills and gain confidence in their abilities. Answers can be found in Appendix A.

1.4 Problem Set

Write the following numbers using standard notation.

1. 6.8×10^4
2. 1.87×10^6
3. 1.03×10^7
4. 8.4×10^{-4}
5. 7.68×10^{-3}
6. 6.239×10^{-5}

Write the following numbers using scientific notation.

7. 0.00000000329

Identify the number of significant figures in the following numbers. Assume that all final zeros in numbers without decimals are not significant. *Note:* The abbreviation *mL* means "milliliters"; the abbreviation *mg* means "milligrams"; the abbreviation *mcg* means "micrograms"; and the abbreviation *kg* means "kilograms."

13. 15.4324 grains
14. 1,500 mL
15. 0.21 mg
16. $1.07
17. 100,000 mcg
18. 507.2 mg
19. 1.01 kg

Chapter Summaries

Each chapter ends with a summary to reinforce key points.

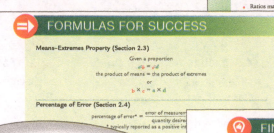

Formulas for Success

The Formulas for Success resource highlights new formulas introduced in each chapter.

FORMULAS FOR SUCCESS

Means–Extremes Property (Section 2.3)

Given a proportion

$$\frac{a}{b} = \frac{c}{d}$$

the product of means = the product of extremes

or

$$b \times c = a \times d$$

Percentage of Error (Section 2.4)

$$\text{percentage of error*} = \frac{\text{error of measurement}}{\text{quantity desired}}$$

* typically reported as a positive integer

CHAPTER SUMMARY

- Ratios are used to describe the amount of medication per dose or unit.
- Ratios may be expressed by using a colon (1:100 or 100:1) or by formatting as a fraction ($^1/_{100}$ or $^{100}/_1$).
- Ratios may be multiplied when a larger ... led when a smaller
- ... of parts per 100
- ...ons, and decimals ...ss the same value.
- ...cent to a numerical ... move the decimal ... left.
- ...merical value to ...100, or move the

- A proportion with one missing value may be solved if three of the four values are known.
- When using the ratio-proportion method to solve for a missing value, the numerators must have the same unit of measurement, and the denominators must have the same unit of measurement.
- The ratio-proportion method may be used to convert between units of measure by setting the ratio desired to be converted equal to a unit of 1.
- Percentage of error is calculated by dividing the error of measurement by the quantity desired, and then multiplying by 100.
- Error of measurement is the difference between the measured value and the quantity desired.

FIND SOLUTIONS

Take a moment to consider what you have learned in this chapter and respond thoughtfully to the prompts.

Note: To indicate your answer for Scenario A, Question 1, ask your instructor for the handout depicting measuring devices.

Scenario A: A patient who has poison ivy has been taking over-the-counter (OTC) diphenhydramine (Benadryl) for itching. The doctor has told the patient to take 50 ... as needed. The medi-...

Scenario C: You receive a prescription for an antibiotic suspension of amoxicillin 125 mg/5 mL. This medication is for a pediatric patient weighing 20 kg, and it is determined that each dose should be 25 mg.

5. How many milliliters are needed for each ... dose?

Appendices

Appendices provide important resources for pharmacy technician student.

Chapter Assessments

Assessments include quick Check Your Understanding multiple-choice quizzes and Find Solutions activities that present challenging situations and real-world scenarios for each chapter.

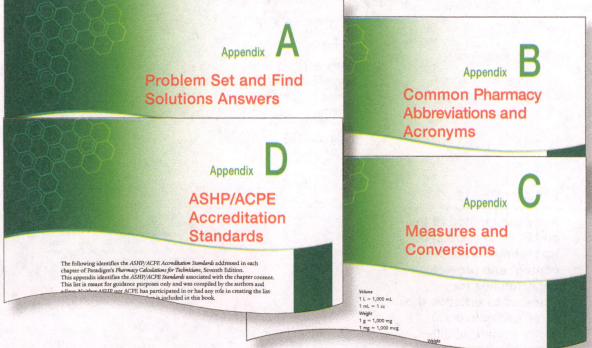

Appendix **A**

Problem Set and Find Solutions Answers

Appendix **B**

Common Pharmacy Abbreviations and Acronyms

Appendix **D**

ASHP/ACPE Accreditation Standards

The following identifies the *ASHP/ACPE Accreditation Standards* addressed in each chapter of Paradigm's *Pharmacy Calculations for Technicians*, Seventh Edition. This appendix identifies the *ASHP/ACPE Standards* associated with the chapter content. This list is meant for guidance purposes only and was compiled by the authors and ... Neither ASHP nor ACPE has participated in or had any role in creating the list ... is included in this book.

Appendix **C**

Measures and Conversions

Volume
1 L = 1,000 mL
1 mL = 1 cc
Weight
1 g = 1,000 mg
1 mg = 1,000 mcg

Weight

Index

Terms and topics can be found quickly using this location guide.

The Cirrus Learning Environment

Elevating student success and instructor efficiency

Cirrus provides a digital courseware solution to meet the learning needs of pharmacy technician students and the teaching needs of their instructors. Cirrus delivers complete course content in a cloud-based learning environment that is platform-independent, ensuring that students and instructors receive the same online learning experience whether they are using PCs, Macs, or Chromebooks. This course content can integrate with a school's preferred learning management system, such as Canvas, Blackboard, D2L, or Moodle, or can be accessed directly in the Cirrus learning environment.

Cirrus provides Student Resources and Instructor Resources to accompany the *Pharmacy Calculations for Technicians*, Seventh Edition, textbook. These resources are outlined below.

Student Resources

Student Resources allow students to access all relevant course content, submit graded assignments and assessments to the grade book, obtain feedback on practice exams, and test their understanding of chapter concepts.

- **Student eBook** allows the textbook content to be accessed through any device (desktop computer, laptop computer, tablet, or smartphone).
- **Learning Objectives** set goals for student learning.
- **Watch and Learn Lessons** provide chapter content in easily digestible sections. Follow-up questions ensure student comprehension.
- **Flash Cards** test students' recall of key terms and their definitions that are critical to student understanding of chapter content.
- **Chapter Summary** provides students with a study tool to review key chapter concepts.
- **Student Practice Exam** offers 30 objective questions to test students' understanding of chapter concepts.
- **Glossary of Key Terms** provides a book-wide resource of important key terms from all chapters in a searchable format.

Instructor Resources

Instructor Resources, visible only to instructors, allow instructors to plan their curriculum, schedule assignments, track student progress, and manage the grade book. The Instructor Resources are organized into three sections: Planning, Delivery, and Assessment.

Planning

- **Planning the Course** document helps instructors plan their course curriculum and create a syllabus.
- **Teaching Objectives** set goals that enable student learning.

- **ASHP/ACPE Accreditation Standards** guide chapter content. These entry-level and advanced-level competencies are correlated to each chapter, providing assurance that the curriculum materials are preparing students for the pharmacy technician externship, certification exam, and workforce.
- **Lesson Plans** offer activities, tips, and resources for shaping high-interest lessons for student learning.

Delivery

- **PowerPoint Presentations** reinforce key chapter concepts and can be used by instructors in their course delivery or can be accessed by students (at instructor discretion) as a supplement to instruction.
- **Handouts** depict devices used to measure medication doses, such as a dosing spoon, dosing cup, and oral syringe. These handouts accompany several end-of-chapter exercises and test students' ability to measure volumes accurately.
- **Answer Keys** for Problem Sets, Check Your Understanding, Find Solutions, and Handouts are available for instructor use during course delivery.

Assessment

- **Instructor-Controlled Exam** offers 40 objective questions and can be used as a final chapter assessment.
- **Additional Chapter Assessments** offer supplemental questions to test student comprehension of chapter content.

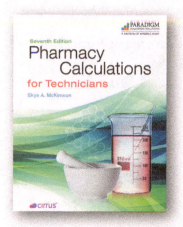

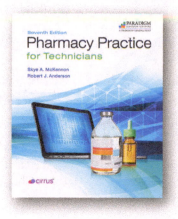

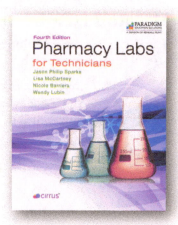

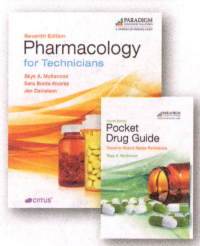

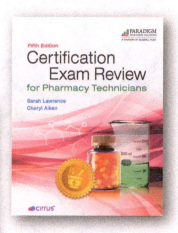

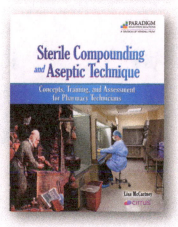

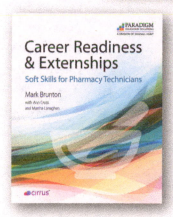

Paradigm's Comprehensive Pharmacy Technician Series

In addition to *Pharmacy Calculations for Technicians*, Seventh Edition, Paradigm Education Solutions offers additional courseware designed specifically for the pharmacy technician curriculum.

- *Pharmacy Practice for Technicians,* Seventh Edition

- *Pharmacy Labs for Technicians,* Fourth Edition

- *Pharmacology for Technicians,* Seventh Edition

- *Pocket Drug Guide: Generic-Brand Name Reference*

- *Certification Exam Review for Pharmacy Technicians,* Fifth Edition

- *Sterile Compounding and Aseptic Technique*

- *Career Readiness & Externships: Soft Skills for Pharmacy Technicians*

Related Health Career Courseware

Paradigm Education Solutions offers additional health career courseware that is particularly useful for pharmacy technicians.

- *What Language Does Your Patient Hurt In? A Practical Guide to Culturally Competent Care*, Third Edition

- *Medical Terminology: Connecting through Language*, First Edition

- *Exploring Electronic Health Records*, Second Edition

- *Emergency & Disaster Preparedness for Health Professionals*, Second Edition

- *Pharmacists and Pharmacy Technicians* eChapter

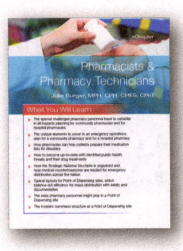

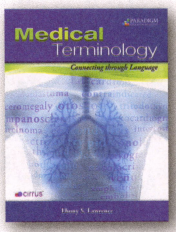

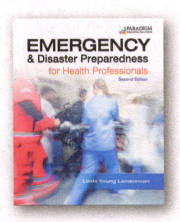

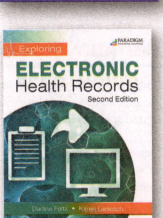

About the Author

Dr. Skye A. McKennon is a licensed pharmacist, board-certified pharmacotherapy specialist (BCPS), educator, and certified preventionist. Dr. McKennon completed her bachelor's degree and doctor of pharmacy (PharmD) degree from Washington State University. She completed postdoctoral residency training at Swedish Medical Center in Seattle, Washington and received a teaching certificate from the University of Washington.

Dr. McKennon has practice experience in the community, institutional, and ambulatory pharmacy settings. Her passion for teaching and education led her to faculty positions at the University of Washington School of Pharmacy and at the Washington State University College of Pharmacy, where she has received honors for teaching, interprofessional education, mentorship, scholarship, and community service.

Dr. McKennon has published in multiple peer-reviewed journals (including the *American Journal of Pharmacy Education and Currents in Pharmacy Teaching and Learning*) and co-authored six pharmacy textbooks. She has presented her work at international and national symposiums such as the Seventh International Conference on Interprofessional Practice and Education, the American Association of Colleges of Pharmacy annual meeting, the Academy of Integrative Health and Medicine annual meeting, and the Pharmacy Technicians Educators Council conference.

Courses designed and directed by Dr. McKennon include applied pharmacotherapeutics, institutional pharmacy practice, diabetes prevention, and evidence-based preventive health. She has been both an instructor and a guest lecturer for various courses for pharmacy and other health science students, including calculations, therapeutics, pharmacotherapy for older adults, global health brigades, and law and ethics.

About the Experts

Several exceptional instructors and content specialists reviewed and contributed to this program's courseware to help ensure accuracy and appropriate institutional approaches. Special thanks are due to these individuals who shared their vast expertise and passion for the profession.

Expert Reviewers

Anne LaVance, BS, CPhT, Delgado Community College
Andrea R. Redman, PharmD, BCPS, Emory Healthcare

Assessment Banks Writer

Francesca Morris, MHA, CPhT

Special Thanks

A special thank you to **Don A. Ballington, Tova Wiegand-Green,** and the many experts and contributors who contributed to earlier editions of this courseware.

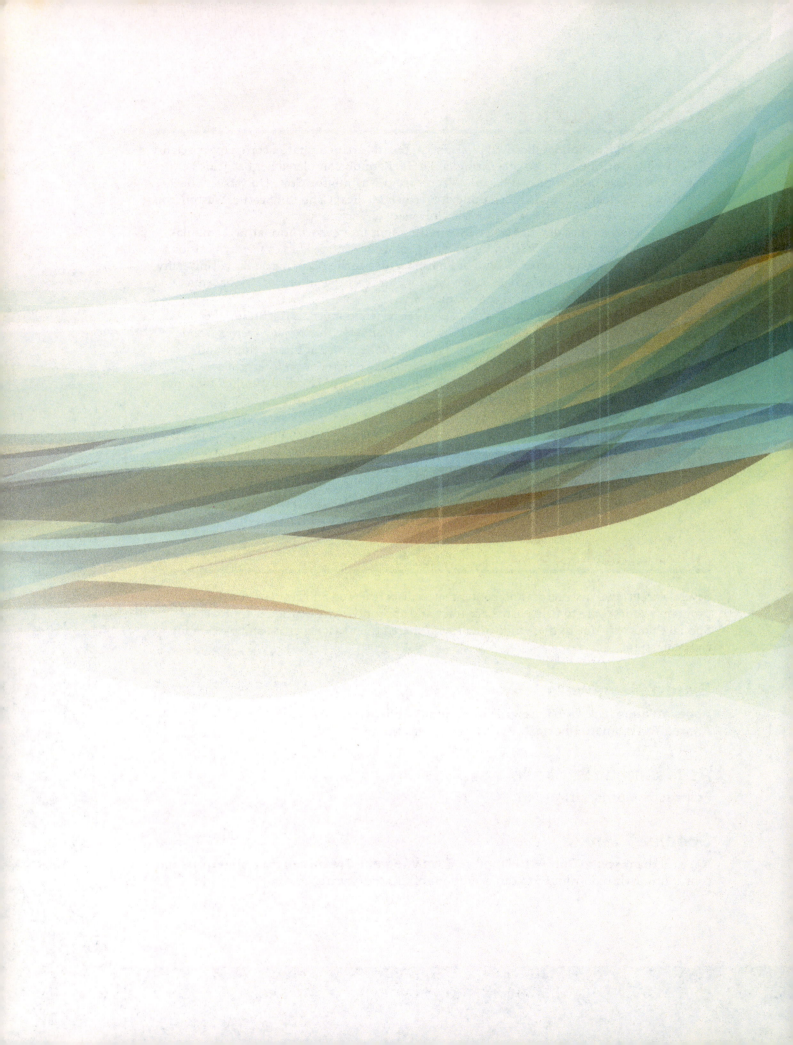

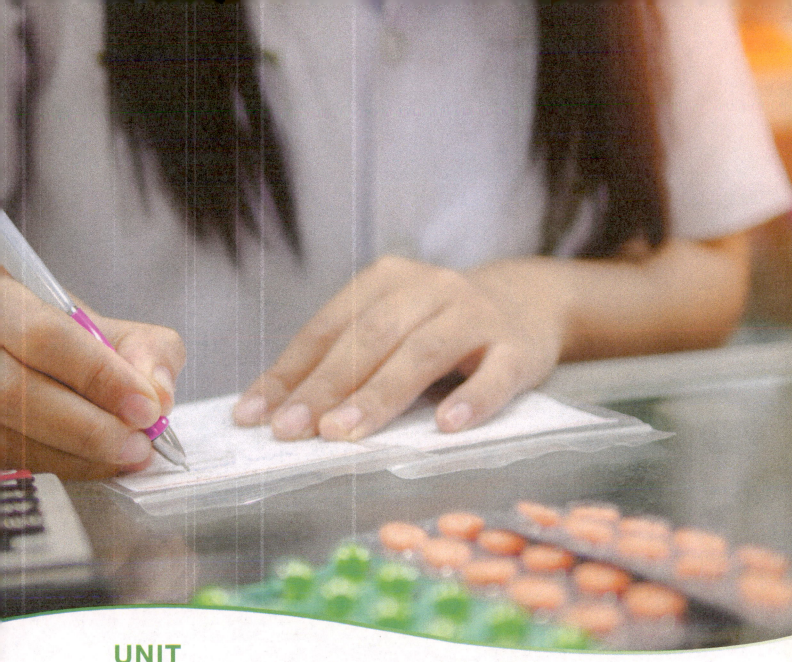

UNIT

1 Fundamentals of Pharmacy Calculations

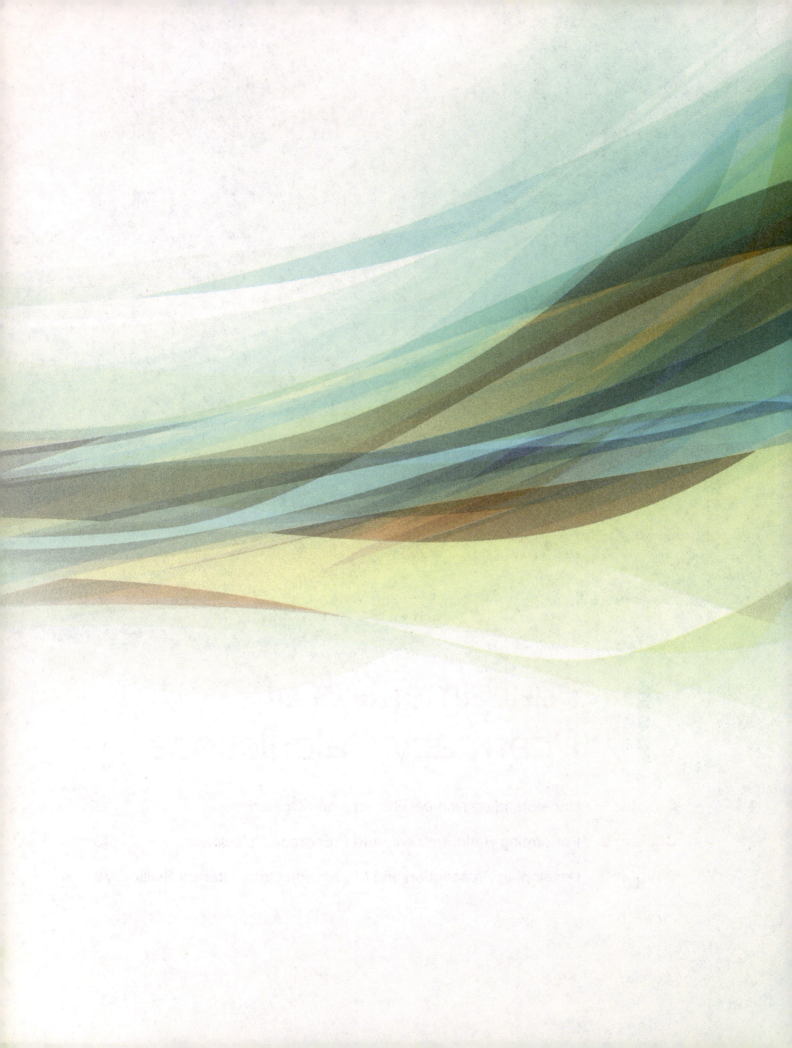

1

Understanding Number Systems and Operations

Learning Objectives

1 Interpret the Arabic number system and the Roman numeral system. (Section 1.1)

2 Analyze fractions and be able to compare fractions, express fractions as decimals, and find common denominators. (Section 1.2)

3 Manipulate fractions by adding, subtracting, multiplying, and dividing them. (Section 1.2)

4 Discuss the place values of decimals as well as how to write and read decimals. (Section 1.3)

5 Manipulate decimals by adding, subtracting, multiplying, and dividing them. (Section 1.3)

6 Demonstrate the rounding of decimals. (Section 1.3)

7 Describe scientific notation, significant figures, and measurement accuracy. (Section 1.4)

8 Perform pharmacy calculations while retaining accuracy and the correct number of significant figures. (Section 1.4)

9 Use estimation to verify whether a calculated drug dose is reasonable. (Section 1.5)

For a key to the body system icons that appear in each chapter of this textbook, refer to the Preface.

ASHP/ACPE Accreditation Standards

To view the *ASHP/ACPE Accreditation Standards* addressed in this chapter, refer to Appendix D.

Working in a healthcare setting often requires you to have **number sense**, or the ability to know what numbers and symbols mean, understand how numbers relate to one another, and apply your knowledge of numbers to real-world settings. Number sense is the foundation for understanding number systems, fractions, decimals, scientific notation, significant figures, and estimation. These skills are critical to the preparation, filling, and dispensing of medications.

1.1 Number Systems

Two types of number systems are used in pharmacy calculations: Arabic numbers and Roman numerals. The Arabic number system uses numbers, fractions, and decimals, whereas the Roman numeral system uses letters to represent quantities or amounts. The Arabic number system is more commonly used in the healthcare setting.

Understanding the Arabic Number System

The **Arabic number system** has its roots in India and consists of 10 digits: 0, 1, 2, 3, 4, 5, 6, 7, 8, and 9. When these digits are combined, they represent every possible number. In expressions using Arabic numbers, whole numbers are to the left of a decimal point, whereas fractions are to the right of a decimal point.

Understanding the Roman Numeral System

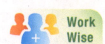

Work Wise

Pharmacy technicians should ask for clarification for any Arabic numbers or Roman numerals that are difficult to read or understand. Engaging in this confirmation process can help to prevent a medication error.

The **Roman numeral system** can be traced back to ancient Rome and includes seven main symbols: *I* (equal to 1), *V* (equal to 5), *X* (equal to 10), *L* (equal to 50), *C* (equal to 100), *D* (equal to 500), and *M* (equal to 1,000). Being able to interpret Roman numerals when used on prescriptions and medication orders is important for the accurate preparation and dispensing of medications (see Table 1.1).

Roman numerals are expressed as either uppercase letters or lowercase letters. The most frequently used uppercase letters are the Roman numerals *I*, *V*, and *X*, which represent 1, 5, and 10, respectively. For example, tablet quantities of ampicillin may be written in uppercase letters, such as *ampicillin 250 mg XXX tabs*, indicating 30 tablets. The lowercase letter *i* is used to represent 1, the lowercase letter *ii* to represent 2, and so on. For example, *aspirin gr iii* indicates 3 grains of aspirin. To prevent errors in interpretation, a line is drawn above the lowercase letters, with the dot above the line (for example: *i, ii, iii*). Another lowercase letter you may see in pharmacy practice is the lowercase letter *s*. For example, the abbreviation *ss* or *s̄s̄* means ½.

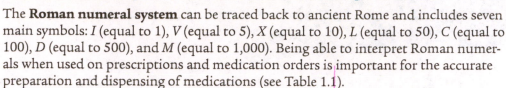

TABLE 1.1 Guidelines for Interpreting Roman Numerals

1. When a numeral is repeated or a smaller numeral follows a larger one, the numerals are added.

   II = 1 + 1 = 2
   VII = 5 + 1 + 1 = 7
   XXI = 10 + 10 + 1 = 21
   LVII = 50 + 5 + 1 + 1 = 57
   LXV = 50 + 10 + 5 = 65
   CXIII = 100 + 10 + 1 + 1 + 1 = 113

2. When a smaller numeral comes before a larger numeral, the smaller numeral is subtracted from the larger numeral.

   IV = 5 − 1 = 4
   IX = 10 − 1 = 9
   CD = 500 − 100 = 400

3. Numerals are never repeated more than three times in sequence.

   III = 3
   IV = 4
   XXX = 30
   XL = 40

4. When a smaller numeral comes between two larger numerals, the smaller numeral is subtracted from the numeral that follows.

   XIX = 10 + (10 − 1) = 19
   XIV = 10 + (5 − 1) = 14

Table 1.2 compares commonly used Roman numerals and their equivalent Arabic numbers. The examples that follow the table show the use of Roman numerals in both dosing instructions and quantity to dispense.

TABLE 1.2 **Comparison of Roman Numerals and Arabic Numbers**

Roman Numeral		Arabic Number	Roman Numeral		Arabic Number
ss or s̄s̄	=	½ or 0.5	L or l	=	50
I or i or i̇	=	1	C or c*	=	100
V or v	=	5	D or d	=	500
X or x	=	10	M or m	=	1,000

*Be aware that cubic centimeter is abbreviated as *cc*. However, the use of this abbreviation is discouraged due to the risk of misinterpretation.

Example 1.1.1

A prescription is received in the pharmacy and includes the following notation: *Disp: C tablets*. How many tablets are to be dispensed?

Answer: The quantity of tablets to dispense is 100 tablets, indicated by the Roman numeral *C*.

Roman numerals may be grouped together to express different quantities. To interpret these numbers, addition and subtraction must be used, as specified in the guidelines shown in Table 1.1. Example 1.1.2 demonstrates how to read groups of Roman numerals.

Example 1.1.2

The following prescription is received in the pharmacy. How many tablets are in the ordered dose, and how many tablets are to be dispensed?

 ℞ **Diphenhydramine XXV mg**

Dosing instructions: Take ï tablets by mouth each night.

Quantity to dispense: XXXII tablets

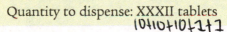

To begin, determine the number of tablets in the ordered dose that the patient will take each night.

$$\text{ï tablets} = 1 + 1 = 2 \text{ tablets}$$

Then calculate the number of tablets to dispense by adding the Roman numerals on the prescription.

$$\text{XXXII tablets} = 10 + 10 + 10 + 1 + 1 = 32 \text{ tablets}$$

Answer: For this prescription, there are 2 tablets of diphenhydramine in the ordered dose, and 32 tablets must be dispensed.

1.1 Problem Set *odds only!*

Provide the equivalent Arabic number for each of the following Roman numerals.

1. X
2. V
3. DCXXIV
4. MML
5. XLVIII

Provide the equivalent Roman numeral for each of the following Arabic numbers.

6. 17
7. 67
8. 1,995

Solve the following problems and provide your answers in Roman numerals.

9. 7 + 6 =
10. 354 − 27 =
11. 2 × 45 =
12. 150 ÷ 2 =

Solve the following problems and provide your answers in Arabic numbers.

13. VIIss + XV + IV =
14. XLVII − XIX =
15. XVII × IV =
16. XLII ÷ III =

Applications

17. A patient is to take "VIIss tablets three times daily." How many tablets are to be taken at each dose?

18. Using the prescription below, answer the following questions. *Note:* The abbreviation *gr* means "grains," and the abbreviation *po* means "by mouth."

> **R͓   Aspirin gr X**
> Dosing instructions: ï po daily
> Quantity to dispense: C

a. What is the strength of the tablet?
b. What is the daily dose?
c. What is the quantity to be dispensed?

19. Using the prescription below, answer the following questions. *Note:* The abbreviation *po* means "by mouth," and the abbreviation *TID* means "three times a day."

> **R͓   Erythromycin 250 mg**
> Dosing instructions: ï po TID with food
> Quantity to dispense: XXVII

a. How many tablets will be taken at each dose?
b. How many days will the prescription last?

20. Using the prescription below, answer the following questions. *Note:* The abbreviation *po* means "by mouth."

> **R͓   Glipizide tablet 5 mg**
> ïï po every morning
> ï po with lunch
> ïï po with dinner
> Quantity to dispense: CL

a. How many tablets are taken each day?
b. How many tablets will be dispensed?

Self-check your work in Appendix A.

1.2 Fractions

When an object is divided into parts, each part is a **fraction** of the whole. For example, a pie might be divided into eight equal slices, each of which is a fraction, or $^1/_8$, of the whole pie. The pie is still whole but has been divided into eight slices. If you select one slice, it is one-eighth of the whole pie, or 1 (the number of slices in the selection) over 8 (the number of slices in the whole pie). In the fraction $^3/_8$, the selection is 3 of the 8 slices (see Figure 1.1).

FIGURE 1.1
Fractions of a Whole Pie

8 slices = $\frac{8}{8}$ of the whole pie   3 slices = $\frac{3}{8}$ of the whole pie   1 slice = $\frac{1}{8}$ of the whole pie

Quick Study

The orientation of the numerator and the denominator in a fraction can be remembered with this catchphrase: The **d**enominator is **d**own below the line in a fraction.

A common fraction consists of a **numerator** (top number) and a **denominator** (bottom number). For example, in the fraction $^1/_8$, the numerator represents the number of pieces that are selected from the pie (1 piece), and the denominator represents the total number of pieces in the pie (8 pieces).

$$\text{numerator} \longrightarrow \frac{1}{8} \longleftarrow \text{denominator}$$

Just as a pie can be divided into parts, so can a tablet. Splitting a **scored tablet** is a common procedure for both pharmacy personnel and patients. Figure 1.2 shows how splitting a 1,000 milligram (mg) tablet into smaller parts relates to fractions.

FIGURE 1.2
Fractions of a Tablet

1 tablet = 1,000 mg $\frac{1}{2}$ tablet = 500 mg $\frac{1}{4}$ tablet = 250 mg

A fraction with the same numerator and denominator has a value of 1.

$$\frac{8}{8} \quad \frac{3}{3} \quad \frac{10}{10} \quad \frac{15}{15}$$

A fraction with a value less than 1 (numerator less than denominator) is called a *proper fraction*.

$$\frac{1}{4} \quad \frac{2}{3} \quad \frac{7}{8} \quad \frac{9}{10}$$

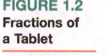
Math Morsel

Proper fractions always have a value less than 1, or less than the "whole" of the pie, tablet, or other object.

A fraction with a value greater than or equal to 1 (numerator greater than or equal to denominator) is called an *improper fraction*.

$$\frac{6}{5} \quad \frac{7}{5} \quad \frac{9}{6} \quad \frac{15}{8}$$

The combination of a whole number and a fraction is called a **mixed number**. A mixed number can be converted into an improper fraction by multiplying the whole number by the denominator and adding the numerator.

$$5\frac{1}{2} = \frac{(5 \times 2) + 1}{2} = \frac{11}{2}$$

An improper fraction can be converted into a mixed number by dividing the numerator by the denominator. The whole number is maintained, and the remainder becomes the new numerator (which is placed over the original denominator).

$$\frac{11}{2} = 11 \div 2 = 5\frac{1}{2}$$

A fraction in which the numerator, the denominator, or both the numerator and the denominator contain a fraction is called a **complex fraction**.

$$\frac{\frac{1}{4}}{\frac{1}{8}}$$

Two fractions that appear different but have the same value are called **equivalent fractions**. The following examples are equivalent fractions: $\frac{1}{2} = \frac{2}{4}$ and $\frac{3}{5} = \frac{15}{25}$. Two fractions are equivalent (equal) only if the product of the numerator (*a*) of the first fraction and the denominator (*d*) of the second fraction are equal to the product of the denominator (*b*) of the first fraction and the numerator (*c*) of the second fraction.

$$\text{If } \frac{a}{b} = \frac{c}{d} \text{ then } a \times d = b \times c$$

Consider the fractions $\frac{3}{4}$ and $\frac{9}{12}$. These fractions are equal if $3 \times 12 = 4 \times 9$. When you multiply the numbers, you see that $3 \times 12 = 36$ and $4 \times 9 = 36$. Therefore, $\frac{3}{4}$ and $\frac{9}{12}$ are equivalent or proportional fractions. The concept and relationship of equivalent fractions and proportions are important principles in pharmacy calculations.

Comparing Fractions

When comparing fractions with the same numerator, the fraction with the smaller denominator has the larger value.

$$\frac{1}{10} > \frac{1}{25}$$

If two fractions have the same denominator, the fraction with the larger numerator has the larger value.

$$\frac{3}{6} > \frac{2}{6}$$

Example 1.2.1

 Which nitroglycerin tablet is the smallest dose?

$$\frac{3}{10} \text{ mg tablet} \qquad \frac{4}{10} \text{ mg tablet} \qquad \frac{6}{10} \text{ mg tablet}$$

Answer: The $\frac{3}{10}$ mg tablet is the smallest dose.

Example 1.2.2

 Which nitroglycerin tablet is the largest dose?

$$\frac{1}{200} \text{ grain tablet} \qquad \frac{1}{150} \text{ grain tablet} \qquad \frac{1}{100} \text{ grain tablet}$$

Answer: The $\frac{1}{100}$ grain tablet is the largest dose.

If two fractions have different numerators and denominators, you must thoughtfully assess their values. This assessment can be performed by converting the fractions to equivalent fractions with the same denominator and then comparing the two fractions. This method is described in detail in the next pages. When medications are dosed using fractions, it is important to recognize which strengths are largest and smallest.

Adding and Subtracting Fractions

Safety Alert

When working with fractions, pharmacy technicians should always include the units (if known) after the number—for example, a $\frac{1}{2}$ mg tablet. Without clearly marked units, serious medication errors can occur.

Addition and subtraction are commonly used mathematical operations in pharmacy practice. A **sum** is the result of adding two or more numbers together. A **difference** is the result of subtracting two or more numbers. As a pharmacy technician, you may find yourself calculating the sum or difference of both whole numbers and fractions.

When adding or subtracting fractions with unlike denominators, it is necessary to create a **common denominator**, or a number into which each of the unlike denominators can be divided evenly. Think of it as making both fractions into "pieces of pies" with equal slices. Creating a common denominator requires transforming each fraction by multiplying it by a fraction that is equal to 1.

Multiplying a number by 1 does not change the value of the number ($5 \times 1 = 5$). Therefore, if you multiply a fraction by a fraction that equals 1 (such as $^5/_5$), you do not change the value of the fraction. This mathematical rule allows for the conversions in the following examples.

Example 1.2.3

Find the sum of $\frac{1}{2} + \frac{3}{5}$.

The lowest number that can be divided evenly by both 2 and 5 is 10. A quick way to determine a possible common denominator is to multiply the denominators ($2 \times 5 = 10$). Thus, 10 will be the common denominator for the two fractions, and each fraction must be converted to tenths.

To convert $\frac{1}{2}$ to tenths, multiply $\frac{1}{2}$ by $\frac{5}{5}$. The product is $\frac{5}{10}$.

$$\frac{1}{2} = \frac{1}{2} \times \frac{5}{5} = \frac{5}{10}$$

To convert $\frac{3}{5}$ to tenths, multiply $\frac{3}{5}$ by $\frac{2}{2}$. The product is $\frac{6}{10}$.

$$\frac{3}{5} = \frac{3}{5} \times \frac{2}{2} = \frac{6}{10}$$

Then add $\dfrac{5}{10}$ and $\dfrac{6}{10}$ and convert the sum into a mixed number.

$$\dfrac{5}{10} + \dfrac{6}{10} = \dfrac{11}{10} = 1\dfrac{1}{10}$$

Answer: The sum of $\dfrac{1}{2} + \dfrac{3}{5}$ is $\dfrac{11}{10}$ or $1\dfrac{1}{10}$.

Example 1.2.4

Find the sum of $\dfrac{1}{4} + \dfrac{3}{7}$.

A possible common denominator is 28 because $4 \times 7 = 28$.

$$\dfrac{1}{4} = \dfrac{1}{4} \times \dfrac{7}{7} = \dfrac{7}{28} \qquad \dfrac{3}{7} = \dfrac{3}{7} \times \dfrac{4}{4} = \dfrac{12}{28}$$

$$\dfrac{7}{28} + \dfrac{12}{28} = \dfrac{19}{28}$$

Answer: The sum of $\dfrac{1}{4} + \dfrac{3}{7}$ is $\dfrac{19}{28}$.

Sometimes, multiplying the denominators is not an efficient way for finding a common denominator. When there are three or more fractions, follow the steps in Table 1.3.

TABLE 1.3 Steps for Finding a Common Denominator

Step 1. Find the prime number* factors for each denominator.

$$\dfrac{1}{15} \qquad \dfrac{5}{6} \qquad \dfrac{11}{36}$$

Denominator	Prime Number Factors
15	3, 5
6	2, 3
36	2, 2, 3, 3

$15 = 3 \times 5 \qquad 6 = 2 \times 3 \qquad 36 = 2 \times 2 \times 3 \times 3$

Step 2. Determine the quantity of prime number factors for each denominator.

- The denominator 15 has two prime number factors: *one* 3 and *one* 5.
- The denominator 6 has two prime number factors: *one* 2 and *one* 3.
- The denominator 36 has four prime number factors: *one* 2, *one* 2, *one* 3, and *one* 3, or *two* 2s and *two* 3s.

Step 3. For each prime number factor in column 2 of the table above, take the highest of these counts.

- The highest count of the 2s is two, as shown in the bottom cell of column 2.
- The highest count of the 3s is two, as shown in the bottom cell of column 2.
- The highest count of the 5s is one, as shown in the top cell of column 2.

Step 4. The least common denominator is the product of the individual prime number factors multiplied by the count, as listed in Step 3.

$$2 \times 2 \times 3 \times 3 \times 5 = 180$$

*A prime number is a number that is divisible only by 1 and itself (such as 2, 3, 5, 7, etc.).

Once two fractions have been converted to fractions with a common denominator, the numerators can be added together. After the numerators have been added, it may be necessary to reduce the resulting fraction. Typically, fractions should be reduced to their lowest terms at the end of a calculation. This process of reducing fractions to their lowest terms requires **cancellation**, or the crossing out of common factors or **like terms** in both the numerators and the denominators. Once the largest number possible has been canceled out of the numerator and the denominator, the fraction is simplified or reduced to its lowest terms. For example, consider the fraction $^2/_{12}$. This fraction can be simplified or reduced to its lowest terms.

$$\frac{2}{12} = \frac{1 \times 2}{2 \times 6}$$

The common factor in the numerator and in the denominator is the number 2. You can cancel the number 2 from the numerator and the denominator, as shown below.

$$\frac{2}{12} = \frac{1 \times \cancel{2}}{\cancel{2} \times 6} = \frac{1}{6}$$

After cancellation, the fraction $^1/_6$ remains.

Example 1.2.5

Reduce $\frac{3}{27}$ to its lowest terms.

$$\frac{3}{27} = \frac{1 \times \cancel{3}}{9 \times \cancel{3}} = \frac{1}{9}$$

Another way to reduce $^3/_{27}$ to its lowest terms is to divide both the numerator and the denominator by a common factor (in this case, 3).

$$\frac{3}{27} = \frac{3 \div 3}{27 \div 3} = \frac{1}{9}$$

Answer: The lowest terms of the fraction $\frac{3}{27}$ is $\frac{1}{9}$.

Example 1.2.6

Reduce $\frac{2}{18}$ to its lowest terms.

$$\frac{2}{18} = \frac{1 \times \cancel{2}}{\cancel{2} \times 9} = \frac{1}{9}$$

Another way to reduce $^2/_{18}$ to its lowest terms is to divide both the numerator and the denominator by a common factor (in this case, 2).

$$\frac{2}{18} = \frac{2 \div 2}{18 \div 2} = \frac{1}{9}$$

Answer: The lowest terms of the fraction $\frac{2}{18}$ is $\frac{1}{9}$.

When adding or subtracting fractions that have the same denominator, add or subtract the numerators and place the number over the common denominator. It may be necessary to reduce the answer if it is not in its lowest terms.

Example 1.2.7

Find the difference of $\dfrac{5}{6} - \dfrac{3}{6}$.

Because these fractions have a common denominator of 6, subtract the numerators and place the difference over the common denominator.

$$\frac{5}{6} - \frac{3}{6} = \frac{2}{6}$$

Then reduce $\dfrac{2}{6}$ to its lowest terms.

$$\frac{2}{6} = \frac{2 \times 1}{2 \times 3} = \frac{1}{3}$$

Answer: The difference of $\dfrac{5}{6} - \dfrac{3}{6}$ is $\dfrac{2}{6}$, reduced to $\dfrac{1}{3}$.

When subtracting fractions that have different denominators, find a common denominator and convert to equivalent fractions. Then subtract the numerators and place the number over the common denominator. It may be necessary to reduce the answer to its lowest terms.

Example 1.2.8

Find the difference of $\dfrac{3}{4} - \dfrac{2}{3}$.

To begin, find the least common denominator (in this case, 12). To convert to equivalent fractions, multiply ¾ by ⅓ and ⅔ by 4/4.

$$\frac{3}{4} \times \frac{3}{3} = \frac{9}{12}$$

$$\frac{2}{3} \times \frac{4}{4} = \frac{8}{12}$$

Then replace the original fractions with the equivalent fractions, subtract the numerators, and place the difference over the common denominator.

$$\frac{9}{12} - \frac{8}{12} = \frac{1}{12}$$

Answer: The difference of $\dfrac{3}{4} - \dfrac{2}{3}$ is $\dfrac{1}{12}$.

When adding or subtracting a mixed fraction, first convert the mixed fraction to an improper fraction. Then, if necessary, find the common denominator and convert to equivalent fractions. Last, add or subtract the numerators and place the number over the common denominator. It may be necessary to reduce the answer to its lowest terms.

Math Morsel

A mixed number has a whole number in front of a fraction.

Example 1.2.9

Find the difference of $3\frac{3}{4} - \frac{1}{2}$.

To begin, change the mixed number to an improper fraction.

$$3\frac{3}{4} = \frac{(3 \times 4) + 3}{4} = \frac{15}{4}$$

Then replace the mixed number with the improper fraction in the original problem.

$$\frac{15}{4} - \frac{1}{2}$$

Because the second fraction ($^1/_2$) has a denominator of 2, this fraction must be changed to a fraction that has a denominator of 4. To do this, multiply the numerator and denominator of $^1/_2$ by 2.

$$\frac{1}{2} \times \frac{2}{2} = \frac{2}{4}$$

Next, replace the second fraction with $\frac{2}{4}$.

$$\frac{15}{4} - \frac{2}{4}$$

Then subtract the numerators and place the difference over the common denominator.

$$\frac{15}{4} - \frac{2}{4} = \frac{13}{4}$$

Finally, change the improper fraction to a mixed number by dividing 13 by 4.

$$\frac{13}{4} = 3\frac{1}{4}$$

Answer: The difference of $3\frac{3}{4} - \frac{1}{2}$ is $\frac{13}{4}$, or $3\frac{1}{4}$.

Example 1.2.10

Find the difference of $2\frac{1}{2} - \frac{6}{3}$.

To begin, change the mixed number to an improper fraction.

$$2\frac{1}{2} = \frac{(2 \times 2) + 1}{2} = \frac{5}{2}$$

Then replace the mixed number in the original problem with the improper fraction.

$$2\frac{1}{2} - \frac{6}{3} = \frac{5}{2} - \frac{6}{3}$$

Next, find the least common denominator (in this case, 6). Convert to equivalent fractions.

$$\frac{5}{2} \times \frac{3}{3} = \frac{15}{6}$$

$$\frac{6}{3} \times \frac{2}{2} = \frac{12}{6}$$

Then replace the original fractions with the equivalent fractions, subtract the numerators, and place the difference over the common denominator.

$$\frac{15}{6} - \frac{12}{6} = \frac{3}{6}$$

Finally, reduce $\frac{3}{6}$ to its lowest terms.

$$\frac{3}{6} = \frac{1}{2}$$

Answer: The difference of $2\frac{1}{2} - \frac{6}{3}$ is $\frac{3}{6}$, reduced to $\frac{1}{2}$.

Multiplying and Dividing Fractions

In pharmacy practice, you may need to multiply fractions prior to filling a prescription or a medication order. For example, you may have to determine the number of tablets a patient will need to last for a certain period. When you multiply fractions together, you multiply numerators by numerators and denominators by denominators. The result, called a ***product***, is then reduced to its lowest terms (see Table 1.4).

TABLE 1.4 Guidelines for Multiplying Fractions

1. Multiplying the numerator by a number, while multiplying the denominator by 1, increases the value of a fraction.

$$\frac{1}{4} \times \frac{2}{1} = \frac{1 \times 2}{4 \times 1} = \frac{2}{4} = \frac{1}{2}$$

2. Multiplying the denominator by a number, while multiplying the numerator by 1, decreases the value of a fraction.

$$\frac{1}{4} \times \frac{1}{2} = \frac{1 \times 1}{4 \times 2} = \frac{1}{8}$$

3. The value of a fraction is not altered by multiplying both the numerator and the denominator by the same number.

$$\frac{1}{4} \times \frac{4}{4} = \frac{1 \times 4}{4 \times 4} = \frac{4}{16} = \frac{1}{4}$$

Consider this example of two proper fractions being multiplied.

$$\frac{1}{8} \times \frac{1}{2} = \frac{1 \times 1}{8 \times 2} = \frac{1}{16}$$

When more than two fractions are multiplied, all the numerators are multiplied by one another and all the denominators are multiplied by one another.

$$\frac{1}{8} \times \frac{1}{2} \times \frac{2}{3} = \frac{1 \times 1 \times 2}{8 \times 2 \times 3} = \frac{2}{48}$$

The product $^2/_{48}$ can be reduced to $^1/_{24}$. Alternatively, the 2 in the numerator and the 2 in the denominator could have been canceled out prior to multiplication.

$$\frac{1}{8} \times \frac{1}{2} \times \frac{2}{3} = \frac{1 \times 1 \times \cancel{2}}{8 \times \cancel{2} \times 3} = \frac{1}{24}$$

When a whole number is multiplied by a fraction, rewrite the whole number as a fraction. In the following example, the whole number (in this case, 5) is rewritten as a fraction with a denominator of 1 or $^5/_1$.

$$5 \times \frac{3}{4} = \frac{5}{1} \times \frac{3}{4} = \frac{5 \times 3}{1 \times 4} = \frac{15}{4} = 3\frac{3}{4}$$

Example 1.2.11

Find the product of $2 \times \dfrac{1}{2} \times \dfrac{1}{3}$. Then reduce the product to its lowest terms.

X=? **Math Morsel**

A whole number can be written as an improper fraction in order to multiply fractions.

To begin, rewrite the whole number as a fraction.

$$\frac{2}{1} \times \frac{1}{2} \times \frac{1}{3}$$

Next, multiply all the numerators together and all of the denominators together.

$$\frac{2 \times 1 \times 1}{1 \times 2 \times 3} = \frac{2}{6}$$

Finally, reduce the fraction $\dfrac{2}{6}$ to its lowest terms.

$$\frac{2}{6} = \frac{\cancel{2}}{1} \times \frac{1}{\cancel{2}} \times \frac{1}{3} = \frac{1}{3}$$

Answer: The product of $2 \times \dfrac{1}{2} \times \dfrac{1}{3}$ is $\dfrac{2}{6}$, reduced to $\dfrac{1}{3}$.

In pharmacy practice, you may also need to divide fractions to find the **quotient**. To divide fractions, you change the division sign (÷) to a multiplication sign (×) and invert the number (create a **reciprocal**) to the right of the multiplication sign. Then you multiply the numerators together and the denominators together and reduce the answer to its lowest terms. You can use this same method if only the numerator is a fraction or if only the denominator is a fraction (see Table 1.5).

TABLE 1.5 Guidelines for Dividing Fractions

1. Dividing the denominator by a number is the same as multiplying the numerator by that number.

$$3 \div \frac{20}{7} = \frac{3}{1} \div \frac{20}{7} = \frac{3}{1} \times \frac{7}{20} = \frac{21}{20}$$

2. Dividing the numerator by a number is the same as multiplying the denominator by that number.

$$\frac{3}{4} \div 6 = \frac{3}{4} \div \frac{6}{1} = \frac{3}{4} \times \frac{1}{6} = \frac{3}{24} = \frac{1}{8}$$

Consider this example of two proper fractions being divided.

$$\frac{1}{2} \div \frac{1}{3}$$

You begin by changing the division sign to a multiplication sign. Then you create the reciprocal of the fraction to the right of the multiplication sign. The reciprocal of $^1/_3$ is $^3/_1$.

$$\frac{1}{2} \times \frac{3}{1}$$

Then you multiply the fractions by multiplying the numerators and the denominators.

$$\frac{1}{2} \times \frac{3}{1} = \frac{1 \times 3}{2 \times 1} = \frac{3}{2}$$

The quotient is an improper fraction and should be reduced to its lowest terms, which is a mixed fraction.

$$\frac{3}{2} = 1\frac{1}{2}$$

<hr />

Example 1.2.12

Find the quotient of $\dfrac{2}{3} \div \dfrac{3}{5}$.

To begin, change the division sign to a multiplication sign and create the reciprocal of the fraction to the right of the multiplication sign.

$$\frac{2}{3} \times \frac{5}{3}$$

Next, multiply the numerators and the denominators of the fractions.

$$\frac{2 \times 5}{3 \times 3} = \frac{10}{9}$$

Finally, reduce the improper fraction to its lowest terms, which is a mixed number.

$$\frac{10}{9} = 1\frac{1}{9}$$

Answer: The quotient of $\dfrac{2}{3} \div \dfrac{3}{5}$ is $\dfrac{10}{9}$, reduced to $1\dfrac{1}{9}$.

<hr />

Using Dimensional Analysis to Multiply and Divide Fractions

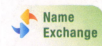

Name Exchange

Dimensional analysis is also known as the *factor label method* or the *unit factor method.*

Dimensional analysis is a problem-solving method that uses the math principle that any number can be multiplied by 1 without changing its value. For that reason, this method is often used in the multiplication and division of fractions. (Refer to Chapter 4 for further instruction on the use of dimensional analysis.)

To understand dimensional analysis, you must first understand equivalent fractions.

$$\text{If } a = b, \text{ then } \frac{a}{b} = 1 \text{ and } \frac{b}{a} = 1.$$

Therefore, any equality ($a = b$) can form two fractions ($^a/_b = 1$, $^b/_a = 1$).

This principle allows you to solve problems by setting them up as fractions that are multiplied by other fractions. You must set up the problems so that the starting units cancel out one another and, consequently, you are left with the desired units.

$$\text{starting units} \times \frac{\text{desired units}}{\text{starting units}} = \text{desired units}$$

For example, you can use the dimensional analysis format above to calculate the number of minutes in one hour. The starting units (the units you are given) are hours, and the desired units (the units you want to find) are minutes. The starting units of hours are canceled out and leave the desired units as minutes.

$$1 \text{ hour} \times \frac{60 \text{ minutes}}{1 \text{ hour}} = 60 \text{ minutes}$$

Consider calculating the number of minutes in one day. There are 24 hours in one day and 60 minutes in one hour. The desired units are minutes per day (minutes/day). Set up fractions to solve for minutes/day by canceling out the hour units.

$$\frac{24 \text{ hours}}{1 \text{ day}} \times \frac{60 \text{ minutes}}{1 \text{ hour}} = \frac{1{,}440 \text{ minutes}}{\text{day}} = 1{,}440 \text{ minutes/day}$$

You can use this method to solve more complex calculations. Consider calculating the number of seconds in one day. There are 60 seconds in one minute, 60 minutes in one hour, and 24 hours in one day. The desired units are seconds per day (seconds/day), and the units that must be canceled out are minutes and hours.

$$\frac{60 \text{ seconds}}{1 \text{ minute}} \times \frac{60 \text{ minutes}}{1 \text{ hour}} \times \frac{24 \text{ hours}}{1 \text{ day}} = \frac{86{,}400 \text{ seconds}}{\text{day}} = 86{,}400 \text{ seconds/day}$$

Dimensional analysis is useful in performing many types of pharmacy calculations. For example, dimensional analysis may be useful when partial doses, such as 1/2 tablet or 3/4 teaspoonful, are prescribed. The following example demonstrates this calculation.

Example 1.2.13

How many milligrams are in $^1/_2$ of a furosemide tablet shown in the label?

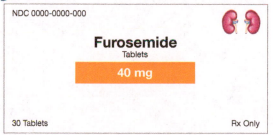

NDC 0000-0000-000

Furosemide
Tablets

40 mg

30 Tablets   Rx Only

You can solve this problem using either the dimensional analysis method or the division method.

Dimensional Analysis Method

$$\frac{40 \text{ mg}}{1 \text{ tablet}} \times \frac{\frac{1}{2} \text{ tablet}}{1} = \frac{40 \text{ mg}}{1} \times \frac{1}{2} = \frac{40 \text{ mg}}{2} = 20 \text{ mg}$$

Division Method

Alternatively, you can divide the strength of the tablet (40 mg) by 2 because $^2/_1$ is the reciprocal (or inverse) of $^1/_2$.

$$40 \text{ mg} \div 2 = 20 \text{ mg}$$

Answer: For this medication label, there are 20 mg in $^1/_2$ of a furosemide tablet.

1.2 Problem Set   odd only! 1-36

Indicate which number is the numerator in the following fractions.

1. $\dfrac{1}{2}$

2. $\dfrac{2}{3}$

3. $\dfrac{5}{5}$

4. $\dfrac{15}{16}$

5. $\dfrac{20}{23}$

Indicate which number is the denominator in the following fractions.

6. $\dfrac{1}{3}$

7. $\dfrac{2}{5}$

8. $\dfrac{4}{4}$

9. $\dfrac{11}{12}$

10. $\dfrac{23}{100}$

Circle the fraction with the highest value.

11. $\dfrac{1}{2},$ $\dfrac{1}{3}$ $\dfrac{1}{4}$

12. $\dfrac{3}{10}$ $\dfrac{3}{12}$ $\dfrac{3}{8}$

13. $\dfrac{1}{4}$ $\dfrac{9}{10}$ $\dfrac{2}{3}$

14. $\dfrac{1}{15}$ $\dfrac{14}{15}$ $\dfrac{15}{15}$

15. $\dfrac{4}{5}$ $\dfrac{2}{3}$ $\dfrac{1}{4}$

Circle the fraction with the lowest value.

16. $\dfrac{3}{1}$ $\dfrac{4}{1}$ $\dfrac{2}{1}$

17. $\dfrac{2}{6}$ $\dfrac{3}{6}$ $\dfrac{4}{6}$

18. $\dfrac{1}{10}$ $\dfrac{1}{8}$ $\dfrac{1}{6}$

19. $\dfrac{4}{5}$ $\dfrac{1}{4}$ $\dfrac{2}{3}$

20. $\dfrac{1}{15}$ $\dfrac{15}{15}$ $\dfrac{14}{15}$

Find the sum of the following fractions.

21. $\dfrac{1}{6} + \dfrac{2}{6} + \dfrac{3}{6} =$

22. $\dfrac{2}{10} + \dfrac{5}{10} + \dfrac{1}{10} =$

23. $\dfrac{16}{100} + \dfrac{12}{100} + \dfrac{51}{100} =$

24. $\dfrac{5}{6} + \dfrac{7}{10} + \dfrac{2}{5} =$

25. $\dfrac{21}{32} + \dfrac{1}{12} + \dfrac{31}{48} =$

Find the difference of the following fractions.

26. $\dfrac{9}{10} - \dfrac{2}{10} - \dfrac{1}{10} =$

27. $\dfrac{30}{50} - \dfrac{10}{50} - \dfrac{8}{50} =$

28. $\dfrac{65}{100} - \dfrac{25}{100} - \dfrac{16}{100} =$

29. $\dfrac{9}{10} - \dfrac{1}{25} - \dfrac{2}{100} =$

30. $\dfrac{3}{5} - \dfrac{2}{50} - \dfrac{7}{25} =$

Reduce the following fractions to their lowest terms and rewrite the fractions as mixed numbers if necessary.

31. $\dfrac{25}{100}$

32. $\dfrac{67}{10}$

33. $\dfrac{11}{5}$

34. $\dfrac{27}{30}$

35. $\dfrac{12}{30}$

36. $\dfrac{90}{100}$

Applications

37. A patient has taken $\frac{1}{4}$ tablet, $\frac{1}{2}$ tablet, $1\frac{1}{2}$ tablets, and $\frac{3}{4}$ tablet. In total, how many tablets has the patient taken?

38. Which dose contains the largest amount of medication: one tablet containing $\frac{1}{150}$ grain or two tablets containing $\frac{1}{100}$ grain in each tablet?

39. You are to measure $\frac{1}{4}$ grain of medication into individual containers. Your bulk container holds 375 grains. How many individual containers can be prepared from one bulk container?

Table sugar is needed for making simple syrup. The first formula calls for $\frac{1}{2}$ pound (lb) of sugar to make enough syrup; the second formula requires $\frac{4}{5}$ lb of sugar; the third formula requires $\frac{1}{4}$ lb of sugar; and the fourth formula requires $2\frac{1}{2}$ lb of sugar. You need to use all four formulas to create one batch of simple syrup.

40. How many bags of sugar must be purchased if it is packaged in 2 lb bags?

41. How many bags of sugar must be purchased if it is packaged in 5 lb bags?

Self-check your work in Appendix A.

1.3 Decimals

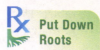
An understanding of the decimal system is crucial to pharmacy calculations because most medication orders are written in decimals. The decimal system is based on the Arabic number system that you learned earlier in this chapter. In the decimal system, 10 Arabic numbers are used: 0, 1, 2, 3, 4, 5, 6, 7, 8, and 9. The placement of these numbers in a decimal is important to the interpretation of the decimal.

A **decimal** is an Arabic number that has two components: a zero *or* a whole number component (which has a value of 1 or greater) and a fractional component (which has a value of less than 1, or parts of a whole). These two components are separated by a **decimal point**.

The position or placement of each digit in a decimal determines its **place value**. The position of each digit to the left of the decimal point signals a tenfold increase in its value, and the position of each digit to the right of the decimal point signals a tenfold decrease in its value. Figure 1.3 illustrates the relative place value of each digit in a decimal. Memorize these place values so that you can correctly write and read decimals.

FIGURE 1.3
Decimal Units and Values

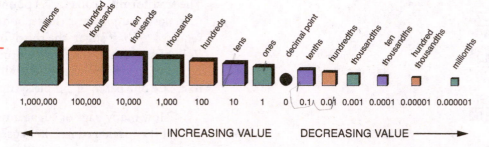

millions	hundred thousands	ten thousands	thousands	hundreds	tens	ones	decimal point	tenths	hundredths	thousandths	ten thousandths	hundred thousandths	millionths
1,000,000	100,000	10,000	1,000	100	10	1	0	0.1	0.01	0.001	0.0001	0.00001	0.000001

← INCREASING VALUE   DECREASING VALUE →

Writing Decimals

You can write any fraction as a decimal. When writing a decimal, you place the whole number component to the left of the decimal point, and the fractional component to the right of the decimal point. To determine the fractional component, divide the numerator by the denominator. For example, the fraction $1\,^2/_{10}$ can be written as the decimal 1.2. Inversely, you can write any decimal as a fraction. For example, the decimal 2.33 can be written as the fraction $^{233}/_{100}$.

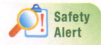
When you are writing a decimal and there is no whole number component, you must place a zero to the left of the decimal point. This zero is called a *leading zero*. Healthcare personnel must consistently use leading zeros in the practice setting because their placement helps to avoid medication errors from the misinterpretation of decimals.

Table 1.6 provides guidelines on how to interpret decimals and determine their values. As you can see by the examples, decimal values are determined by the place values of their digits.

TABLE 1.6 **Guidelines for Interpreting Decimals**

1. The digits to the left of the decimal point represent the whole number component of the fraction. If there is no number to the left of the decimal point, place a 0 to the left of the decimal point. This is called a *leading zero*.

2. If the whole number components of two decimals are different, whichever decimal has the larger whole number component has the greater value.

   8.2 > 6.2

   20.1 > 14.6

   3.08 > 0.39

3. If the whole number components of two decimals are identical (including if both are zeros), the digits in the tenths place of both decimals are examined.

4. If the digits in the tenths place of two decimals are different, the digit with the higher value determines which decimal has the greater value.

   0.4 > 0.3

   2.41 > 2.39

5. If the digits in the tenths place of two decimals are identical, the digits in the hundredths place of both decimals are examined.

6. If the digits in the hundredths place of two decimals are different, the digit with the higher value determines which decimal has the greater value.

   0.17 > 0.15

   0.35 > 0.30

   10.66 > 10.64

7. If the digits in the hundredths place of two decimals are identical, the digits in the thousandths place of both decimals are examined.

8. If the digits in the thousandths place of two decimals are different, the digit with the higher value determines which decimal has the greater value—and so on.

   0.125 > 0.124

   7.0097 > 7.0092

9. The total value of a decimal is the sum of the different components.

467.43 represents	400.00	=	four hundreds
	+60.00	=	six tens
	+ 7.00	=	seven ones
	+ 0.40	=	four tenths
	+ 0.03	=	three hundredths

   You say this number as "four hundred sixty-seven and forty-three hundredths."

Reading Decimals

A decimal is read from left to right. First, you read the whole number component to the left of the decimal point. Then you say "and" or "point" to refer to the decimal point. Finally, you read the fractional component to the right of the decimal point. For example, the decimal *2.375* is read as "two point three seven five" or "two and three hundred seventy-five thousandths."

Table 1.7 provides a summary of interpreting decimals. The table reveals how to express fractions as decimals as well as how to read the decimals.

Safety Alert

Medication labels for certain drugs, such as nitroglycerin used to treat chest pain, may contain either decimals or fractions. Therefore, pharmacy technicians should be sure to check labels carefully before preparing medications.

TABLE 1.7 Writing and Reading Decimals

Fraction	Writing the Decimal	Reading the Decimal
$1\frac{1}{2}$ or $\frac{3}{2}$	1.5	"one point five" or "one and five tenths"
$\frac{3}{4}$	0.75*	"zero point seven five" or "seventy-five hundredths"
$\frac{1}{8}$	0.125*	"zero point one two five" or "one hundred twenty-five thousandths"

*Note the presence of the leading zero.

Adding and Subtracting Decimals

When adding or subtracting decimals, place the numbers in columns so that the decimal points are aligned vertically. You may need to add zeros after the decimal point to correctly align the decimal points. Add or subtract from the far-right column to the far-left column.

$$
\begin{array}{r} 20.4 \\ + 21.8 \\ \hline 42.2 \end{array}
\qquad
\begin{array}{r} 11.2 \\ 13.6 \\ + 16.0 \\ \hline 40.8 \end{array}
\qquad
\begin{array}{r} 15.36 \\ - 3.80 \\ \hline 11.56 \end{array}
$$

Multiplying and Dividing Decimals

Unlike adding and subtracting decimals, the multiplication of decimals does not require you to align the decimal points. You simply multiply decimals the same way that you multiply whole numbers. However, you will omit the decimal places until the last step of the calculation. When you arrive at your answer, you then add the total number of decimal places that are in the two numbers being multiplied (which is the number of decimal places in your answer), count that number of places from right to left in the answer, and insert a decimal point.

$$
\begin{array}{r} 1.23 \\ \times\, 2.3 \\ \hline 369 \\ + 2460 \\ \hline 2.829 \end{array}
$$

(two decimal places)
(one decimal place)

(A zero is added to align the columns.)
(Answer has three decimal places.)

To divide decimals, change both the **divisor** (the number you are dividing by) and the **dividend** (the number being divided) to whole numbers by moving their decimal points the same number of places to the right. If the divisor and the dividend have a different number of digits after the decimal point, choose the one that has more digits and move its decimal point a sufficient number of places to make it a whole number. Then move the decimal point in the other number the same number of places, adding a zero at the end if necessary.

In the first example below, the divisor (3.625) has more digits after the decimal point than the dividend (1.45). Therefore, you would move the divisor's decimal point three places to the right to make it a whole number. You would then move the decimal point in the dividend the same number of places and add a zero at the end (as shown below). In the second example below, the dividend (1.617) has more digits after the decimal point than the divisor (2.31). Therefore, you would move the dividend's decimal point three places to the right to make it a whole number. You would then move the decimal point in the divisor three places to the right and add a zero at the end (as shown below).

$$1.45 \div 3.625 = 0.4 \qquad 1.617 \div 2.31 = 0.7$$

$$\frac{1.45}{3.625} = \frac{1450}{3625} = 0.4 \qquad \frac{1.617}{2.31} = \frac{1617}{2310} = 0.7$$

Rounding Decimals

Rounding is the process of replacing a number by another number of approximately the same value but with fewer digits. Rounding numbers is essential in pharmacy calculations and, in the rounding examples in this textbook, is performed as the last step in the calculations process. The purpose of rounding is to keep the numbers that you are working with to a manageable size. It is important to recognize, however, that rounding will affect the *accuracy* to which a medication can be measured. In some cases, it may be appropriate to calculate a dose to the nearest whole milliliter and, in other cases, to round to the nearest tenth or hundredth of a milliliter. Depending on the medication and strength prescribed, it may not be possible to accurately measure a very small quantity such as a hundredth of a milliliter.

When numbers with decimals are used to calculate a volumetric (volume-related) dose, a number with multiple digits beyond the decimal often results. It is not practical to retain all of these digits, as a dose cannot be accurately measured beyond the hundredths or thousandths place for most medications. Most commonly, a volumetric dose is rounded to the nearest tenth. For doses that are measured in weight, it is common practice to round to the hundredths or thousandths place, or as precisely as the particular measuring device (or medication) will permit.

To round an answer to the nearest tenth, carry the calculation out two places or to the hundredths place. If the digit in the hundredths place is 5 or greater, add 1 to the tenths place number. If the digit in the hundredths place is less than 5, round the number down by omitting the digit in the hundredths place.

$$5.65 \text{ becomes } 5.7 \qquad 4.24 \text{ becomes } 4.2$$

The same procedure may be used when rounding to the nearest hundredths place or thousandths place.

$$3.8421 = 3.84 \qquad \text{(hundredths place)}$$
$$41.2674 = 41.27 \qquad \text{(hundredths place)}$$
$$0.3928 = 0.393 \qquad \text{(thousandths place)}$$
$$4.1111 = 4.111 \qquad \text{(thousandths place)}$$

The following example shows how an exact dose can be rounded to the nearest tenths, hundredths, and thousandths place.

exact dose calculated: 0.08752 g
rounded to nearest tenth place: 0.1 g
rounded to nearest hundredth place: 0.09 g
rounded to nearest thousandth place: 0.088 g

 WORKPLACE WISDOM

In pharmacy practice, leading zeros are always used before a decimal point. For example, a one-half milligram should be written as 0.5 mg instead of .5 mg. The use of a leading zero helps to prevent medication errors. In fact, the US Food and Drug Administration has received reports of tenfold drug dosing errors due to prescriptions omitting a leading zero.

Example 1.3.1

Find the product of 3.46 × 7.1. Then round the answer to the nearest tenth.

$$3.46 \times 7.1 = 24.566$$

Answer: The product of 3.46 × 7.1 is 24.566, rounded to 24.6.

Example 1.3.2

Find the product of 0.3563 × 1.3. Then round the answer to the nearest tenth.

$$0.3563 \times 1.3 = 0.46319$$

Answer: The product of 0.3563 × 1.3 is 0.46319, rounded to 0.5.

In most cases, a zero occurring at the end of a string of digits after the decimal point is not written. This zero is called a *trailing zero*. An exception to this rule may occur when rounding results in a zero as the last place value. When the last digit resulting from rounding is a zero, there are cases in which this zero should be written because it is considered significant to that particular problem or dosage. In such cases, the amount can be measured out to an exact zero as the place value.

Example 1.3.3

Round 9.98 to the nearest tenth.

Answer: The decimal 9.98 rounded to the nearest tenth is 10.0.

Example 1.3.4

Round 0.599 to the nearest hundredth.

Answer: The decimal 0.599 rounded to the nearest hundredth is 0.60.

1.3 Problem Set   1-40 odd only!

Write the following decimals.

1. seven hundred eighty-four and thirty-six hundredths

2. nine tenths

Express the following fractions in decimal form.

3. $\dfrac{1}{5}$

4. $\dfrac{1}{20}$

5. $4\dfrac{2}{4}$

6. $\dfrac{30}{100}$

7. $\dfrac{1}{200}$

8. $\dfrac{1}{500}$

9. $1\dfrac{8}{10}$

10. $\dfrac{1}{25}$

11. $\dfrac{1}{125}$

In each group of decimals, circle the decimal with the highest value.

12. 3.1   1.7   4.1

13. 0.5   0.56   0.6

In each group of decimals, circle the decimal with the lowest value.

14. 2.02   2.12   2.1

15. 0.16   0.167   0.017

Identify the digit in the designated place value of the number below.

92,375.046

16. tenths place

17. thousandths place

18. hundredths place

State the place value of the underlined digit.

19. 18,240.6

20. 7.2391

21. 621.508

22. 0.98

23. 40. 023

Find the sum of the following decimals.

24. 0.34 + 1.54 =

25. 1.39 + 1.339 =

Find the difference of the following decimals.

26. 15.36 − 0.987 =

27. 3.09875 − 0.00045 =

28. 12.901 − 0.903 =

Find the product of the following decimals and round to the nearest hundredth.

29. 21.62 × 21.62 =

30. 0.9 × 500 =

Find the quotient of the following decimals and round to the nearest thousandth.

31. 12 ÷ 6.5 =

32. 0.8 ÷ 0.6 =

Round the following decimals to the nearest hundredth.

33. 3.872

34. 0.138

35. 0.076

Round the following decimals to the nearest thousandth.

36. 0.1961

37. 0.0488

Find the product of the following decimals and round to the nearest tenth.

38. $6.7 \times 5.21 =$

39. $0.45 \times 3.1 =$

Applications

40. Using the prescription below, answer the following questions. *Note:* The abbreviation *po* means "by mouth," and the abbreviation *TID* means "three times a day."

> ℞ **Alprazolam 0.25 mg**
>
> Dosing instructions: 3 tablets po TID
>
> Quantity to dispense: 100 tablets

a. How many milligrams is the patient taking with each dose?

b. How many milligrams is the patient taking each day?

c. How many tablets will the patient need for 14 days?

d. Is the prescription written for enough tablets to last the patient until the next office visit in two weeks?

e. The pharmacy plans to charge $7.59 plus the cost of the medication. The available products include the following:

alprazolam 0.25 mg 100 tablets/$14.95
alprazolam 0.5 mg 100 tablets/$17.46
alprazolam 1 mg 100 tablets/$23.87

Select the appropriate product and calculate the price for the patient. Based on the prescription provided, the pharmacy can dispense only 100 tablets.

41. The physician changes the prescription at the patient's next visit. The new prescription is shown below. *Note:* The abbreviation *po* means "by mouth," and the abbreviation *TID* means "three times a day."

> ℞ **Alprazolam 0.25 mg**
>
> Dosing instructions: 4 tablets po TID
>
> Quantity to dispense: 175 tablets

The available products include the following:

alprazolam 0.25 mg 100 tablets/$14.95
alprazolam 0.5 mg 100 tablets/$17.46
alprazolam 1 mg 100 tablets/$23.87

a. How many milligrams is each dose?

b. How much would 125 tablets of alprazolam 0.5 mg cost the pharmacy?

c. How much would 50 tablets of alprazolam 1 mg cost the pharmacy?

d. How many days would 50 tablets of alprazolam 1 mg taken TID last?

42. Sterile water is available in a 1 liter (L) container. You need to pour out 120 milliliter (mL) bottles for each patient.

a. How many 120 mL bottles will you get from a 1 L bottle? (1 L = 1,000 mL)

b. How many milliliters will be left over?

43. How many total milliliters need to be dispensed for the following prescription? Round your answer to the nearest whole milliliter. *Note:* The abbreviation *mg* means "milligrams"; the abbreviation *mL* means "milliliters"; and the abbreviation *BID* means "twice a day."

> ℞ **Augmentin 125 mg/5 mL suspension**
>
> 8.5 mL BID days 1–2
>
> 5.75 mL BID days 3–7

44. Round the following amounts to the nearest whole dollar.

   a. $46.92

   b. 12 @ $1.26

   c. $7.37 ÷ 2 =

45. Calculate the following dollar amounts and round to the nearest cent.

   a. $5.84 × 12 =

   b. $0.415 × 269 =

46. Find the quotient and round your answer to the nearest hundredth.

   a. 34 ÷ 38 =

   b. 51 ÷ 60 =

   c. 83 ÷ 90 =

Self-check your work in Appendix A.

1.4 Scientific Notation, Significant Figures, and Measurement Accuracy

Precision and accuracy are extremely important when performing pharmacy calculations. To maintain precision and accuracy, you should be aware of three important concepts: scientific notation, significant figures, and measurement accuracy.

Expressing Numbers in Scientific Notation

Standard notation is when a numeral is completely written out using Arabic numbers. An example of a number written in standard notation is 0.624 or 624. There are times when expressing a number in standard notation is inconvenient. It is not practical to write out numbers that have a large number of zeros (such as 5,200,000,000,000) or very small numbers (such as 0.00000025) in standard notation because of space issues as well as readability. In these cases, scientific notation may be utilized. **Scientific notation** is a method used to write numbers that have very large or very small numerical values.

 Math Morsel

Exponents can be positive (10^2) or negative (10^{-2}). The positive exponent $10^2 = 100$, and the negative exponent $10^{-2} = 0.01$.

To change a number written in standard notation to scientific notation, you can rewrite the number as a group of significant figures multiplied by 10 with an exponent. **Significant figures** are all the digits of a number that signify accuracy. An **exponent** is a number placed above and to the right of another number to show that it has been raised to a power. The number in the exponent indicates how many places the decimal has been moved, and the sign of the exponent (positive or negative) indicates the direction the decimal was moved. A **positive exponent** indicates a number greater than 1, and a **negative exponent** indicates a number less than 1.

Consider the following examples that use scientific notation.

$$6.24 \times 10^{17} \qquad 5.19 \times 10^{-84}$$

In the first example, the group of significant figures is 6.24, and the exponent is 17. Because 17 is a positive number, it is considered a positive exponent. In the second example, the group of significant figures is 5.19, and the exponent is −84. Because −84 is a negative number, it is considered a negative exponent.

Table 1.8 shows examples of values written in standard notation and their equivalence in scientific notation.

TABLE 1.8 Standard Notation and Scientific Notation Equivalence

Standard Notation	Decimal Place Movement	Scientific Notation
6,500	6,500 (3 places to the left)	6.5×10^3
120,000	120,000 (5 places to the left)	1.2×10^5
921,000,000	921,000,000 (8 places to the left)	9.21×10^8
4,800,000,000,000	4,800,000,000,000 (12 places to the left)	4.8×10^{12}
0.109	0.109 (1 place to the right)	1.09×10^{-1}
0.000587	0.000587 (4 places to the right)	5.87×10^{-4}
0.00000026	0.00000026 (7 places to the right)	2.6×10^{-7}
0.000000000049	0.000000000049 (11 places to the right)	4.9×10^{-11}

Counting Significant Figures

As mentioned earlier, significant figures are the digits of a number, often a measurement, that contribute to the degree of accuracy of the value. The number of significant figures is equal to the number of digits that are known with some degree of confidence plus the last digit (which is an estimate). The last digit is known as the ***lowest known place value***. The lowest known place value is approximate because of many sources of error (including limitations of the measuring instrument, temperature variation, and the need to round at a certain point to make the number practical for calculations). For example, consider the number 8.16. There are three significant figures in this number (8, 1, and 6). The lowest known place value in 8.16 is 6.

In pharmacy practice, there are rules that determine how significant figures are counted. These rules are outlined in Table 1.9.

Safety Alert

Pharmacy technicians should not use a trailing zero unless it is a significant figure that determines the accuracy of a number.

TABLE 1.9 Rules for Counting Significant Figures

Rule 1. Begin counting at the first nonzero digit.

Rule 2. Continue counting to the right until you reach the place value that is last (or rounded).

Rule 3. Count zeros that are located between digits as significant.

Rule 4. Do not count zeros that are placed to the left of the first digit. These zeros only mark the place of the decimal.

Rule 5. Recognize that one or more trailing zeros may or may not be significant, depending on the accuracy to which the number is held.

Consider the number 0.01023. You begin counting significant figures at the first *nonzero* digit. For this example, you would begin counting the significant figures at the first 1.

0.01023

Next, you continue counting to the right until you reach the lowest known place value. In this example, the lowest known place value is 3.

0.01023

Zeros that are located between digits are significant figures and should be counted. In this example, the zero between the 1 and 2 should be counted.

0.01023

Do not count zeros that are placed to the left of the first digit. These zeros are considered place markers. In this example, the zeros that precede 1 are not counted.

0.01023

Therefore, based on these rules, the number 0.01023 has four significant figures.

0.01023

Table 1.10 shows several numerals and their number of significant figures.

TABLE 1.10 Counting Significant Figures

Numeral	Number of Significant Figures
1.8	2
18.3	3
183	3
1.832	4
1,832	4
0.183	3 (not the leading zero)
0.108	3 (not the leading zero)
0.0108	3 (not the leading zero or the zero before the first digit)
0.01	1 (not the leading zero or the zero before the first digit)
0.8	1 (not the leading zero)
8	1
10	2

Determining Measurement Accuracy

Accuracy is the degree to which a measurement matches the actual value of the quantity being measured. The degree of accuracy may be expressed as the number of significant figures or as a percent. A measurement with two-figure accuracy measures a value to within 5% of the actual value. Likewise, a measurement with three-figure accuracy measures a value to within 0.5% of the actual value. **Accuracy range** is the extent (upper and lower limits) that a value can be measured (see Table 1.11).

TABLE 1.11 Significant Figures and Degree of Accuracy

Number of Significant Figures	Degree of Accuracy	Accuracy Range for 100 mg
2	within 5%	95–105 mg
3	within 0.5%	99.5–100.5 mg
4	within 0.05%	99.95–100.05 mg
5	within 0.005%	99.995–100.005 mg

When the degree of accuracy is known to a certain place value, the significant figures are counted only to that place value. Knowing the level of accuracy is important when considering the weighing capacity and sensitivity of a scale or balance in the pharmacy. More significant figures indicate a greater accuracy of known values.

Numbers greater than 100 have significant figures based on the relative accuracy of the measurement. If a number greater than 100 is accurate to the nearest 10, the zero in the ones place is considered an estimate and not significant. Only the digits to the left of that place value are considered significant. Significant figures are counted similarly for numbers that are accurate to the nearest 100 or larger. For example, if the following numbers are accurate to the nearest 10, they will have the indicated number of significant figures.

200 has two significant figures

1,800 has three significant figures

30,000 has four significant figures

Similarly, if the following numbers are accurate to the nearest 100, they will have the indicated number of significant figures.

200 has one significant figure

1,800 has two significant figures

30,000 has three significant figures

When multiplying or dividing, the answer should have the same number of significant figures as the original inexact number that has the fewest significant figures.

Example 1.4.1

An item is weighed on a balance with a degree of accuracy to the nearest tenth when measuring milligrams. The balance indicates that the item weighs 1.459 mg. How many significant figures does this weight have? What would the rounded value be?

Answer: Because the accuracy of the scale can be relied on only to the tenths place, the number of significant figures is two. The "5" and the "9" in the item's weight are not considered significant figures because of the sensitivity of the scale being used. The weight should be rounded to 1.5 mg.

Example 1.4.2

Determine the product of 6.75 × 3 using the appropriate number of significant figures for accuracy.

Note the number of significant figures and the level of accuracy for each number: 6.75 has three significant figures and is accurate to the tenths place, whereas 3 has one significant figure and is accurate to the ones place.

Now, determine the actual product of the two numbers.

$$6.75 \times 3 = 20.25$$

Answer: The product of 6.75 × 3 is 20.25. Because 3 has one significant figure, the product needs to be rounded to the tens place: 20.

Example 1.4.3

Determine the product of 12.59 × 1,572 using the appropriate number of significant figures for accuracy.

When you multiply two numbers together, the answer should have the same number of significant figures as the number that has the lesser number of significant figures in the equation. In this example, both numbers have four significant figures.

Now, determine the actual product of the two numbers.

$$12.59 \times 1{,}572 = 19{,}791.48$$

Answer: The product of 12.59 × 1,572 is 19,791.48. Because both numbers in the problem have four significant figures, the answer can have only four significant figures: 19,790.

Using Exact Numbers

In pharmacy applications, it is typical to consider certain values as exact numbers. **Exact numbers** can be thought of as having infinitely many significant figures. The number of items is considered an exact number in pharmacy practice. For example, the number of tablets or the number of days are considered exact numbers. Consequently, you count only the significant figures in the measured (inexact) quantities, such as dosages.

1.4 Problem Set

Write the following numbers using standard notation.

1. 6.8×10^4

2. 1.87×10^6

3. 1.03×10^7

4. 8.4×10^{-4}

5. 7.68×10^{-3}

6. 6.239×10^{-5}

Write the following numbers using scientific notation.

7. 0.00000000329

8. 390,000,000,000

9. 0.0038

10. 52,000,000,000,000,000

11. 3,779,000

12. 0.000000000202

Identify the number of significant figures in the following numbers. Assume that all final zeros in numbers without decimals are not significant.
Note: The abbreviation *mL* means "milliliters"; the abbreviation *mg* means "milligrams"; the abbreviation *mcg* means "micrograms"; and the abbreviation *kg* means "kilograms."

13. 15.4324 grains

14. 1,500 mL

15. 0.21 mg

16. $1.07

17. 100,000 mcg

18. 507.2 mg

19. 1.01 kg

20. 0.001 mg

21. 21,204.075 mcg

22. 100 mL

Round the following numbers to three significant figures.

23. 42.75

24. 10.091

25. 0.04268

26. 18.426

27. 0.003918

Round the following numbers to the hundredths place and state how many significant figures each number has.

28. 0.3479

29. 0.056921

30. 1.9947

31. 0.00986

32. 1.0277

Calculate the following products and retain the correct number of significant figures in the answers.

33. $0.67 \times 95.2 =$

34. $1.26 \times 24 =$

35. $325 \times 0.5 =$

Applications

36. You are to prepare capsules that contain 0.125 gram (g) of a drug. You have four partial containers of medication, which weigh 3.2 g, 1.784 g, 2.46 g, and 5.87 g. Assume that you have weighed each of the four containers with the same scale, and the accuracy is known to the hundredth gram.

   a. Which amount will need to be rounded?

   b. Which amount is not as accurate as it should be?

   c. What amount of medication will be left over after making as many 0.125 g capsules as possible?

37. A unit dose of an oral medication requires 21.65 mg. You are to prepare 45 doses.

   a. How many milligrams will you need?

   b. How many significant figures does this amount have?

   Self-check your work in Appendix A.

1.5 Estimates

Estimation is the process of finding an approximate solution or answer, known as an *estimate*, to a mathematical problem *prior to* performing the actual calculation. Determining an estimate allows you to verify whether your calculated solution is reasonable. Estimation can be used in both simple mathematical equations and more-complicated algebraic equations. This method may also be used in everyday tasks, such as rounding to the nearest whole dollar while shopping.

There are no set mathematical rules for estimation; however, it is commonly performed by rounding to the nearest whole unit that makes sense for the numbers involved. This whole unit may be the ones place, tens place, hundreds place, or even larger.

Estimating Sums and Differences

When estimating sums and differences, it is common practice to round the numbers to the nearest tens place, hundreds place, or thousands place, and then to add or subtract the rounded numbers. When rounding and then adding or subtracting, the values in the ones place and lower are often ignored. The following calculations compare an actual sum or difference with a corresponding estimate.

actual sum:	$73.8 + 42.03 + 18.3 + 87.32 = 221.45$
estimated sum:	$70 \ \ + 40 \ \ \ + 20 \ \ + 90 \ \ \ = 220$
actual sum:	$623 + 1{,}493 + 1{,}631 + 794 + 86 \ \ = 4{,}627$
estimated sum:	$600 + 1{,}500 + 1{,}600 + 800 + 100 = 4{,}600$
actual difference:	$8{,}425 - 2{,}652 - 2{,}328 - 1{,}490 = 1{,}955$
estimated difference:	$8{,}000 - 3{,}000 - 2{,}000 - 1{,}000 = 2{,}000$

Safety Alert

Estimation can be used to double-check doses but should *never* be relied on for accuracy.

Estimation is a process that becomes easier with practice. A short list of numbers will often generate a fairly accurate estimate, whereas a longer list of numbers may require more practice and may be less accurate. The sum or difference determined by estimation cannot be relied on for accuracy when filling prescriptions or medication orders.

Estimating Products and Quotients

One commonly used method to estimate products or quotients is to round each of the original numbers. If any of the rounded numbers have zeros at the end of the numbers, you can temporarily drop the zeros before performing multiplication or division. Then the rounded numbers can be quickly multiplied or divided. In the case of multiplication, the appropriate number of zeros can be added to the answer. In the case of division, the number of zeros dropped from the divisor can be subtracted from the number of zeros dropped from the dividend. The following examples walk you through these steps.

Example 1.5.1

Estimate the product of 325 × 618. Then compare the estimated product to the actual product.

To begin, round the two numbers: 325 is closer to 300 than 400 and should be rounded to 300; 618 is closer to 600 than 700 and should be rounded to 600.

Next, temporarily drop the zeros from both values. You will replace these zeros once you arrive at the estimated answer.

300 becomes 3
600 becomes 6

Then multiply the rounded numbers.

$$3 \times 6 = 18$$

Next, replace the appropriate number of zeros in the answer. Two zeros should be added for 300, and two zeros should be added for 600. As a result, you will add four zeros to 18.

180,000

Finally, calculate the actual product of 325 × 618.

Answer: The estimated product of 325 × 618 is 180,000; the actual product of this problem is 200,850.

Example 1.5.2

Estimate the product of 843 × 41. Then compare the estimated product to the actual product.

To begin, round the two numbers: 843 should be rounded to 800, and 41 should be rounded to 40.

Next, you can temporarily drop the zeros from both values. You will replace these zeros once you arrive at the estimated answer.

800 becomes 8
40 becomes 4

Then multiply the rounded numbers.

$$8 \times 4 = 32$$

Next, replace the appropriate number of zeros in the answer. Two zeros should be added for 800, and one zero should be added for 40. As a result, a total of three zeros should be added.

32,000

Finally, calculate the actual product of 843 × 41.

Answer: The estimated product of 843 × 41 is 32,000; the actual product of this problem is 34,563.

Example 1.5.3

Estimate the quotient of 953 ÷ 52. Then compare the estimated quotient to the actual quotient.

To begin, round the two numbers: 953 should be rounded to 1,000, and 52 should be rounded to 50.

Next, temporarily drop the zeros from both values. You will replace these zeros once you arrive at the estimated answer.

$$1,000 \text{ becomes } 10$$
$$50 \text{ becomes } 5$$

Then divide the rounded numbers.

$$10 \div 5 = 2$$

Next, replace the appropriate number of zeros in the answer. To do so, subtract the number of zeros dropped from the divisor (in this case, one zero) from the number of zeros dropped from the dividend (in this case, two zeros). As a result, a total of one zero should be added to the estimated answer.

$$20$$

Finally, calculate the actual quotient of 953 ÷ 52.

Answer: The estimated quotient of 953 ÷ 52 is 20; the actual quotient of this problem is 18.3.

Example 1.5.4

Estimate the quotient of 5,355 ÷ 4.79. Then compare the estimated quotient to the actual quotient.

To begin, round the two numbers: 5,355 is closer to 5,000 than 6,000 and should be rounded to 5,000; 4.79 is closer to 5 than 4 and should be rounded to 5.

Next, temporarily drop the zeros, as necessary. You will replace these zeros once you arrive at the estimated answer.

$$5,000 \text{ becomes } 5$$
$$5 \text{ remains } 5$$

Then divide the rounded numbers.

$$5 \div 5 = 1$$

Next, subtract the number of zeros dropped from the divisor (in this case, no zeros) from the number of zeros dropped from the dividend (in this case, three zeros). As a result, a total of three zeros should be added to the estimated answer.

$$1,000$$

Finally, calculate the actual quotient of 5,355 ÷ 4.79.

Answer: The estimated quotient of 5,355 ÷ 4.79 is 1,000; the actual quotient of this problem is 1,117.95.

Example 1.5.5

A patient needs to take 3.75 mL of an oral liquid medication daily for 30 days. Estimate the total number of milliliters needed to fill this order. Then compare your estimated number of milliliters to the actual number. Finally, determine which bottle you will need to fill this order: a 120 mL bottle or a 180 mL bottle.

To begin, round 3.75 mL to 4 mL.

Next, multiply 4 mL by the number of days needed (30 days).

$$4 \text{ mL} \times 30 \text{ days} = 120 \text{ mL}$$

Finally, use the actual number (3.75 mL) in your calculation.

$$3.75 \text{ mL} \times 30 \text{ days} = 112.5 \text{ mL}$$

Answer: The estimated product of 4 mL × 30 days is 120 mL; the actual product of this problem is 112.5 mL. For that reason, you will select the 120 mL bottle to dispense 112.5 mL of this medication.

Estimating a Drug Dose

Math Morsel

Estimation can help to prevent dispensing errors by providing an approximation of the amount of product to dispense. Significant differences in the estimated and actual amounts should prompt pharmacy technicians to double-check their work for accuracy.

Estimating a drug dose before calculating the actual dose is helpful because the estimate can be used to double-check the accuracy of the actual dose. If the actual dose is not close to the estimated dose, then the calculations should be rechecked. When estimating a drug dose, the first step is to round the dose to a number you can easily divide by the available drug strength. Next, divide the rounded number by the available drug strength.

Example 1.5.6

An order for 12.5 mg of a drug needs to be filled. The pharmacy has 5 mg tablets in stock. Estimate the number of tablets needed for this dose and compare this estimated number to the actual number of tablets needed.

Because the order is for 12.5 mg of the drug, the dose to be measured out will be larger than one 5 mg tablet.

To begin, simplify the estimation by rounding down 12.5 mg to 10 mg. This rounding will make it easier to use the available dose to estimate the required number of tablets.

$$10 \text{ mg (estimated requested amount)} \times \frac{1 \text{ tablet}}{5 \text{ mg}} \text{ (available amount)} = 2 \text{ tablets}$$

Now calculate the number of tablets needed for a 12.5 mg dose.

$$12.5 \text{ mg (actual requested amount)} \times \frac{1 \text{ tablet}}{5 \text{ mg}} \text{ (available amount)} = 2.5 \text{ tablets}$$

The calculated actual dose of 2.5 tablets can then be checked by comparing it with the estimated dose. In this case, the estimated dose was 2 tablets. Because the two tablet doses are similar, you can be more confident in the accuracy of your calculated dose.

Answer: The estimated number of tablets needed for 12.5 mg of this drug is 2 tablets, and the actual number of tablets needed is 2.5 or $2^1/_2$ tablets.

In addition to drug doses, the volume to be dispensed and the size of the container needed can be useful estimates when preparing a drug for dispensing. For example, when dispensing a liquid medication, it is important to round up and overestimate the amount of liquid your patient will need. This action ensures that the individual receives enough medication.

Example 1.5.7

The pharmacy receives an order for a 10 days' supply of a liquid antibiotic to be taken in a dose of 8.5 mL of medication three times a day. The pharmacy has 100 mL, 200 mL, and 300 mL bottles of this antibiotic in stock. Which size bottle of antibiotic should be dispensed?

To begin, round the dose: 8.5 mL/dose to 10 mL/dose. Recall that it is important to round up to make sure the patient has enough medication.

Then use this rounded value (estimated dose) to calculate the amount of medication needed per day. To do so, multiply the estimated dose by the number of doses each day.

$$\frac{10 \text{ mL}}{1 \text{ dose}} \times \frac{3 \text{ doses}}{1 \text{ day}} = \frac{30 \text{ mL}}{1 \text{ day}}$$

Consequently, the patient will need about 30 mL of the medication per day.

Because the patient needs to take this medication for 10 days, multiply the amount of medication per day by the number of days of therapy.

$$\frac{30 \text{ mL}}{1 \text{ day}} \times 10 \text{ days} = 300 \text{ mL}$$

Now, determine the actual amount the patient will need for a 10 days' supply.

$$\frac{8.5 \text{ mL}}{1 \text{ dose}} \times \frac{3 \text{ doses}}{\text{day}} \times 10 \text{ days} = 255 \text{ mL}$$

Therefore, the patient will need about 300 mL of the medication. The actual amount needed is 255 mL.

Answer: Because the patient will need 255 mL of medication, the 300 mL bottle is necessary to fill the prescription.

1.5 Problem Set

Round dollar amounts to the nearest whole dollar to find the estimated value. Then calculate the actual value.

1. $12.53 − $6.15 =

2. $6.28 + $1.99 + $3.98 =

3. $40 − $34.81 =

4. $100 − $18.29 =

5. $100 − $17.52 − $31.90 =

Round the two numbers and multiply them to find the estimated product. Then calculate the actual product.

6. 6.8 × 7,656 =

7. 4.02 × 350.07 =

8. 598.4 × 0.015 =

9. 4,569 × 0.0972 =

10. 6,183 × 18 =

11. 1,253 × 9.1 =

Round the two numbers and divide them to find the estimated quotient. Then calculate the actual quotient.

12. $185 \div 18 =$

13. $18,015 \div 56 =$

14. $584.0 \div 8 =$

15. $844.23 \div 4.4 =$

16. $123 \div 14 =$

Applications

Use rounding and estimation to solve the following problems.

17. A compounding pharmacy requires last-minute supplies. If the following items are needed, estimate how much the total cost will be.

food dye	$1.89
sugar, 2 bags	$4.25/bag
baking soda	$0.79
cherry flavoring	$2.39
bleach, 1 gal	$1.97
distilled water, 4 gal	$0.89/gal

18. Estimate how much sterile water for injection (SWFI) you will need for the following reconstitutions: 3.2 mL, 7.6 mL, 1.6 mL, and 4.1 mL. Choose from the following available vials (15 mL SWFI, 30 mL SWFI, and 50 mL SWFI).

19. A patient is receiving the following fluids: intravenous (IV) fluids, 1,723 mL; juice, 150 mL; and coffee, 126 mL. Estimate the patient's intake to the nearest 10 mL.

20. A patient's parenteral fluid intake for the first 24 hours after hospital admission includes the following: 780 mL normal saline (NS), three 50 mL piggybacks, 250 mL NS, three 1,000 mL bags of NS. Estimate the total to the nearest 100 mL amount.

Self-check your work in Appendix A.

Review and Assessment

CHAPTER SUMMARY

- Arabic numbers use a decimal point to show the place value of digits in the numbers.

- Roman numerals may be used on prescriptions, and they may be written as either uppercase or lowercase letters.

- Roman numerals are never repeated more than three times in sequence.

- Roman numerals that have a smaller value in front of Roman numerals that have a larger value should be subtracted to determine the final value.

- Fractions are part of a whole.

- The upper number in a fraction is the numerator.

- The lower number in a fraction is the denominator.

- When adding or subtracting fractions, you need to have a common denominator.

- Common denominators can be found by factoring the denominators and comparing them.

- When multiplying fractions, you multiply the numerators together and the denominators together.

- When dividing fractions, you multiply the first fraction by the reciprocal of the second fraction.

- Decimals may use a leading zero in front of the decimal point to avoid calculation errors.

- Scientific notation is a way to write very large or very small numbers using a power of 10 and an exponent.

- Exponents, or superscript numbers placed to the right of numbers, are used in scientific notation to show that numbers have been raised to a power; exponents can be positive or negative numbers.

- Significant figures can be used to determine accuracy.

- Accuracy is the degree to which a measurement matches the actual value of the quantity being measured.

- A trailing zero should be used only when it is a significant figure that determines the accuracy of a number.

- Estimation is helpful in double-checking results, but an estimate should never be considered accurate.

CHECK YOUR UNDERSTANDING

Take a moment to review what you have learned in this chapter and answer the following questions.

1. When adding or subtracting fractions with unlike denominators, you should
    a. create a common denominator.
    b. multiply by the reciprocal of the second fraction.
    c. subtract the numerators.
    d. add the denominators.

2. When multiplying fractions, you should
    a. always change mixed numbers into improper fractions first.
    b. multiply the denominators by the least common denominator.
    c. multiply the first fraction by the reciprocal of the second fraction.
    d. reduce all fractions so that a 1 is in the numerator.

3. To divide fractions, you should
    a. add the numerators.
    b. find a common denominator.
    c. switch the numerator and denominator of the fraction to the right of the division sign and multiply.
    d. switch the numerator and denominator of the fraction to the left of the division sign and multiply.

4. In the number 1.23578, which digit is in the hundredths place?
    a. 1
    b. 2
    c. 3
    d. 5

5. Scientific notation is used to write
    a. Roman numerals that need to be converted.
    b. standard notation numbers that are very large or very small.
    c. notes to the pharmacist about an estimated dose.
    d. drug doses when they are very small.

6. Significant figures are used for
    a. determining accuracy.
    b. estimating a drug dose.
    c. eliminating zeros to the left of a decimal.
    d. calibrating the sensitivity of a pharmacy scale.

7. Which decimal has an underlined digit in the tenths place?
    a. 4$\underline{1}$2.678
    b. 41$\underline{2}$.678
    c. 412.$\underline{6}$78
    d. 412.6$\underline{7}$8

8. Which decimal value represents the fraction $^1/_5$?
    a. 0.05
    b. 0.15
    c. 0.2
    d. 1.5

9. Sterile water is purchased in containers of 1,000 mL. How many 125 mL containers could be poured out of the large container?
    a. 5
    b. 8
    c. 10
    d. 12

10. If a 100-count bottle of alprazolam 1 mg costs the pharmacy $23.87, how much would 75 tablets cost the pharmacy?
    a. $12.56
    b. $17.90
    c. $21.45
    d. $27.91

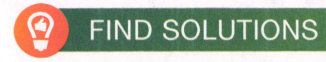

Take a moment to consider what you have learned in this chapter and respond thoughtfully to the prompts.

Note: *To indicate your answer for Scenario C, Question 8, ask your instructor for the handout depicting a dosing spoon.*

Scenario A: A patient brings the following prescription to you.

> ℞ **Lasix 40 mg**
>
> Dosing instructions: Take ȋ tablet by mouth each Monday, Wednesday, and Friday, and ȋȋ tablets on other days.
>
> Quantity to dispense: 30 days' supply
>
> Refills: 2

1. How many tablets per day does the patient take on each Monday, Wednesday, and Friday?

2. Estimate how many tablets the patient will need to last 30 days.

3. Calculate exactly how many tablets the patient will need in a 30-day period if the patient picks up the medication on a Sunday.

Scenario B: The maximum dose for an over-the-counter medication is 4,000 mg per day. A patient reports taking 4 whole tablets and $\frac{1}{2}$ tablet today but wants to take more, if possible. The package indicates that there are 500 mg in each tablet.

4. How many milligrams of medication did the patient receive from the ingestion of the whole tablets?

5. How many milligrams did the patient receive from the ingestion of the $\frac{1}{2}$ tablet?

6. How many total milligrams of medication did the patient take?

7. How many more tablets can the patient take before the patient exceeds the maximum dose? Calculate to the nearest $\frac{1}{2}$ tablet.

Scenario C: A mother has come to the pharmacy and is confused about the markings on a dosing spoon. The prescription drug label states that she is to give $\frac{3}{4}$ of a teaspoon to her daughter.

8. On the handout that you obtained from your instructor, indicate the amount of medication that should be measured out in the dosing spoon.

Scenario D: A patient brings the following prescription to you.

> ℞ **Warfarin 5 mg**
>
> Dosing instructions: Take ï tablet by mouth on Tuesday, Thursday, and Saturday. Take ss tablets on all other days.
>
> Quantity to dispense: 30 days' supply
>
> Refills: 5

9. How many tablets per day does the patient take on Monday, Wednesday, Friday, and Sunday?

10. How many tablets does the patient take on Tuesday, Thursday, and Saturday?

11. How many milligrams are ingested with Monday's dose?

12. Calculate exactly how many tablets the patient will need in a 30-day period if the patient begins taking the medication on Sunday.

Scenario E: A patient brings the following prescription to you.

> ℞ **Levothyroxine 125 mcg**
>
> Dosing instructions: Take ï tablet by mouth on Monday, Wednesday, Friday, and Saturday.
>
> Quantity to dispense: 90 days' supply
>
> Refills: 1

13. How many tablets does the patient take per week?

14. How many milligrams of levothyroxine are taken each week?

15. How many tablets should you dispense if the patient first fills the prescription on a Tuesday?

16. How many tablets would be dispensed if the patient received a 30 days' supply and first filled the prescription on a Tuesday?

 The online course includes additional review and assessment resources.

Performing Ratio, Percent, and Proportion Calculations

2

Learning Objectives

1 Define *ratios* and describe their use in the pharmacy setting. (Section 2.1)

2 Utilize ratios to calculate medication doses or volumes. (Sections 2.1, 2.3)

3 Define *percent* as it pertains to pharmacy calculations. (Sections 2.2, 2.4)

4 Convert ratios to percents, percents to ratios, percents to decimals, and decimals to percents. (Sections 2.1, 2.2, 2.3)

5 Utilize percents to calculate medication doses or volumes. (Section 2.2)

6 Define *proportion* and the three ways it can be expressed in a pharmacy calculation. (Section 2.3)

7 Explain the rules and steps for using the ratio-proportion method in pharmacy calculations. (Sections 2.1, 2.3)

8 Describe the applications and calculations associated with percentage of error and error tolerance. (Section 2.4)

For a key to the body system icons that appear in each chapter of this textbook, refer to the Preface.

ASHP/ACPE Accreditation Standards
To view the *ASHP/ACPE Accreditation Standards* addressed in this chapter, refer to Appendix D.

Whether you plan to practice in a community setting or an institutional setting, you will be required to perform calculations in your role as a pharmacy technician. This chapter introduces you to concepts that are fundamental to pharmacy calculations: ratios, percents, and proportions. Mastering ratios, percents, and proportions will allow you to complete a myriad of pharmacy calculations that are pertinent to the interpretation of prescriptions and medication orders, the conversions between measurement systems, and the computation of doses.

2.1 Ratios

A **ratio** is a numerical representation of the relationship between two parts of a whole or of the relationship of one part to the whole. Ratios may be written with a colon (:) between the numbers, which may be read as *per*, *of*, *to*, or *in*. The ratio 1:2 could mean that the second part has twice the value (e.g., size, number, weight, volume) of the first part, or the ratio could indicate that one part is something within a total of two parts. Ratios may also be written as fractions, and it is the ratio in fraction form that is commonly used in pharmacy calculations.

Math Morsel

A ratio written in the form of a fraction is commonly used in pharmacy calculations.

1:2	is read as	1 part to 2 parts	and may also be written as	$\frac{1}{2}$
3:4	is read as	3 parts to 4 parts	and may also be written as	$\frac{3}{4}$
1:20	is read as	1 part to 20 parts	and may also be written as	$\frac{1}{20}$
1:10	is read as	1 part to 10 parts	and may also be written as	$\frac{1}{10}$

Math Morsel

Ratios of drugs are usually written as the concentration of a drug per dose or the weight of a drug in a unit of measurement.

A ratio can be any numerical relation you need to show. With medications, you commonly use a ratio to express the weight or strength of a drug per dose or volumetric measurement. Ratios are commonly used to express concentrations of a medication in solution. For example, a 1:100 concentration of a medication means that there is 1 part of the medication in 100 parts of the solution (1 g per 100 mL). It is also common to reverse the order of the values written in a ratio.

250 mg:1 tablet	or	1 tablet:250 mg
1 g:100 mL	or	100 mL:1 g
500 mg:20 mL	or	20 mL:500 mg

A ratio may be manipulated by multiplying or dividing both parts of the ratio by the same factor. Pharmacists and pharmacy technicians use this process when calculating the volume of a medication to be administered or, in some cases, the amount of a drug per volume of the medication administered.

Some medication labels, especially those of injectable medications, have more than one ratio listed. For example, the aminophylline label (see Figure 2.1) includes three ratios, each descriptive of the medication's concentration. The first ratio, shown within the green bar of the medication label, is 500 mg/20 mL and represents the total amount of medication in the entire ampule. The second ratio on the medication label is 25 mg/mL and represents the amount of medication in 1 mL. The third ratio is 19.7 mg/mL and describes the concentration of the medication in its anhydrous-theophylline state. The pharmacist may use this concentration to further analyze the dosage. The ratio indicating the total amount of medication in the ampule is of the most importance to a pharmacy technician. Typically, this ratio is the most prominent one on the label, as is the case for this label.

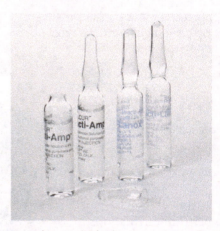

Ampules are single-dose containers of medication that are opened at the time of use.

FIGURE 2.1
Ratios on an Ampule Label

When more than one ratio appears on a medication label, the most prominent ratio—in this case, 500 mg/20 mL—is typically the most important.

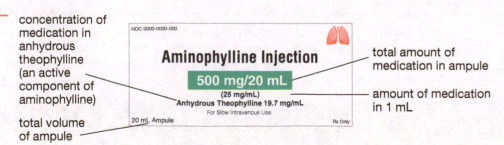

concentration of medication in anhydrous theophylline (an active component of aminophylline)

total volume of ampule

total amount of medication in ampule

amount of medication in 1 mL

Medication labels indicate the ratio of the active ingredient, and, as described in Chapter 1, the ratio may be manipulated by multiplying or dividing both parts of the ratio by the same factor. If the dose needs to be increased, you multiply the ratio by a factor. If the dose needs to be decreased, you divide the ratio by a factor.

Example 2.1.1

 Using the label shown in Figure 2.1, how many milligrams of aminophylline were ordered if two ampules were administered and each ampule contained 500 mg/20 mL?

For two ampules, you multiply both parts of the ratio by 2.

$$\frac{500 \text{ mg} \times 2}{20 \text{ mL} \times 2} = \frac{1,000 \text{ mg}}{40 \text{ mL}}$$

Answer: The order was for 1,000 mg of aminophylline.

Example 2.1.2

 Using the label shown in Figure 2.1, how many milligrams of aminophylline were ordered if half of an ampule was administered and each ampule contained 500 mg/20 mL?

To determine the number of milligrams in half of an ampule, you can either divide both parts of the ratio by 2 or multiply both parts of the ratio by $\frac{1}{2}$.

Division Method

$$\frac{500 \text{ mg} \div 2}{20 \text{ mL} \div 2} = \frac{250 \text{ mg}}{10 \text{ mL}}$$

Multiplication Method

$$\frac{500 \text{ mg} \times \frac{1}{2}}{20 \text{ mL} \times \frac{1}{2}} = \frac{250 \text{ mg}}{10 \text{ mL}}$$

Answer: The order was for 250 mg of aminophylline.

Pharm Fact

Pharmacy technicians should be aware that some drug manufacturers always capitalize the name of the drug on a medication label, regardless of whether the medication is a generic product or a brand name. For that reason, they should be sure to memorize both the generic and brand names of drugs.

Example 2.1.3

A physician has ordered that a patient take $\frac{1}{2}$ of a 137 microgram (mcg) tablet of levothyroxine. How many micrograms will the patient take?

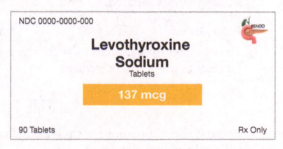

NDC 0000-0000-000

Levothyroxine Sodium
Tablets

137 mcg

90 Tablets   Rx Only

This label does not overtly indicate the ratio. However, you can determine a ratio because the label says each tablet contains 137 mcg of levothyroxine. Therefore, the ratio is 137 mcg/1 tablet. You can use either multiplication or division to solve the problem. You can also use the dimensional analysis method you learned in Chapter 1.

Multiplication Method

$$\frac{137 \text{ mcg} \times \frac{1}{2}}{1 \text{ tablet} \times \frac{1}{2}} = \frac{68.5 \text{ mcg}}{\frac{1}{2} \text{ tablet}}$$

Division Method

$$\frac{137 \text{ mcg} \div 2}{1 \text{ tablet} \div 2} = \frac{68.5 \text{ mcg}}{\frac{1}{2} \text{ tablet}}$$

Dimensional Analysis Method

$$\frac{137 \text{ mcg}}{1 \text{ tablet}} \times \frac{0.5 \text{ tablet}}{1} = 68.5 \text{ mcg}$$

Answer: The patient will take ½ tablet of levothyroxine, which contains 68.5 mcg.

Some medications are ordered in concentrations that are expressed as a ratio. Typically, these medications are available in a very small percentage (less than 1%). The dosage form influences the ratio. A common dosage form is a **solution** (a liquid mixture in which the minor component, the **solute**, is uniformly distributed within the major component, the **solvent**). A similar dosage form is a **suspension**, or a mixture in which solute particles are mixed with, but not dissolved in, a fluid. The following examples use a 1:10,000 ratio.

1 g active ingredient:10,000 g of a solid, such as a cream

1 g active ingredient:10,000 mL of a solution

1 mL active ingredient:10,000 mL of a liquid

Example 2.1.4

A 1:100 solution has 1 g active ingredient in 100 mL. How much active ingredient is present in 300 mL of this solution?

You can either set up a ratio to solve this problem, or you can use the dimensional analysis method.

Ratio Method

To begin, set up a ratio to solve for the unknown variable x. In this problem, x represents the active ingredient.

$$\frac{x \text{ g}}{300 \text{ mL}} = \frac{1 \text{ g}}{100 \text{ mL}}$$

Because these fractions are equivalent, you can cross multiply and the equations will still equal one another.

$$x \text{ g} (100 \text{ mL}) = 300 \text{ mL} (1 \text{ g})$$

Then solve for x by dividing each side of the equation by 100 mL and canceling the similar units (like units) in the numerators and in the denominators.

$$\frac{x \text{ g } (\cancel{100 \text{ mL}})}{\cancel{100 \text{ mL}}} = \frac{300 \cancel{\text{ mL}} (1 \text{ g})}{100 \cancel{\text{ mL}}}$$

$$x \text{ g} = \frac{300 (1 \text{ g})}{100}$$

$$x = 3 \text{ g}$$

Dimensional Analysis Method

$$\frac{1 \text{ g}}{100 \cancel{\text{ mL}}} \times \frac{300 \cancel{\text{ mL}}}{1} = 3 \text{ g}$$

Answer: There are 3 g of active ingredient in 300 mL of solution.

2.1 Problem Set   *odd only!!!*

Express the following ratios as fractions and then reduce the fractions to their lowest terms.

1. 3:7

2. 8:6

3. 3:4

4. 4:6

5. 1:7

Reduce the following fractions to their lowest terms and then express these fractions as ratios.

6. $\dfrac{2}{3}$

7. $\dfrac{6}{8}$

8. $\dfrac{5}{10}$

9. $\dfrac{1}{9}$

10. $\dfrac{1}{10,000}$

Applications

State the ratio for the following doses.

11. 30 mg capsule of Cymbalta

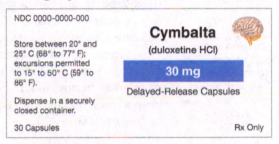

12. 100 mg capsule of Dilantin

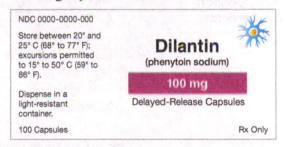

13. 5 mL dose of oral suspension containing 250 mg of amoxicillin

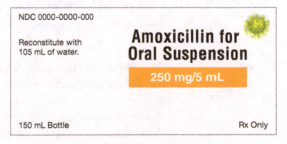

Use the ratios calculated in items 11–13 to calculate the amount of medication in the following doses. Write your answers as ratios.

14. 3 capsules of Cymbalta

15. 2 capsules of Dilantin

16. 15 mL of amoxicillin suspension

Fill in the blanks.

17. A 10:1,000 solution contains _____ g of active ingredient in _____ mL of product, and 100 mL of that solution contains _____ g.

18. A 1:100 solution contains _____ g of active ingredient in _____ mL of product, and 500 mL of that solution contains _____ g.

19. A 1:250 solution contains _____ g of active ingredient in _____ mL of product, and 1,000 mL of that solution contains _____ g.

20. A 1:1,000 solution contains _____ g of active ingredient in _____ mL of product, and 50 mL of that solution contains _____ g.

Self-check your work in Appendix A.

2.2 Percents

Put Down Roots

The word *percent* comes from the Latin term *per centum*, meaning "by the hundred." Therefore, *percent* literally means "per 100."

The word *percent* means "per 100" or "hundredths." Consequently, a **percent** expresses the number of parts compared with a total of 100 parts. A percent is represented by the symbol % and can be written as a ratio, a fraction, or a decimal. For example, 30% can be written as a ratio (30:100), a fraction ($^{30}/_{100}$), or a decimal (0.30). All three forms indicate 30 parts in a total of 100 parts.

A percent can be visualized by comparing a stack of 100 pennies (equivalent to one dollar) next to smaller stacks of pennies (see Figure 2.2). A stack of 40 pennies equals 40% of one dollar, which can also be expressed as 40:100 or $^{40}/_{100}$ or 0.40. Similarly, a stack of 5 pennies equals 5% of one dollar, which can also be expressed as 5:100 or $^{5}/_{100}$ or 0.05.

FIGURE 2.2 Comparison of Percents

100% of one dollar	40% of one dollar	5% of one dollar

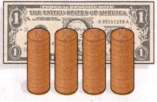 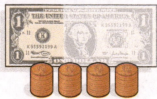 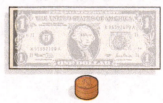

100 pennies	40 pennies	5 pennies

Math Morsel

The higher the percentage of a dissolved substance, the greater the strength.

Percents are often used to describe the strengths or concentrations of intravenous (IV) solutions and topically applied medications. The higher the percentage of dissolved substances in a solution or in a topical medication, the greater the strength. Both examples below may be expressed as 1:100, $^{1}/_{100}$, or 0.01.

A 1% solution contains 1 g of medication per 100 mL of fluid.

A 1% hydrocortisone cream contains 1 g of hydrocortisone per 100 g of cream.

When performing calculations with medications described by percents, it is helpful to rewrite the medication as a fraction or ratio first. Then the ratio may be manipulated by multiplying or dividing both parts of the ratio by the same factor. As mentioned earlier, if the dose needs to be increased, you multiply the ratio by a factor. If the dose needs to be decreased, you divide the ratio by a factor.

Example 2.2.1

A 5% solution contains 5 g of solute per 100 mL of solution. If a patient is to receive 200 mL of solution, how many grams of solute will it contain?

You can either set up a ratio to solve this problem, or you can use the dimensional analysis method.

Ratio Method

$$\frac{x \text{ g}}{200 \text{ mL}} = \frac{5 \text{ g}}{100 \text{ mL}}$$

Because these fractions are equivalent, you can cross multiply and the equations will still equal one another.

$$x \text{ g} (100 \text{ mL}) = 5 \text{ g} (200 \text{ mL})$$

Then solve for x by dividing each side of the equation by 100 mL and canceling the similar units (like units) in the numerators and in the denominators.

$$\frac{x \text{ g} (\cancel{100 \text{ mL}})}{\cancel{100 \text{ mL}}} = \frac{5 \text{ g} (200 \cancel{\text{ mL}})}{100 \cancel{\text{ mL}}}$$

$$x = 10 \text{ g}$$

Dimensional Analysis Method

$$\frac{200 \cancel{\text{ mL}}}{1} \times \frac{5 \text{ g}}{100 \cancel{\text{ mL}}} = 10 \text{ g}$$

Answer: The 200 mL solution contains 10 g of solute.

Example 2.2.2

A 2% solution contains 2 g of solute per 100 mL of solution. How many milliliters of this solution are needed to give a dose of 6 g of solute?

You can either set up a ratio to solve this problem, or you can use the dimensional analysis method.

Ratio Method

$$\frac{2 \text{ g}}{100 \text{ mL}} = \frac{6 \text{ g}}{x \text{ mL}}$$

Because these fractions are equivalent, you can cross multiply and the equations will still equal one another.

$$x \text{ mL} (2 \text{ g}) = 100 \text{ mL} (6 \text{ g})$$

Then solve for x by dividing each side of the equation by 2 g and canceling the similar units (like units) in the numerators and in the denominators.

$$\frac{x \text{ mL} (\cancel{2 \text{ g}})}{\cancel{2 \text{ g}}} = \frac{100 \text{ mL} (6 \cancel{\text{ g}})}{2 \cancel{\text{ g}}}$$

$$x = 300 \text{ mL}$$

Dimensional Analysis Method

$$\frac{6\,\cancel{g}}{1} \times \frac{100\ \text{mL}}{2\,\cancel{g}} = 300\ \text{mL}$$

Answer: A 300 mL solution is needed to give a dose of 6 g of solute.

Example 2.2.3

The medication label shows a 1% solution of Xylocaine. Write the percent as a fraction. Then determine the number of milligrams per milliliter (mg/mL) in a 1% solution of Xylocaine.

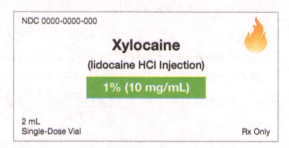

A 1% solution of Xylocaine contains 1 g of Xylocaine per 100 mL of solution. To begin, write the percent as a fraction.

$$1\% = \frac{1\ \text{g}}{100\ \text{mL}}$$

Then convert the fraction from grams per 100 mL to milligrams per 100 mL.

$$\frac{1\ \text{g}}{100\ \text{mL}} = \frac{1{,}000\ \text{mg}}{100\ \text{mL}}$$

Finally, divide to solve the problem.

$$\frac{1{,}000\ \text{mg}}{100\ \text{mL}} = \frac{10\ \text{mg}}{1\ \text{mL}}$$

Answer: A 1% Xylocaine solution contains 10 mg/mL of medication.

When working in a pharmacy, you will need to know equivalent values for different mathematical expressions such as percents, fractions, ratios, and decimals. The examples shown in Table 2.1 show these equivalent mathematical expressions.

TABLE 2.1 Equivalent Mathematical Expressions

Percent	Fraction	Ratio	Decimal
45%	$\frac{45}{100}$	45:100	0.45
0.5%	$\frac{0.5}{100} = \frac{1}{200}$	0.5:100	0.005

Converting a Fraction to a Percent

Fractions compare a number of parts (the numerator) with a total number of parts (the denominator). This comparison is similar to a percent, in which the number of parts is compared with a total of 100 parts. There are two methods you can use to convert a fraction to a percent. One method is to convert the fraction to an equivalent fraction with a denominator of 100.

Consider the fraction $^3/_{10}$.

$$\frac{3}{10} = \frac{3}{10} \times \frac{10}{10} = \frac{30}{100} = 30\%$$

Another way to convert a fraction to a percent is to divide the numerator by the denominator, multiply by 100, and add a percent sign.

Consider the fraction $^2/_{10}$.

$$\frac{2}{10} = 2 \div 10 = 0.2$$

$$0.2 \times 100 = 20\%$$

Example 2.2.4

Convert the fraction $^1/_{50}$ to a percent.

You can solve this problem using two different methods: by making an equivalent fraction with a denominator of 100 or by dividing the numerator by the denominator, multiplying by 100, and adding a percent sign.

Making an Equivalent Fraction with a Denominator of 100

To begin, convert the fraction $^1/_{50}$ to an equivalent fraction with a denominator of 100.

$$\frac{1}{50} \times \frac{2}{2} = \frac{2}{100}$$

Then rewrite the fraction $^2/_{100}$ as a percent.

$$\frac{2}{100} = 2\%$$

Dividing, Multiplying by 100, and Adding a Percent Sign

To begin, divide the numerator (1) by the denominator (50).

$$\frac{1}{50} = 1 \div 50 = 0.02$$

Next, multiply by 100, and add a percent sign.

$$0.02 \times 100 = 2\%$$

Answer: The fraction $^1/_{50}$ is the same as 2%.

Converting a Ratio to a Percent

Recall that percent is the number of parts compared with a total of 100 parts. To convert the ratio 5:1 to a percent, you need to rewrite the ratio as a fraction ($^5/_1$), and then convert the fraction to an equivalent fraction with a denominator of 100. In this case, you must multiply the numerator and denominator by 100 to create a fraction with a denominator of 100.

$$\frac{5}{1} = \frac{5 \times 100}{1 \times 100} = \frac{500}{100} = 500\%$$

Another way to convert a ratio to a percent is to rewrite the ratio as a fraction; then multiply by 100; and, finally, add a percent sign.

$$5{:}1 \qquad \frac{5}{1} \times 100 = \frac{500}{1} = 500\%$$

$$1{:}5 \qquad \frac{1}{5} \times 100 = \frac{100}{5} = 20\%$$

$$1{:}2 \qquad \frac{1}{2} \times 100 = \frac{100}{2} = 50\%$$

Example 2.2.5

A prescriber ordered a 1:1,000 solution. You have a 1% solution, a 0.5% solution, and a 0.1% solution in stock. Which one of these solutions will fill the order?

You can solve this problem using two different methods: by making an equivalent fraction with a denominator of 100 or by multiplying by 100, dividing, and adding a percent sign.

Making an Equivalent Fraction with a Denominator of 100

To begin, rewrite the ratio 1:1,000 as a fraction.

$$1{:}1{,}000 = \frac{1}{1{,}000}$$

Note that the denominator of the fraction is 1,000. To determine the percent solution, $^1/_{1,000}$ needs to be rewritten as an equivalent fraction with a denominator of 100. To do this, divide both the numerator (1) and the denominator (1,000) by 10.

$$\frac{1}{1{,}000} = \frac{1 \div 10}{1{,}000 \div 10} = \frac{0.1}{100} = 0.1\%$$

Multiplying by 100, Dividing, and Adding a Percent Sign

To begin, rewrite the ratio 1:1,000 as a fraction.

$$1{:}1{,}000 = \frac{1}{1{,}000}$$

Next, multiply the fraction by 100.

$$\frac{1}{1{,}000} \times 100 = \frac{100}{1{,}000}$$

Finally, divide the fraction and add a percent sign to your answer.

$$\frac{100}{1,000} = 0.1\%$$

Answer: The 0.1% solution is the same concentration as the ordered 1:1,000 solution.

Converting a Percent to a Ratio

To convert a percent to a ratio, rewrite the percent as a fraction with a denominator of 100. Then reduce the fraction to its lowest terms. Finally, express this fraction as a ratio by making the numerator the first number of the ratio and the denominator the second number of the ratio.

$$2\% = \frac{2}{100} = \frac{1}{50} = 1{:}50$$

$$10\% = \frac{10}{100} = \frac{1}{10} = 1{:}10$$

$$75\% = \frac{75}{100} = \frac{3}{4} = 3{:}4$$

$$\frac{1}{2}\% = \frac{\frac{1}{2}}{100} = \frac{1}{2} \times \frac{1}{100} = \frac{1}{200} = 1{:}200$$

Example 2.2.6

A prescriber ordered a 0.02% solution. You have a 1:1,000 solution; a 1:5,000 solution; and a 1:10,000 solution in stock. Which one of these solutions will fill the order?

To begin, convert the percent to an equivalent fraction. By definition, a percent solution is written in grams per 100 mL (g/100 mL).

$$0.02\% = \frac{0.02 \text{ g}}{100 \text{ mL}}$$

As you know, you can multiply any number by 1 (or a fraction that is equivalent to 1) without changing its value. Therefore, you want to multiply the fraction above by creating a fraction that is equivalent to 1.

$$\frac{0.02 \text{ g}}{100 \text{ mL}} \times \frac{100}{100} = \frac{2 \text{ g}}{10,000 \text{ mL}}$$

Next, you can reduce 2 g/10,000 mL to 1 g/5,000 mL.

Finally, you can convert the fraction 1 g/5,000 mL to a ratio: 1:5,000.

Answer: The 1:5,000 solution can be used to fill the order for a 0.02% solution.

A solution commonly used for cleaning in healthcare facilities is a 1:10 dilution (10%) of bleach and water. This solution is available commercially or may be prepared daily using regular bleach. Figure 2.3 shows a recipe for making a 10% bleach solution. In the recipe, one part bleach is mixed with nine parts of water. The amounts can be adjusted, but the ratio should not change. Because it chemically degrades, a bleach solution prepared according to this recipe expires after one day.

FIGURE 2.3

Recipe for a 10% Bleach Solution

The master formula provides a recipe or a set of instructions for preparing a 10% bleach solution.

10% Bleach Solution

Materials: Storage container, measuring cup or graduated cylinder, bleach, water, label

Instructions: Measure one quantity of bleach (such as 1 cup) and place it into the storage container. Measure the same quantity of water nine times (in this case, 9 cups) and place it into the storage container. Mix well, label, and date the container.

Example 2.2.7

You have been asked to prepare 480 mL of a 10% bleach solution. Convert this percent to an equivalent fraction reduced to its lowest terms. Then determine how much bleach and water you will need to measure.

To begin, convert 10% to an equivalent ratio. Recall that a percent solution, by definition, is listed in grams per 100 milliliters (g/100 mL).

$$10\% = \frac{10 \text{ g}}{100 \text{ mL}}$$

Next, reduce the fraction to its lowest terms.

$$\frac{10 \text{ g}}{100 \text{ mL}} = \frac{1 \text{ g}}{10 \text{ mL}}$$

Now, rewrite this fraction as a ratio.

$$\frac{1 \text{ g}}{10 \text{ mL}} = 1{:}10$$

Next, determine the size of one "part" by dividing 10 parts into the total volume.

$$\text{total volume} \div \text{number of parts} = \text{volume per one part}$$

$$480 \text{ mL} \div 10 \text{ parts} = \frac{48 \text{ mL}}{1 \text{ part}}$$

You know from the recipe in Figure 2.3 that the water-bleach solution (total volume) contains a bleach volume that is equal to one part, or 48 mL. Therefore, determine the amount of water needed by subtracting the known bleach volume from the total volume.

$$\text{total volume} - \text{bleach volume} = \text{water volume}$$

$$480 \text{ mL} - 48 \text{ mL} = 432 \text{ mL}$$

Answer: A 10% bleach solution contains 1 g of bleach per 10 mL. To make 480 mL of 10% bleach solution, combine 48 mL of bleach and 432 mL of water.

Converting a Percent to a Decimal

 Math Morsel

When converting a percent to a decimal, pharmacy technicians should remember to insert zeros—including a leading zero—if necessary.

To convert a percent to a decimal, you drop the percent sign and divide the number by 100. Dividing a number by 100 is equivalent to moving the decimal point two places to the left, inserting zeros if necessary.

$$4\% = 4 \div 100 = 0.04$$
$$15\% = 15 \div 100 = 0.15$$
$$200\% = 200 \div 100 = 2.0$$

Converting a Decimal to a Percent

To change a decimal to a percent, you multiply by 100 or move the decimal point two places to the right. Then add a percent sign.

$$0.25 = 0.25 \times 100 = 25\%$$
$$1.35 = 1.35 \times 100 = 135\%$$
$$0.015 = 0.015 \times 100 = 1.5\%$$

2.2 Problem Set   *odd 1-29 only*

Express the following fractions as percents. Round your answers to the nearest whole percent.

1. $\dfrac{6}{7}$

2. $\dfrac{5}{12}$

3. $\dfrac{1}{4}$

4. $\dfrac{2}{3}$

5. $\dfrac{0.5}{10}$

Express the following ratios as percents. Round your answers to the nearest tenth of a percent.

6. 2:3

7. 1.5:4.65

8. 1:250

9. 1:10,000

10. 1:6

Convert the following percents to fractions; then reduce the fractions to their lowest terms.

11. 50%

12. 2%

Convert the following percents to decimals.

13. 6%

14. 12.5%

15. 126%

Perform the following calculations and round your answers to the nearest hundredth when necessary.

16. 5% of 20

17. 20% of 60

18. 19% of 63

19. 110% of 70

20. 0.2% of 50

Fill in the missing values.

	Percent	Fraction	Ratio	Decimal
21.	33%	$\frac{1}{3}$	_____	_____
22.	2.5%	_____	1:40	_____
23.	_____	$\frac{1}{2}$	_____	0.5
24.	_____	_____	1:100	0.01
25.	90%	_____	_____	0.90
26.	67%	_____	_____	0.67
27.	_____	$\frac{1}{500}$	1:500	_____
28.	0.45%	_____	_____	0.0045
29.	5%	_____	1:20	_____
30.	20%	$\frac{1}{5}$	_____	_____

Applications

Choose the appropriate solution from the available stock solutions.

31. A 1:10,000 solution has been ordered. You have a 0.05% solution, a 0.01% solution, and a 1% solution in stock. Which solution should you choose?

32. A 1:20 solution has been ordered. You have a 5% solution, a 10% solution, and a 20% solution in stock. Which solution should you choose?

33. A 1:25 solution has been ordered. You have a 0.4% solution, a 0.05% solution, and a 4% solution in stock. Which solution should you choose?

34. A 1:800 solution has been ordered. You have a 0.01% solution, a 0.125% solution, and a 1.25% solution in stock. Which solution should you choose?

35. A 1:10 solution has been ordered. You have a 0.09% solution, a 0.01% solution, and a 10% solution in stock. Which solution should you choose?

Self-check your work in Appendix A.

2.3 Proportions

A **proportion** is an expression of equality between two ratios. This expression can be visualized by thinking of two triangles that have the same shape but are different sizes. The triangles in Figure 2.4 have equal proportions.

FIGURE 2.4
Triangles with Equal Proportions

These two triangles have equal proportions because $^{15}/_{20}$ can be reduced to its lowest terms: $^3/_4$.

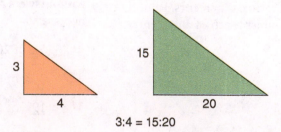

3:4 = 15:20

A proportion can be written three ways: using an equal sign between the ratios, using a double colon (::) between the ratios, or writing the ratios as fractions, as shown below.

$$3:4 = 15:20 \quad \text{or} \quad 3:4 :: 15:20 \quad \text{or} \quad \frac{3}{4} = \frac{15}{20}$$

In a proportion, the first and fourth, or outside, numbers are called the **extremes**. The second and third, or inside, numbers are called the **means**.

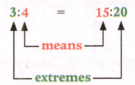

The product of the means must always equal the product of the extremes in a proportion. You can check the accuracy of a proportion by using this formula.

Given a proportion

$$a{:}b = c{:}d$$

the product of means = the product of extremes

or

$$b \times c = a \times d$$

Example 2.3.1

Confirm that the proportion 3:4 equals the proportion 15:20.

If the two proportions are equal, the product of the means should equal the product of the extremes.

To begin, write the proportions as if they were equal to one another.

$$3{:}4 = 15{:}20$$

Next, calculate the product of the means (4 and 15) and the product of the extremes (3 and 20).

$$4 \times 15 = 3 \times 20$$

$$60 = 60$$

Answer: Because the product of the means equals the product of the extremes, the ratios 3:4 and 15:20 are proportional.

Put Down Roots

The word *ratio* is a Latin term meaning "to reason or calculate." The word *proportion* also has its roots in Latin, with the phrase *pro portione* meaning "for or according to the relation of parts." Thus, the ratio-proportion method is based on calculating the relationship of parts to each other.

The **ratio-proportion method** is one of the most frequently used methods for calculating medication doses in a pharmacy. You can use this method any time one ratio is complete and the other ratio has a missing component. In other words, if you know three of the four values in a proportion, you can solve for the missing value. You must also ensure that the numbers remain in the correct proportion to one another and that the numbers have the correct units of measurement in both the numerator and the denominator. Table 2.2 lists the rules for using the ratio-proportion method.

TABLE 2.2 Rules for Using the Ratio-Proportion Method

Rule 1. Three of the four amounts must be known.

Rule 2. The numerators must have the same unit of measurement.

Rule 3. The denominators must have the same unit of measurement.

Once you learn the ratio-proportion method for solving pharmacy calculations, you can use this method to calculate a medication dose. Table 2.3 lists the steps for using the ratio-proportion method to solve for an unknown quantity, typically designated by the letter *x*.

WORKPLACE WISDOM

When performing ratio-proportion calculations, you can choose where to place the unknown variable (typically represented by the letter *x*) in the equivalent proportion. In fact, the unknown variable *x* can appear in all four possible positions, as long as the units in the numerators and the denominators match. However, you may find it helpful to place the unknown variable *x* in the same location. For example, some pharmacy technicians choose to always place the unknown variable *x* in the numerator on the left side of the equal sign. The equivalent proportion below uses this format to determine how many milligrams (mg) are in 2 grams (g). Note that the units in the numerators (milligrams) and the denominators (grams) are the same.

$$\frac{x \text{ mg}}{2 \text{ g}} = \frac{1{,}000 \text{ mg}}{1 \text{ g}}$$

Example 2.3.2

A medication is available as 250 mg/5 mL. How many milliliters represent a dose of 375 mg?

You can solve this problem by using the ratio-proportion method or by using the dimensional analysis method.

Ratio-Proportion Method

To begin, create a proportion by placing the ratios in fraction form and use a variable (the letter *x* in this example) to represent the unknown quantity.

ordered dose ratio = pharmacy stock ratio

$$\frac{375 \text{ mg}}{x \text{ mL}} = \frac{250 \text{ mg}}{5 \text{ mL}}$$

Note that the proportion could be written in several additional ways.

$$\frac{x \text{ mL}}{375 \text{ mg}} = \frac{5 \text{ mL}}{250 \text{ mg}}$$

$$\frac{5 \text{ mL}}{250 \text{ mg}} = \frac{x \text{ mL}}{375 \text{ mg}}$$

$$\frac{250 \text{ mg}}{5 \text{ mL}} = \frac{375 \text{ mg}}{x \text{ mL}}$$

These proportions are all acceptable and could be used to solve for the unknown variable x in this example.

Next, check that the unit of measurement in the numerators is the same and the unit of measurement in the denominators is the same. The numerators have the same unit of measurement (milligrams), and the denominators have the same unit of measurement (milliliters).

Now, use the means–extremes property of proportions to cross multiply and solve for the unknown variable x.

$$x \text{ mL} (250 \text{ mg}) = 5 \text{ mL} (375 \text{ mg})$$

Next, divide each side of the equation by 250 mg to isolate the unknown variable (x mL). Then cancel like terms and solve for x.

$$\frac{x \text{ mL} (250 \text{ mg})}{250 \text{ mg}} = \frac{5 \text{ mL} (375 \text{ mg})}{250 \text{ mg}}$$

$$x = 7.5 \text{ mL}$$

Verify your answer by checking that the product of the means equals the product of the extremes.

$$\frac{375 \text{ mg}}{7.5 \text{ mL}} = \frac{250 \text{ mg}}{5 \text{ mL}}$$

$$375{:}7.5 = 250{:}5$$

$$375 \times 5 = 7.5 \times 250$$

$$1{,}875 = 1{,}875$$

Dimensional Analysis Method

$$\frac{375 \text{ mg}}{1} \times \frac{5 \text{ mL}}{250 \text{ mg}} = 7.5 \text{ mL}$$

Answer: To deliver a dose of 375 mg of medication, you would need 7.5 mL.

Example 2.3.3

The label shown below is the available stock medication for gentamicin. How many milliliters will need to be prepared if a patient is prescribed 50 mg?

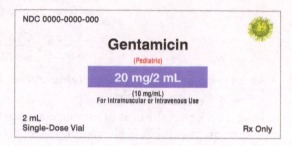

You can solve this problem by using the ratio-proportion method or by using the dimensional analysis method.

Ratio-Proportion Method

To begin, set up a proportion of the ordered dose (50 mg) over the unknown quantity (*x* mL) on the left side of the equation, and the available stock medication (20 mg/2 mL) on the right side of the equation. Check that the units of measurement are the same in the numerators (milligrams) and in the denominators (milliliters).

$$\frac{50 \text{ mg}}{x \text{ mL}} = \frac{20 \text{ mg}}{2 \text{ mL}}$$

Next, use the means–extremes property of proportions to cross multiply.

$$x \text{ mL } (20 \text{ mg}) = 2 \text{ mL } (50 \text{ mg})$$

Then solve for *x* by dividing each side of the equation by 20 mg and canceling the similar units (like units) in the numerators and in the denominators.

$$\frac{x \text{ mL } (20 \text{ mg})}{20 \text{ mg}} = \frac{2 \text{ mL } (50 \text{ mg})}{20 \text{ mg}}$$

$$x = 5 \text{ mL}$$

Verify your answer by checking that the product of the means equals the product of the extremes.

$$\frac{50 \text{ mg}}{5 \text{ mL}} = \frac{20 \text{ mg}}{2 \text{ mL}}$$

$$50{:}5 = 20{:}2$$

$$50 \times 2 = 5 \times 20$$

$$100 = 100$$

Dimensional Analysis Method

$$\frac{50 \text{ mg}}{1} \times \frac{2 \text{ mL}}{20 \text{ mg}} = 5 \text{ mL}$$

Answer: To fulfill an order for 50 mg, you will need to prepare 5 mL of gentamicin.

The label shown below is the available stock medication. How many milligrams of diazepam will need to be dispensed if a patient is prescribed 4 mL?

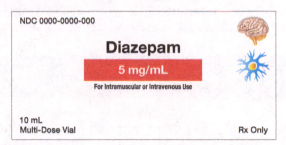

NDC 0000-0000-000

Diazepam

5 mg/mL

For Intramuscular or Intravenous Use

10 mL
Multi-Dose Vial   Rx Only

You can solve this problem by using the ratio-proportion method or by using the dimensional analysis method.

Ratio-Proportion Method

Set up a proportion of the unknown quantity (x mg) over the ordered dose (4 mL) on the left side of the equation, and the available stock (5 mg/1 mL) on the right side of the equation. Be sure to check that the unit of measurement in the numerators is the same (milligrams) and that the unit of measurement in the denominators is the same (milliliters).

$$\frac{x \text{ mg}}{4 \text{ mL}} = \frac{5 \text{ mg}}{1 \text{ mL}}$$

Because these fractions are equivalent, you can cross multiply and the equations will still equal one another.

$$x \text{ mg } (1 \text{ mL}) = 5 \text{ mg } (4 \text{ mL})$$

Then solve for the unknown variable x by dividing each side of the equation by 1 mL and canceling the similar units (like units) in the numerators and in the denominators.

$$\frac{x \text{ mg } (1 \text{ mL})}{1 \text{ mL}} = \frac{5 \text{ mg } (4 \text{ mL})}{1 \text{ mL}}$$

$$x = 20 \text{ mg}$$

Verify your answer by checking that the product of the means equals the product of the extremes.

$$\frac{20 \text{ mg}}{4 \text{ mL}} = \frac{5 \text{ mg}}{1 \text{ mL}}$$

$$20{:}4 = 5{:}1$$

$$20 \times 1 = 4 \times 5$$

$$20 = 20$$

Dimensional Analysis Method

$$\frac{4 \text{ mL}}{1} \times \frac{5 \text{ mg}}{1 \text{ mL}} = 20 \text{ mg}$$

Answer: You will need to dispense 20 mg of diazepam to fill the ordered medication.

In addition to being useful for calculating drug doses in the pharmacy, the ratio-proportion method can be used for converting between units of measurement. To solve a conversion problem, use a conversion factor as one of the proportions. A **conversion factor** is an equivalency equal to 1. For example, because 1 g = 1,000 mg, you can use the conversion factors 1 g/1,000 mg or 1,000 mg/1 g to solve a pharmacy calculations problem. Additional conversion factors are presented in Appendix C.

WORKPLACE WISDOM

Conversion factors are extremely helpful in pharmacy calculations. Although it is not necessary to memorize all the conversion factors in Appendix C, you may find it helpful to memorize the ones commonly used in most practice settings. For example, the conversion factor of 1 kg = 2.2 lb (written as the ratio *1 kg/2.2 lb*) is used in community and institutional pharmacy practice to convert weight. The same can be said for the conversion factor for height: 1 in. = 2.54 cm (written as the ratio *1 in./2.54 cm*).

Example 2.3.5

How many milligrams are equivalent to 3 g?

You can solve this problem by using the ratio-proportion method or by using the dimensional analysis method.

Ratio-Proportion Method

To begin, set up a proportion of the unknown quantity (x mg) over the unit of measurement (3 g) on the left side of the equation, and the conversion factor of milligrams to grams (1,000 mg/1 g) on the right side of the equation. Be sure to check that the unit of measurement in the numerators is the same (milligrams) and that the unit of measurement in the denominators is the same (grams).

When setting up a proportion to solve a conversion, the units in the numerators must match, and the units in the denominators must match.

$$\frac{x \text{ mg}}{3 \text{ g}} = \frac{1,000 \text{ mg}}{1 \text{ g}}$$

Because these fractions are equivalent, you can cross multiply and the equations will still equal one another.

$$x \text{ mg } (1 \text{ g}) = 1,000 \text{ mg } (3 \text{ g})$$

Then solve for x by dividing each side of the equation by 1 g and canceling the similar units (like units) in the numerators and in the denominators.

$$\frac{x \text{ mg } (1\!\!\!/ \text{ g})}{1\!\!\!/ \text{ g}} = \frac{1,000 \text{ mg } (3\!\!\!/ \text{ g})}{1\!\!\!/ \text{ g}}$$

$$x = 3,000 \text{ mg}$$

Verify your answer by checking that the product of the means equals the product of the extremes.

$$\frac{3,000 \text{ mg}}{3 \text{ g}} = \frac{1,000 \text{ mg}}{1 \text{ g}}$$

$$3,000\!:\!3 = 1,000\!:\!1$$

$$3{,}000 \times 1 = 3 \times 1{,}000$$

$$3{,}000 = 3{,}000$$

Dimensional Analysis Method

$$\frac{3\,\cancel{g}}{1} \times \frac{1{,}000\ mg}{1\,\cancel{g}} = 3{,}000\ mg$$

Answer: There are 3,000 mg in 3 g.

Example 2.3.6

Convert 44 lb to kilograms. Refer to Appendix C to determine the conversion from pounds (lb) to kilograms (kg).

This example requires you to convert a unit in the household measurement system (pounds) to a unit in the metric measurement system (kilograms). You can solve this problem by using the ratio-proportion method or by using the dimensional analysis method.

Ratio-Proportion Method

To begin, set up a proportion of the unknown quantity (x kg) over the known measurement (44 lb) on the left side of the equation. Then use the conversion you found in Appendix C (2.2. lb = 1 kg) to create a fraction (1 kg/2.2 lb) on the right side of the equation. Note that you must arrange the conversion factor so that similar units (like units) appear in the numerators (kilograms) and in the denominators (pounds).

$$\frac{x\ kg}{44\ lb} = \frac{1\ kg}{2.2\ lb}$$

Next, cross multiply the equivalent fractions.

$$x\ kg\ (2.2\ lb) = 1\ kg\ (44\ lb)$$

Then solve for x by dividing each side of the equation by 2.2 lb and canceling the similar units (like units) in the numerators and in the denominators.

$$\frac{x\ kg\ (2.2\ \cancel{lb})}{2.2\ \cancel{lb}} = \frac{1\ kg\ (44\ \cancel{lb})}{2.2\ \cancel{lb}}$$

$$x = 20\ kg$$

Verify your answer by checking that the product of the means equals the product of the extremes.

$$\frac{20\ kg}{44\ lb} = \frac{1\ kg}{2.2\ lb}$$

$$20{:}44 = 1{:}2.2$$

$$20 \times 2.2 = 44 \times 1$$

$$44 = 44$$

Dimensional Analysis Method

$$\frac{44 \text{ lb}}{1} \times \frac{1 \text{ kg}}{2.2 \text{ lb}} = 20 \text{ kg}$$

Answer: The weight of 44 lb in the household measurement system converts to 20 kg in the metric measurement system.

The ratio-proportion method can also be used to solve many types of percent problems. When setting up the ratios, remember that a percent may be written in fraction form, with the percent value over 100. For example, 95% is equivalent to $^{95}/_{100}$.

Example 2.3.7

A patient needs to take 75% of a recommended dose before the medication may be discontinued. The recommended dose is 650 mg. How many milligrams of medication must the patient take before it is discontinued?

You can solve this problem by using the ratio-proportion method or by using the dimensional analysis method.

Ratio-Proportion Method

To begin, place the unknown variable (x mg) over the recommended dose (650 mg) on the left side of the equation. Then write the percent (75%) as a fraction ($^{75}/_{100}$) on the right side of the equation.

$$\frac{x \text{ mg}}{650 \text{ mg}} = \frac{75 \text{ mg}}{100 \text{ mg}}$$

Be sure to check that the unit of measurement in the numerators is the same (milligrams) and that the unit of measurement in the denominators is the same (milligrams).

Next, cross multiply the equivalent fractions.

$$x \text{ mg } (100 \text{ mg}) = 650 \text{ mg } (75 \text{ mg})$$

Then solve for x by dividing each side of the equation by 100 mg and canceling the similar units (like units) in the numerators and in the denominators.

$$\frac{x \text{ mg } (100 \text{ mg})}{100 \text{ mg}} = \frac{650 \text{ mg } (75 \text{ mg})}{100 \text{ mg}}$$

$$x = 487.5 \text{ mg}$$

Verify your answer by checking that the product of the means equals the product of the extremes.

$$\frac{487.5 \text{ mg}}{650 \text{ mg}} = \frac{75}{100 \text{ mg}}$$

$$487.5{:}650 = 75{:}100$$

$$487.5 \times 100 = 650 \times 75$$

$$48{,}750 = 48{,}750$$

Dimensional Analysis Method

$$\frac{650 \text{ mg (total amount)}}{1} \times \frac{75 \text{ mg (portion of total)}}{100 \text{ mg (total amount)}} = 487.5 \text{ mg}$$

Answer: To take 75% of the recommended dose, the patient must take 487.5 mg of the medication.

Example 2.3.8

A patient has taken 85% of a recommended dose of medication. If the amount taken is 320 mg, what was the recommended dose?

Another way of phrasing this question is as follows: "320 mg is 85% of what amount?"

You can solve this problem by using the ratio-proportion method or by using the dimensional analysis method.

Ratio-Proportion Method

To begin, set up two equivalent proportions based on the information given.

$$\frac{320 \text{ mg}}{x \text{ mg}} = \frac{85 \text{ mg}}{100 \text{ mg}}$$

Be sure to check that the unit of measurement in the numerators is the same (milligrams of the portion of the whole) and that the unit of measurement in the denominators is the same (milligrams of the total amount).

Next, cross multiply the equivalent fractions.

$$x \text{ mg} \, (85 \text{ mg}) = 320 \text{ mg} \, (100 \text{ mg})$$

Then solve for *x* by dividing each side of the equation by 85 mg and canceling the similar units (like units) in the numerators and in the denominators.

$$\frac{x \text{ mg} \, (85 \text{ mg})}{85 \text{ mg}} = \frac{320 \text{ mg} \, (100 \text{ mg})}{85 \text{ mg}}$$

$$x = 376.5 \text{ mg}$$

Verify your answer by checking that the product of the means equals the product of the extremes.

$$\frac{320 \text{ mg}}{376.5 \text{ mg}} = \frac{85 \text{ mg}}{100 \text{ mg}}$$

$$320{:}376.5 = 85{:}100$$

$$320 \times 100 = 376.5 \times 85$$

$$32{,}000 = 32{,}000$$

Dimensional Analysis Method

$$\frac{320 \text{ mg (portion of total)}}{1} \times \frac{100 \text{ mg (total amount)}}{85 \text{ mg (portion of total)}} = 376.5 \text{ mg}$$

Answer: The recommended dose of the medication was 376.5 mg.

2.3 Problem Set   1-55 odd only.

Solve for the unknown variable x in each of the following proportions. Round your answers to the nearest hundredth when necessary.

1. $\dfrac{x}{10} = \dfrac{20}{40}$

2. $\dfrac{x}{0.6} = \dfrac{0.8}{6.12}$

3. $\dfrac{x}{9} = \dfrac{5}{10}$

4. $\dfrac{x}{1} = \dfrac{0.5}{5}$

5. $\dfrac{x}{50} = \dfrac{0.4}{125}$

6. $\dfrac{13}{15} = \dfrac{5}{x}$

7. $\dfrac{x}{68} = \dfrac{72}{90}$

8. $\dfrac{14}{3} = \dfrac{x}{52}$

9. $\dfrac{x}{27} = \dfrac{49}{51}$

10. $\dfrac{13}{x} = \dfrac{52}{64}$

11. $\dfrac{14}{23} = \dfrac{27}{x}$

12. $\dfrac{31}{13} = \dfrac{51}{x}$

13. $\dfrac{47}{9} = \dfrac{x}{15}$

14. $\dfrac{9}{26} = \dfrac{x}{31}$

15. $\dfrac{37}{x} = \dfrac{11}{23}$

Set up ratio-proportion problems to solve for the unknown variable x. Round your answers to the nearest hundredth.

16. 72 is what percent of 254?

17. 90% of what number is 44?

18. 44% of what number is 100?

19. 28% of what number is 34?

20. 24.5 is what percent of 45?

Change the following weights using the conversion factor 1 g = 1,000 mg.

21. 100 mg = _____ g

22. 247 mg = _____ g

23. 1,420 mg = _____ g

24. 495 mg = _____ g

25. 3,781 mg = _____ g

26. 0.349 g = _____ mg

27. 1.5 g = _____ mg

28. 0.083 g = _____ mg

29. 0.01 g = _____ mg

30. 2.1 g = _____ mg

Change the following weights using the conversion factor 1 kg = 2.2 lb. Round your answers to the tenths place.

31. 6.3 lb = _____ kg

32. 15 lb = _____ kg

33. 97 lb = _____ kg

34. 115 lb = _____ kg

35. 186 lb = _____ kg

36. 7.5 kg = _____ lb

37. 3.6 kg = _____ lb

38. 79.2 kg = _____ lb

39. 90 kg = _____ lb

40. 0.5 kg = _____ lb

Applications

Use the ratio-proportion method to solve the following problems.

41. Progesterone is available as 50 mg/mL. The order calls for 100 mg of progesterone. How many milliliters will you prepare?

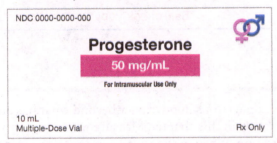

42. Capicillin is available as a 125 mg tablet. How many tablets are needed to provide a dose of 375 mg?

43. Soakamycin is available as a concentration of 20 mg/mL. How many milliliters are needed to prepare a foot soak that contains 300 mg?

44. You are going to buy some folders to file your orders. After doing research, you find that the most cost-effective price is $7.40 per box of 100 folders. You have $15 to spend. How many 100-count boxes can you buy?

45. A patient is to receive an intramuscular injection of 10,000 units of Musclesporin. You have a bottle containing 250,000 units per 15 mL. How many milliliters must be prepared to administer this dose?

46. A prescriber ordered a dose of 30 mg of gentamicin. The medication is available as a 20 mg/2 mL solution. How many milliliters are needed to provide the ordered dose?

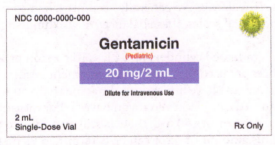

47. A prescriber ordered a dose of 60 mg of famotidine. The medication is available as a 40 mg/4 mL solution. How many milliliters are needed to provide the ordered dose?

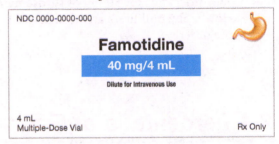

48. A prescriber ordered a dose of 300 mg. The medication is available as a 500 mg/10 mL solution. How many milliliters are needed to provide the ordered dose?

49. A prescriber ordered a dose of 30 mg of lamivudine oral solution. The medication is available as a 5 mg/mL oral solution. How many milliliters are needed to provide the ordered dose?

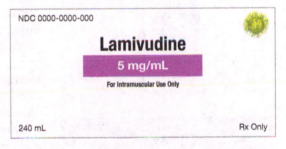

50. A prescriber ordered a dose of 30 mg. The medication is available as a 20 mg/mL solution. How many milliliters are needed to provide the ordered dose?

Use the following medication label to determine the doses needed for questions 51–55.

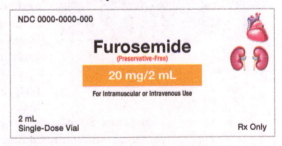

51. The order calls for 5 mL of furosemide. How many milligrams will the patient receive in the ordered amount?

52. The order calls for 80 mg of furosemide. How many milliliters are needed to fill the order?

53. The order calls for 50 mg of furosemide. How many milliliters are needed to fill the order?

54. The order calls for 12.5 mg of furosemide. How many milliliters are needed to fill the order?

55. The order calls for 3.5 mL of furosemide. How many milligrams will the patient receive in the ordered amount?

Self-check your work in Appendix A.

2.4 Percentage of Error

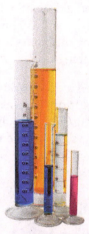

Graduated cylinders are used to accurately measure liquids in the pharmacy.

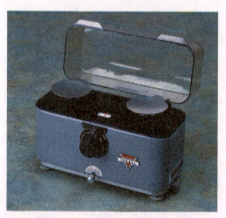

A Class III torsion prescription balance can accurately weigh small quantities.

Percentage has applications in pharmacy beyond what has been discussed previously in this chapter. Measurement accuracy is one such application. When measuring a substance, the measuring device will approximate the actual amount to a certain degree of accuracy. **Percentage of error** is a way of expressing the difference between a known or desired value and its measured value. In other words, percentage of error tells you how close your measured value is to its true value.

Percentage of error is used to determine the accuracy of two measuring devices commonly used in a pharmacy: graduates and prescription balances. Regardless of the measuring device, it is important for you to know the margin of error associated with a particular graduate or prescription balance.

Graduates are instruments used for liquid volume measurements. In pharmacy practice, the graduates may be cylindrical or conical in shape. Graduated cylinders are more commonly used as they are typically more accurate. A graduated cylinder has marks, or graduations, in increments (usually milliliters). Although not all graduated cylinders are equally accurate, these measuring devices are more accurate than the household measuring devices used by patients at home.

Prescription balances are used to measure weights in the pharmacy. The most common balance in pharmacies is the Class III torsion prescription balance. This balance uses a two-pan torsion system that requires both internal and external weights. Typically, this balance may be used only to weigh masses ≥ 120 mg and no more than 60 g or 120 g, depending on the balance. Although Class III balances are generally accurate when compared with other small scales, these balances may exhibit slight variations.

Although graduated cylinders and Class III torsion prescription balances are used to improve measurement accuracy, all measuring instruments have limitations. Imagine that you want to measure 50 mL of water in a graduated cylinder. Even if you have stellar measuring technique and painstakingly attempt to measure 50 mL, there is still error due to the precision of the measuring device. This amount of error can be determined using the percentage of error formula.

$$\text{percentage of error} = \frac{\text{error of measurement}}{\text{quantity desired}} \times 100$$

In the preceding formula, the term *error of measurement* is the difference between the measured value and the quantity desired.

$$\text{error of measurement} = \text{measured value} - \text{quantity desired}$$

In pharmacy calculations, it is typical to report percentage of error as a positive integer.

Consider the following situation. You are to dispense 50 mL of cetirizine solution. The original measurement shows 50 mL. When you verify the amount using a more accurate graduated cylinder, the actual amount is 52 mL. The error of measurement in this example is the difference between the measured value and the quantity desired.

$$52 \text{ mL} - 50 \text{ mL} = 2 \text{ mL}$$

Now that you know the error of measurement, you can calculate the percentage of error.

$$\text{percentage of error} = \frac{2}{50} \times 100 = 4\%$$

The following examples further illustrate how to calculate percentage of error.

Example 2.4.1

You are to dispense 50 mL of cetirizine solution. The original measurement shows 50 mL. When you verify the amount using a more accurate graduated cylinder, the actual amount is 54 mL. What is the error of measurement?

To begin, use the following formula to determine the error of measurement.

$$\text{measured value} - \text{quantity desired} = \text{error of measurement}$$

Then calculate the difference between the measured value (54 mL) and the quantity desired (50 mL) to determine the error of measurement.

$$54 \text{ mL} - 50 \text{ mL} = 4 \text{ mL}$$

Answer: The error of measurement is 4 mL.

Example 2.4.2

You are to dispense 120 mL of a liquid. The original measurement is 120 mL. When you verify the amount using a more accurate graduated cylinder, the measured amount is 126 mL. What is the percentage of error of the original measurement?

To begin, determine the error of measurement by using the following formula.

$$\text{measured value} - \text{quantity desired} = \text{error of measurement}$$

$$126 \text{ mL} - 120 \text{ mL} = 6 \text{ mL}$$

Next, use the percentage of error equation to determine the percentage of error of the measurement.

$$\frac{\text{error of measurement}}{\text{quantity desired}} \times 100 = \frac{6 \text{ mL}}{120 \text{ mL}} \times 100 = 5\%$$

Answer: The percentage of error of the original measurement is 5%.

Example 2.4.3

You are to dispense 30 g of a powder. The original measurement is 30 g. When you verify the amount using a more accurate balance, the actual amount is 31.8 g. What is the percentage of error of the original measurement?

To begin, calculate the difference in the two amounts to determine the error of measurement.

$$31.8 \text{ g} - 30 \text{ g} = 1.8 \text{ g}$$

Then use the percentage of error equation to determine the percentage of error of the measurement.

$$\frac{\text{error of measurement}}{\text{quantity desired}} \times 100 = \frac{1.8 \text{ g}}{30 \text{ g}} \times 100 = 6\%$$

Answer: The percentage of error of the original measurement is 6%.

Example 2.4.4

You are to dispense 453 mg of a powder. The original measurement is 453 mg. When you verify the amount using a more accurate balance, the actual amount is 438 mg. What is the percentage of error of the original measurement?

To begin, calculate the difference in the two measurements to determine the error of measurement.

$$438 \text{ mg} - 453 \text{ mg} = -15 \text{ mg}$$

Next, take the absolute value of −15, which is 15.

Finally, use the percentage of error equation to determine the percentage of error of the measurement.

$$\frac{\text{error of measurement}}{\text{quantity desired}} \times 100 = \frac{15 \text{ mg}}{453 \text{ mg}} \times 100 = 3.3\%$$

Answer: The percentage of error of the original measurement is 3.3%.

A concept related to percentage of error is error tolerance. **Error tolerance** is the acceptable amount of error allowed in measurements. The range of error tolerance varies based on your practice setting.

Consider a setting with a 5% range of error tolerance. This range means that a measured quantity must be within 5% of the desired quantity. For a desired quantity of 100 g, the measured quantity must be between 95 g and 105 g to be acceptable within the 5% range of error tolerance. The following examples utilize error tolerance and its application in pharmacy practice.

Example 2.4.5

You are to weigh 60 g of a cream base for a topical compound. Your error tolerance range is 3%. What will be the lower weight limit (in grams) and the upper weight limit (in grams) that would be within the 3% error tolerance range?

To begin, convert the error tolerance range (3%) to a decimal: 0.03. Then multiply the target weight (60 g) by the error tolerance range.

$$60 \text{ g} \times 0.03 = 1.8 \text{ g}$$

Next, determine the lower and upper limits of the error range by subtracting and adding 1.8 g to your target weight of 60 g.

$$60 \text{ g} - 1.8 \text{ g} = 58.2 \text{ g} \qquad 60 \text{ g} + 1.8 \text{ g} = 61.8 \text{ g}$$

Answer: To be within the 3% error tolerance range, your lower weight limit for the cream base would be 58.2 g, and your upper weight limit would be 61.8 g.

Example 2.4.6

You are preparing an order by measuring 800 mL from a 1 liter (L) normal saline IV bag. When you verify the volume of the fluid in a graduated cylinder, the amount measured is actually 820 mL. What is the percentage of error in this measurement? If your error tolerance range is 2%, is your measurement acceptable?

To begin, find the difference in the two measurements to determine the error of measurement.

$$820 \text{ mL} - 800 \text{ mL} = 20 \text{ mL}$$

Then use the percentage of error equation to determine the percentage of error of the measurement.

$$\frac{\text{error of measurement}}{\text{quantity desired}} \times 100 = \frac{20 \text{ mL}}{800 \text{ mL}} \times 100 = 2.5\%$$

Answer: Because 2.5% is larger than the acceptable error tolerance range of 2%, the target range was not met.

2.4 Problem Set   1-23 odd only!

Calculate the percentage of error for the following measurements. Then round your answers to the nearest hundredth when necessary.

1. The desired weight is 185 mg, but the measured weight is 189 mg.

2. The desired weight is 500 mg, but the measured weight is 476 mg.

3. The desired weight is 1,200 mg, but the measured weight is 1,507 mg.

4. The desired weight is 15 mg, but the measured weight is 12.5 mg.

5. The desired weight is 400 mcg, but the measured weight is 415 mcg.

6. The desired volume is 5 mL, but the measured volume is 6.3 mL.

7. The desired volume is 15 mL, but the measured volume is 13 mL.

8. The desired volume is 15 mL, but the measured volume is 20 mL.

9. The desired volume is 1.5 L, but the measured volume is 1.45 L.

10. The desired volume is 700 mL, but the measured volume is 726 mL.

Determine the percentage of error for the following measurements, and identify whether or not your answers fall within the error tolerance range of 3%.

11. The desired volume is 3 mL, but the measured volume is 2.6 mL.

12. The desired volume is 12.5 mL, but the measured volume is 12.1 mL.

13. The desired volume is 1.8 mL, but the measured volume is 1.5 mL.

14. The desired volume is 3.2 mL, but the measured volume is 3.29 mL.

Determine the percentage of error for the following measurements, and identify whether or not your answers fall within the error tolerance range of 5%.

15. The desired weight is 150 mg, but the measured weight is 149 mg.

16. The desired weight is 200 mg, but the measured weight is 192 mg.

17. The desired weight is 30 mg, but the measured weight is 31.5 mg.

18. The desired weight is 454 mg, but the measured weight is 450 mg.

State the acceptable error tolerance range for the following measurements. Round your answers to the nearest hundredth as needed.

19. The desired volume is 200 mL, and the error tolerance is 0.5%.

20. The desired volume is 10.3 mL, and the error tolerance is 0.75%.

21. The desired volume is 830 mL, and the error tolerance is 2%.

22. The desired weight is 18 g, and the error tolerance is 0.15%.

23. The desired weight is 750 mg, and the error tolerance is 0.4%.

Applications

24. If a generic drug manufacturer meets a bioavailability (the degree to which a drug becomes available to the target tissue after administration) comparison to within 20%, and a drug typically has a bioavailability of 100 mg, what is the acceptable range?

25. The drug manufacturer of a new brand of vitamin C tablets claims that its product has a bioavailability within 12% of an established brand of vitamin C tablets. The established brand has 500 mg of vitamin C per tablet. What is the acceptable range of vitamin C contained in the new brand of tablet?

Self-check your work in Appendix A.

Review and Assessment

CHAPTER SUMMARY

- Ratios are used to describe the amount of medication per dose or unit.

- Ratios may be expressed by using a colon (1:100 or 100:1) or by formatting as a fraction ($\frac{1}{100}$ or $\frac{100}{1}$).

- Ratios may be multiplied when a larger dose is desired or divided when a smaller dose is desired.

- Percent is the number of parts per 100 parts.

- Ratios, percents, fractions, and decimals may all be used to express the same value.

- When converting a percent to a numerical value, divide by 100, or move the decimal point two places to the left.

- When converting a numerical value to a percent, multiply by 100, or move the decimal point two places to the right.

- Proportions are an expression of equivalency between two ratios (or fractions).

- A proportion with one missing value may be solved if three of the four values are known.

- When using the ratio-proportion method to solve for a missing value, the numerators must have the same unit of measurement, and the denominators must have the same unit of measurement.

- The ratio-proportion method may be used to convert between units of measure by setting the ratio desired to be converted equal to a unit of 1.

- Percentage of error is calculated by dividing the error of measurement by the quantity desired, and then multiplying by 100.

- Error of measurement is the difference between the measured value and the quantity desired.

- Error tolerance is the acceptable amount of error allowed in measurements.

FORMULAS FOR SUCCESS

Means–Extremes Property (Section 2.3)

Given a proportion

$a:b = c:d$

the product of means = the product of extremes

or

$b \times c = a \times d$

Percentage of Error (Section 2.4)

$$\text{percentage of error*} = \frac{\text{error of measurement}}{\text{quantity desired}} \times 100$$

* typically reported as a positive integer

Error of Measurement (Section 2.4)

error of measurement = measured value − quantity desired

CHECK YOUR UNDERSTANDING

Take a moment to review what you have learned in this chapter and answer the following questions.

1. The term *percent* when applied to medications means
   a. the amount of medication per 100 doses.
   b. the amount of medication per 100 parts (grams or milliliters).
   c. the amount of medication purchased for $100.
   d. the ratio strength of 100 mg of medication.

2. The ratio-proportion method is used in pharmacy calculations when
   a. all four values are known.
   b. three of the four values are known.
   c. the units of measurement are all the same.
   d. the unknown value is in a unit not written on the medication label.

3. You can check the accuracy of your ratio-proportion calculations by
   a. verifying that the product of the means equals the product of the extremes.
   b. subtracting the product of the means from the product of the extremes.
   c. inverting one ratio in the proportion and recalculating.
   d. converting all of the units to one common unit of measurement.

4. Percentage of error is
   a. calculated by dividing the error of measurement by the quantity desired.
   b. calculated by multiplying the quantity desired by 5%.
   c. always expressed as a negative value.
   d. determined by comparing a weighed amount of medication to an estimated amount of medication.

5. Which ratio of components corresponds to a medication labeled as a 5% solution?
   a. 5 mg of solute per 100 mL of solution
   b. 5 mg of solute per 1,000 mL of solution
   c. 5 g of solute per 100 mL of solution
   d. 5 g of solute per 1,000 mL of solution

6. A proportion is best described as
   a. a calculation of percent.
   b. an expression of equality between two ratios.
   c. the product of the means of a ratio.
   d. the product of the extremes of a ratio.

7. A conversion factor is best described as
   a. the number of parts per 100.
   b. a numerical representation of the relationship between two parts of the whole.
   c. the percentage by which a measurement is inaccurate.
   d. an equivalency equal to 1.

8. A medication label reads 300 mg/5 mL. How many milligrams of medication are in 15 mL?
   a. 150 mg
   b. 450 mg
   c. 500 mg
   d. 900 mg

9. How many grams of medication are in 200 g of a 1% ointment?
   a. 0.2 g
   b. 1 g
   c. 1.2 g
   d. 2 g

10. A solution that is 1:20 is also the concentration of
    a. 1.2%.
    b. 2%.
    c. 5%.
    d. 20%.

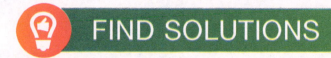

FIND SOLUTIONS

Take a moment to consider what you have learned in this chapter and respond thoughtfully to the prompts.

Note: *To indicate your answer for Scenario A, Question 1, ask your instructor for the handout depicting measuring devices.*

Scenario A: A patient who has poison ivy has been taking over-the-counter (OTC) diphenhydramine (Benadryl) for itching. The doctor has told the patient to take 50 mg every six hours as needed. The medication is available in a 12.5 mg/5 mL solution.

1. On the handout that you obtained from your instructor, indicate how many milliliters the patient will need for each dose.

2. If the patient takes three doses per day, how many milliliters will the patient need to last three days?

3. How many 4 fluid ounce bottles (120 mL/bottle) will the patient need to purchase?

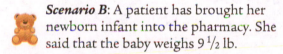

Scenario B: A patient has brought her newborn infant into the pharmacy. She said that the baby weighs 9 ½ lb.

4. What is the infant's weight in kilograms?

Scenario C: You receive a prescription for an antibiotic suspension of amoxicillin 125 mg/5 mL. This medication is for a pediatric patient weighing 20 kg, and it is determined that each dose should be 25 mg.

5. How many milliliters are needed for each 25 mg dose?

6. The patient needs to take two doses per day for a total of 50 mg. How many milliliters are needed for 50 mg of medication?

7. The total prescription requires that 500 mg of medication be dispensed. How many milliliters are needed to equal 500 mg of amoxicillin?

8. How would you express the concentration of amoxicillin in mg/10 mL?

Scenario D: You are compounding a diluted bleach solution that requires 50 mL of bleach. You use a graduated cylinder and measure 50 mL. When you verify the amount using a more accurate graduated cylinder, the actual amount is 48 mL.

9. What is the percentage of error?

10. Is this percentage of error within an error tolerance range of 5%?

The online course includes additional review and assessment resources.

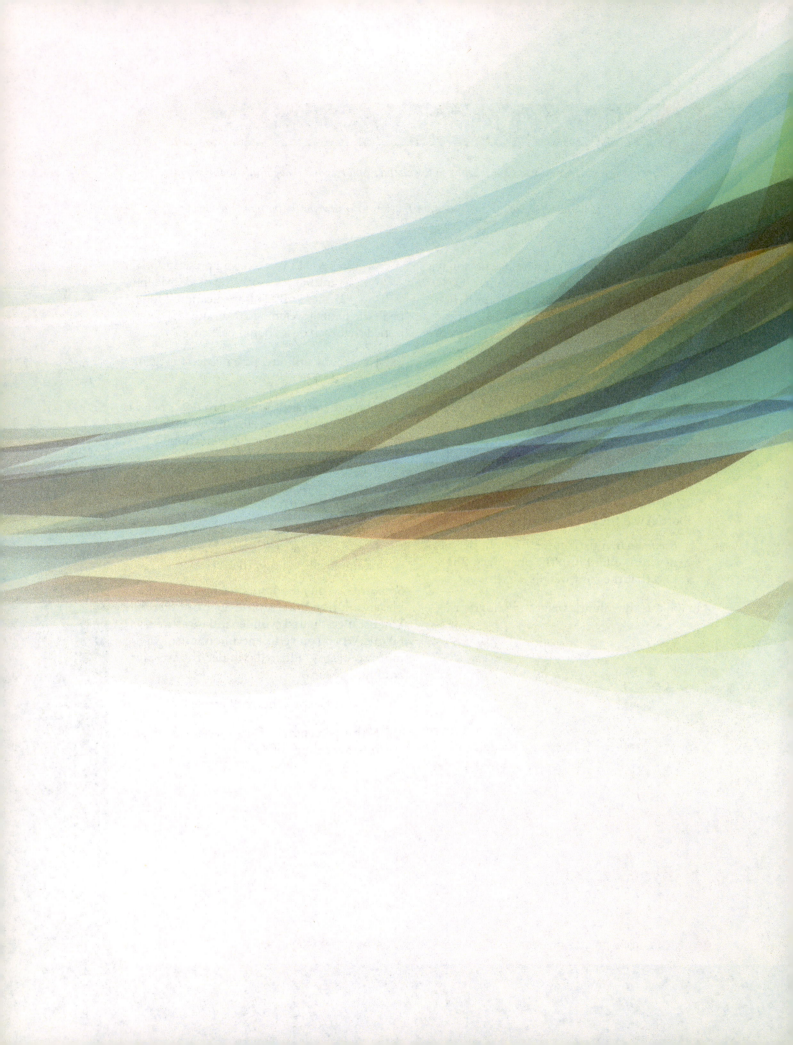

Developing Prescription and Medication Order Literacy Skills

3

Learning Objectives

1 Define *prescription* and understand the types of prescriptions. (Sections 3.1, 3.3, 3.4)

2 Identify the components of a prescription. (Sections 3.1, 3.3, 3.4)

3 Perform the check digit verification process. (Sections 3.1, 3.4)

4 Calculate days' supply and quantity to dispense.(Section 3.1)

5 Define *medication order* and understand the types of medication orders. (Sections 3.2, 3.3, 3.4)

6 Identify the components of a medication order. (Sections 3.2, 3.3, 3.4)

7 Convert between standard time and 24-hour time. (Section 3.2)

8 List common medical abbreviations, acronyms, and symbols used in prescriptions and medication orders. (Sections 3.1, 3.2, 3.3, 3.4)

9 Apply calculation operations in handling prescriptions and medication orders. (Section 3.4)

For a key to the body system icons that appear in each chapter of this textbook, refer to the Preface.

ASHP/ACPE Accreditation Standards
To view the *ASHP/ACPE Accreditation Standards* addressed in this chapter, refer to Appendix D.

In both community and institutional pharmacy settings, you will be receiving, interpreting, calculating, and filling prescriptions and medication orders routinely. In light of these responsibilities, this chapter addresses the types and components of prescriptions and medication orders as well as the common medical abbreviations, acronyms, and symbols that prescribers use as shorthand communication tools in these orders. Your correct interpretation of prescriptions and medication orders and your accurate pharmacy calculations based on these orders are critical to the health and safety of patients.

3.1 Prescriptions

A **prescription** is an order of medication for a patient that is issued by a physician or another licensed healthcare prescriber, such as a nurse practitioner or a dentist, for a valid medical condition. Prescriptions are written for patients and are typically relayed from prescribers to pharmacies for dispensing to patients.

Understanding Different Types of Prescriptions

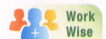

Put Down Roots

The word *prescription* comes from the Latin word *praescriptus*, with the prefix *pre–* meaning "before" and the root word *script* meaning "written." Thus, the word *prescription* means "to write before," alluding to the fact that an order must be written down before a medication is prepared.

Work Wise

A written prescription is often referred to as the "hard copy" in community pharmacy settings.

Prescriptions may be received by the pharmacy by several means, including written prescriptions, faxed prescriptions, telephone prescriptions, and e-prescriptions. You need to interpret the prescription to determine the types of calculations that are necessary to fill the order correctly and appropriately. The requirements for information that appears on a prescription are regulated by state law and, therefore, vary among states. However, the following elements appear on every prescription: patient information, prescriber information, and medication information. In addition, controlled-substance prescriptions must follow specific regulations regarding their method of delivery.

Written Prescriptions

A **written prescription** is recorded by a licensed healthcare professional on a preprinted form bearing the name, address, and telephone and fax numbers of the prescriber; information about the patient; the date; and the medication prescribed. A written prescription is typically given to the patient, who then submits the form to a pharmacy for filling.

Faxed Prescriptions

A **faxed prescription** is written by a prescriber and then faxed to the appropriate pharmacy. This order contains the necessary patient demographic, prescriber, and medication information to fill the prescription. Faxed orders are entered into the patient's medication profile by a pharmacy technician and then verified by a pharmacist.

Telephone Prescriptions

A **telephone prescription** is phoned into a pharmacy. A telephone order, sometimes called a *verbal order*, must be transcribed into a written prescription and verified for accuracy prior to being entered into the computerized patient profile. In states allowing pharmacy technicians to receive verbal orders, the order must be checked by a pharmacist prior to computer entry.

E-prescriptions

An **electronic prescription (e-prescription)** is transmitted electronically from a prescriber to a pharmacy, typically via a personal computer in an examination room or from

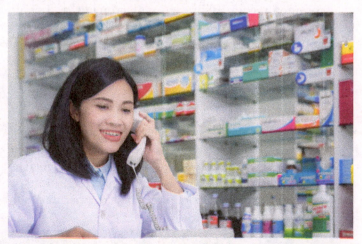

This pharmacist is receiving a verbal prescription over the telephone, which will be transcribed into a written prescription.

a handheld device such as a tablet or a smartphone. E-prescriptions have become the most common prescribing method for healthcare practitioners. For prescribers and pharmacy personnel, e-prescriptions streamline the prescription-filling process, improve billing, minimize the potential for prescription forgeries, and reduce medication errors. For patients, e-prescriptions increase accuracy, improve safety, and decrease filling wait times.

Controlled-Substance Prescriptions

A **controlled-substance prescription** must follow specific regulations for delivery. Controlled substances in Schedules III–V can be written, faxed, or communicated verbally. Traditionally, prescriptions for Schedule II controlled substances were primarily delivered as written prescriptions with few exceptions. However, federal law now allows electronic transmission of controlled-substance prescriptions (Schedules II–V). The law stipulates that electronically transmitted prescriptions for controlled substances are valid only if both the prescriber and the pharmacy that fills the prescription use software that is compliant with the security requirements outlined in the Electronic Prescriptions for Controlled Substances (EPCS) program of the US Drug Enforcement Administration (DEA). When such a prescription is transmitted, the pharmacist sees an EPCS logo appear on the computer screen that verifies the validity of the prescription. Some pharmacies and physicians' offices do not yet have the software required to transmit these prescriptions.

Learning the Components of Prescriptions

As mentioned earlier, the following elements appear on every prescription: patient information, prescriber information, and medication information. You must diligently verify and interpret this prescription information in order to accurately perform calculations, provide patients with the correct quantity of medication, and bill insurance companies appropriately.

Patient Information

Every prescription order must have enough information to uniquely identify a patient. In addition to the patient's full name (first and last), most states also require an **outpatient prescription** (a prescription for a patient who is not in a hospital or other medical institution) to include the patient's address.

A prescription must also contain the patient's birth date, which is used by the pharmacy to distinguish between patients with the same name and to bill the patient's insurance provider. Knowing the patient's age also helps the pharmacist evaluate the appropriateness of the drug, its quantity, and the dosage form prescribed, thus minimizing medication errors.

Many pharmacies require that the patient's height and weight be available, either on the prescription itself or in the patient's profile. A patient's height is generally measured in centimeters (cm) or inches (″ or in.). A patient's weight may be measured in either kilograms (kg) or pounds (# or lb). If height and weight are included in the patient information, these measurements must include the units because metric units of measurement are quite different from household units of measurement. For example, a 76 cm patient is most likely a child under three years of age, whereas a 76″ patient is a very tall adult; a 100 kg patient is more than twice the size of a 100 lb patient. (To learn more about height and weight conversions, refer to Chapter 4.)

Figures 3.1 and 3.2 illustrate components of a written prescription and an e-prescription. Patient information such as the patient's name, birth date, and address is included in both examples.

FIGURE 3.1
Components of a Written Prescription

All prescriptions should be legible, be written in ink (if hand-written), and include a leading zero before any number that is less than one (in this case, 0.5 mg). If appropriate, the prescription should also include the indication (in this case, *anxiety*).

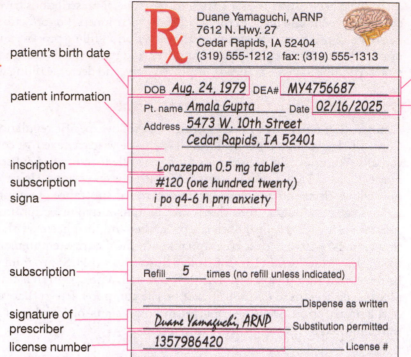

patient's birth date

patient information

DEA number for controlled drug and insurance

date of prescription

inscription
subscription
signa

subscription

signature of prescriber
license number

R𝑥

Duane Yamaguchi, ARNP
7612 N. Hwy. 27
Cedar Rapids, IA 52404
(319) 555-1212 fax: (319) 555-1313

DOB _Aug. 24, 1979_ DEA# _MY4756687_

Pt. name _Amala Gupta_ Date _02/16/2025_
Address _5473 W. 10th Street_
Cedar Rapids, IA 52401

Lorazepam 0.5 mg tablet
#120 (one hundred twenty)
i po q4-6 h prn anxiety

Refill ___5___ times (no refill unless indicated)

_____ Dispense as written
Duane Yamaguchi, ARNP Substitution permitted
1357986420 License #

FIGURE 3.2
Components of an E-prescription

E-prescriptions are transmitted electronically to pharmacies. This example shows the e-prescription sent from the prescriber to the pharmacy on the right side of the computer screen. The left side of the screen shows how the e-prescription is integrated into the pharmacy's order entry and dispensing software. Note that the abbreviation *mg* means "milligrams"; the abbreviation *po* means "by mouth"; and the abbreviation *qhs* means "at bedtime."

Patient Profile

Patient	KELLY DENIS	Birth Date	08/13/1953
Address	19 WALNUT STREET PITTSBURGH, PA 15807	Birth Sex	MALE
Phone	555-217-0624	Self-Identified Gender Identity	MALE

New Prescription

Rx Number	12597
Drug	rosuvastatin 20 mg tablet
Quantity	90 tablets
Sig Code	1 po qhs
Sig	Take 1 tablet by mouth every night at bedtime
Refills	4
Date Written	04/15/2025
Rx Expiration	04/15/2026
Rx Origin	Electronic
Prescriber	Stanley Fray
DEA Number	BF3456781
DAW 0, No DAW	No DAW

Date Written _04/15/2025_

Doctor _Stanley Fray_ Doctor _555-636-4200_

Address _3333 Burnet Avenue_ DEA _BF3456781_
Location A, 8th Floor
Pittsburgh, PA 15809

Patient Name _Kelly Denis_ Phone _555-217-0624_

Address _19 Walnut Street_ Birth Date _08/13/1953_
Pittsburgh, PA 15807

R𝑥 _rosuvastatin 20 mg tablet_

Instructions _1 po qhs_

Refills _4_

DAW _No_

Prescriber Information and DEA Numbers

In most states, outpatient prescription orders must include the name, authority (such as medical doctor, doctor of osteopathy, nurse practitioner, physician assistant, dentist, etc.), and address of the prescribing practitioner. Frequently, the prescription order includes the prescriber's telephone number.

Work Wise

If needed, a pharmacy technician can always look up a prescriber's NPI number on the NPI registry website at https://npiregistry .cms.hhs.gov.

Other prescriber identification information, such as a **National Provider Identifier (NPI) number** and a **US Drug Enforcement Administration (DEA) number**, may also be included on a prescription. An NPI number is a 10-digit, unique identification number for healthcare providers. This number is required by the Health Insurance Portability and Accountability Act (HIPAA) for all administrative and financial healthcare transactions. A DEA number is a carefully regulated registration code that signifies the authority of the holder to prescribe or handle controlled substances. Sometimes, the DEA number of the prescriber is handwritten (rather than preprinted) on a paper prescription to prevent forgeries.

A DEA number is *always* two letters followed by seven digits. The first two letters of the DEA number provide information about the prescriber:

- The first letter in the DEA number usually (but not always) designates the level of authority of the holder. For example, the letters *A*, *B*, and *F* are used for primary-level practitioners such as physicians and dentists, and the letter *M* is used to indicate mid-level practitioners such as nurse practitioners, nurse midwives, nurse anesthetists, clinical nurse specialists, and physician assistants.

- The second letter in the DEA number represents the first letter of the prescriber's last name at the time of DEA number application. There are instances where the second letter in a DEA number does not match the first letter of the prescriber's last name. This mismatch occurs most frequently when a prescriber's last name is legally changed after the DEA number was assigned (for example, in the case of marriage or divorce).

Therefore, the first two letters of the DEA number for a family medicine physician named *Dr. Mary Smith* might be *AS*, *BS*, or *FS*, whereas the first two letters for a nurse practitioner named *David Jones* might be *MJ*.

As mentioned earlier, these first two letters are followed by seven digits. The first six digits are used to calculate a sum known as a *checksum* (outlined in Table 3.1). The last of the seven digits is called a *check digit*. The checksum and check digit give pharmacists and pharmacy technicians one way to confirm whether a DEA number is fraudulent. A DEA number that does not have a correct check digit (as determined by the steps in Table 3.1) is invalid. However, be aware that passing the check digit verification process does not necessarily mean that a DEA number is valid. If you discover an invalid DEA number or suspect a problem with the authenticity of a prescription, you must notify a pharmacist immediately.

TABLE 3.1 DEA Check Digit Verification Process

Step 1. Add the first, third, and fifth digits of the DEA number.

Step 2. Add the second, fourth, and sixth digits of the DEA number.

Step 3. Double the sum obtained in Step 2 (i.e., multiply it by 2).

Step 4. Add the results of Steps 1 and 3. This sum is known as the *checksum*. The last digit of the checksum should match the check digit, or the last digit of the DEA number.

The following examples demonstrate how the steps in Table 3.1 can be used to check for fraudulent DEA numbers.

Example 3.1.1

A patient brings a prescription for methylphenidate tablets to the pharmacy. The prescription is signed by Anders Karl Johnson, MD, and bears a DEA number of BJ2345678. Could this be a valid DEA number?

To begin, review the letters of the DEA number. The first letter is consistent with the prescriber's level of authority (the letters A, B, or F for a primary-level practitioner), and the second letter (the letter J) matches the last name of the physician.

Next, check the validity of the check digit by following the steps outlined in Table 3.1.

Step 1. Add the first, third, and fifth digits of the DEA number.

$$2 + 4 + 6 = 12$$

Step 2. Add the second, fourth, and sixth digits of the DEA number.

$$3 + 5 + 7 = 15$$

Step 3. Multiply the sum obtained in Step 2 by 2.

$$15 \times 2 = 30$$

Step 4. Add the results of Steps 1 and 3. The last digit of this sum, or the checksum, should match the check digit, the last digit of the DEA number.

$$12 + 30 = 4\textcolor{red}{2}$$

Answer: Because the check digit is 8, not 2, this DEA number is invalid.

Example 3.1.2

A patient brings a prescription for oxycodone to the pharmacy. The prescription is signed by nurse practitioner Ann Jefferson and bears a DEA number of MJ3456781. (In the state where the prescription is received, nurse practitioners are authorized to prescribe narcotic analgesics.) Could this be a valid DEA number?

To begin, review the letters of the DEA number. The first letter is consistent with the prescriber's level of authority (the letter M for a nurse practitioner), and the second letter (the letter J) matches the last name of the prescriber.

Now, check the validity of the check digit.

Step 1. Add the first, third, and fifth digits of the DEA number.

$$3 + 5 + 7 = 15$$

Step 2. Add the second, fourth, and sixth digits of the DEA number.

$$4 + 6 + 8 = 18$$

Step 3. Multiply the sum obtained in Step 2 by 2.

$$18 \times 2 = 36$$

Step 4. Add the results of Steps 1 and 3. The last digit of this sum, or the checksum, should match the check digit, the last digit of the DEA number.

$$15 + 36 = 5\textcolor{red}{1}$$

Answer: Because the check digit is 1, this DEA number could be valid.

The signature of the prescriber must be present on a prescription. For a paper prescription, the signature must be in ink. An electronic signature may be utilized on a faxed prescription for all medications except for controlled substances. E-prescriptions must include an electronic signature.

In many states, a prescriber can use the signature line of a prescription to specify that a pharmacy must dispense the brand-name drug (rather than the less-expensive generic drug). In some states, there are two signature lines at the bottom of a prescription: one stating *dispense as written*, or *DAW*, and the other stating *substitution permitted*. If the *dispense as written* line is signed, then a pharmacy cannot substitute a generic equivalent when filling the prescription.

Medication Information

The date a prescription is written or ordered must appear on the document. Most prescriptions are valid for one year. Prescriptions for Schedule III and Schedule IV controlled substances are valid for six months. In addition, the date a prescription is written may be important to a pharmacist for therapeutic reasons. For example, if a prescription for an antibiotic was written several weeks ago, a pharmacist may need to determine whether the patient still needs to take the medication.

A prescription order must always designate the medication that is intended for the patient. The **inscription** is the part of the prescription that lists the medication prescribed, including the dosage form and strength or amount. Sometimes, the drug will be identified by its **generic name**, the name by which it was approved by the US Food and Drug Administration (FDA) as a unique chemical product safe and effective for its approved indication or use. The generic name of a drug is the same, regardless of the company that manufactures it or the dosage form or packaging in which it is supplied. Other times, a prescriber will specify a brand name. The **brand name** is a registered trademark of the manufacturer and may indicate the dosage form or packaging of the drug as well. For example, Prinivil and Zestril are two brand names under which the generic drug lisinopril is marketed by pharmaceutical companies. Generic drugs are often less expensive than brand-name drugs and are often automatically substituted for brand-name drugs in the pharmacy software under regulations now existing in every state. If a prescription for a brand-name drug is filled with a generic equivalent, then the name, strength, and manufacturer of the generic substitution may be included on the dispensed medication container label. In other situations, the pharmacy must supply the exact brand-name drug prescribed, unless the pharmacist has discussed a substitution with the prescriber.

WORKPLACE WISDOM

As a pharmacy technician, it is important that you understand how generic drugs and brand-name drugs are similar and how they are different. You may also be asked by patients to explain the distinctions between these two drug products. Generic drugs are required to have the same active ingredient(s), strength, dosage form, and route of administration as brand-name drugs. Generic drug manufacturers must also prove that the efficacy of their medications is equivalent to that of brand-name products. However, the inactive ingredients of generic drugs do not have to be the same as those of brand-name products. A small amount of variability may be present, which is permitted and monitored by the FDA.

Figure 3.3 identifies the standard parts of a drug label for Cleocin Phosphate. As shown in this example, the label of a brand-name drug indicates both the brand name and the generic name. Medications with a given name (brand or generic) are frequently available in a variety of strengths, doses, or dosage forms, and information about the particular strength, dose, and dosage form is clearly stated on the drug label. Because drugs present a similar array of choices (brand names, strengths, doses, and dosage forms), the proper product to select must be clear in the prescription order.

Figure 3.4 shows labels for the drug furosemide in different dosage forms and strengths. Note how the labels use color to help distinguish the unique information.

FIGURE 3.3 **Parts of a Drug Label**

Although medication labels from different manufacturers vary slightly in format, the labels' components remain the same. As a pharmacy technician, you must be able to identify and interpret all parts of a drug label.

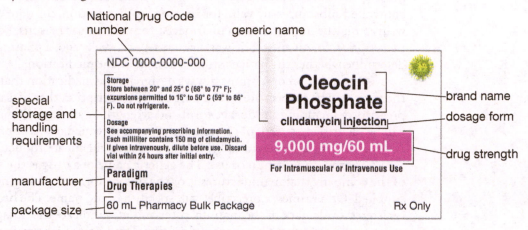

FIGURE 3.4
Comparison of Dosage Forms

These medication labels indicate 20 mg tablets, 40 mg tablets, and a 40 mg/4 mL solution.

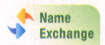

Name Exchange

Furosemide, a diuretic, is the generic name for the brand-name drug Lasix.

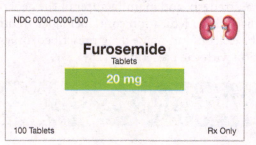

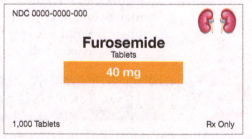

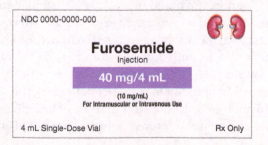

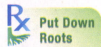

Put Down Roots

The term *signa* comes from the Latin verb *signare*, meaning "to mark, write, or indicate." A prescription's signa provides instruction for patient use.

The **signa** (commonly referred to as the "sig") is the part of the prescription that communicates the directions for use. This information is transferred from the prescription onto the label that is placed on the medication container for patient use.

The **subscription** is the part of the prescription that lists the instructions to the pharmacist about dispensing the medication, including quantity to dispense, compounding instructions, labeling instructions, information about the appropriateness of dispensing drug equivalents, and refill information. A **refill** is an approval by the prescriber to dispense the medication again without requiring a new prescription. If the refill section on the prescription is left blank, the prescription cannot be refilled. The words *no refill* (sometimes abbreviated *NR*) will appear on the medication container label, and *no refill* will be entered into the patient's profile. Even if the refill blank on the prescription indicates a *prn* (or "as needed") order, unlimited duration is not allowed. Most pharmacies and state laws require at least yearly updates on *prn* (also written *PRN*) prescriptions.

Quantity to Dispense

Every outpatient prescription order must indicate to the pharmacist what quantity to dispense. Sometimes, as in Figure 3.1, a prescriber writes the number of tablets to dispense next to "#" (used as a number symbol). This number is often written as a Roman numeral or spelled out ("thirty" for #30) on written prescriptions. Using a word rather than a number to indicate the quantity makes it more difficult to obtain a greater quantity than prescribed because a number is easier to alter. Other times, a prescriber indicates the number of doses the patient is to take or the number of days the therapy is to last. The pharmacy staff, in turn, calculates the quantity to dispense from the information on the prescription.

Calculating quantity to dispense can be done using the ratio-proportion method or the dimensional analysis method. The following examples show how to calculate the quantity to dispense utilizing these methods.

Example 3.1.3

A prescription for amoxicillin 125 mg chewable tablets twice daily is written for a patient in your pharmacy. How many chewable tablets should be dispensed for a 10-day supply?

You can solve this problem by using the ratio-proportion method or by using the dimensional analysis method.

Ratio-Proportion Method

To begin, set up a ratio.

$$\frac{x \text{ tablets}}{10 \text{ days}} = \frac{2 \text{ tablets}}{1 \text{ day}}$$

Then use the means–extremes property of proportions to cross multiply.

$$x \text{ tablets (1 day)} = 2 \text{ tablets (10 days)}$$
$$x = 20 \text{ tablets}$$

Verify your answer by checking that the product of the means equals the product of the extremes.

Dimensional Analysis Method

To begin, you know the desired units are tablets. Set up the dimensional analysis calculation with tablets in the numerator. Then cancel out the units *dose(s)* and *day(s)*.

$$\frac{1 \text{ tablet}}{\cancel{\text{dose}}} \times \frac{2 \cancel{\text{ doses}}}{\cancel{\text{day}}} \times \frac{10 \cancel{\text{ days}}}{1} = 20 \text{ tablets}$$

Answer: The pharmacy should dispense 20 tablets for a 10-day supply.

Example 3.1.4

A prescription for an antacid states, "Take 1 oz three times a day," and instructs the pharmacy to dispense a 5-day supply. What volume should be dispensed?

You can use a multi-step or a one-step dimensional analysis method to solve this problem.

Dimensional Analysis Multi-Step Method

To begin, you know that the patient takes 1 ounce (oz) three times a day. Using that information, determine the number of ounces taken in one day. Note that the units cancel out, as shown below.

$$\frac{1 \text{ oz}}{\cancel{\text{dose}}} \times \frac{3 \cancel{\text{ doses}}}{\text{day}} = 3 \text{ oz per day}$$

Next, determine the amount to dispense by multiplying the daily dose by the number of days.

$$\frac{3 \text{ oz}}{\cancel{\text{day}}} \times \frac{5 \cancel{\text{ days}}}{1} = 15 \text{ oz}$$

Dimensional Analysis One-Step Method

You can also perform these calculations in one step.

$$\frac{1 \text{ oz}}{\cancel{\text{dose}}} \times \frac{3 \cancel{\text{ doses}}}{\cancel{\text{day}}} \times \frac{5 \cancel{\text{ days}}}{1} = 15 \text{ oz}$$

Answer: A 15 oz volume should be dispensed for a 5-day supply.

Example 3.1.5

A prescription for Dificid states, "Take 200 mg every 12 hours," and instructs the pharmacy to dispense a 7-day supply. The pharmacy has the following medication in stock. How many tablets are dispensed?

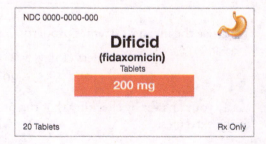

You can solve this problem by using the ratio-proportion method or by using the dimensional analysis method.

Ratio-Proportion Method

To begin, you know that 1 tablet contains 200 mg and that each dose is 200 mg. Therefore, each dose is 1 tablet. You also know that the patient is to take 2 doses per day, which means that the patient takes 2 tablets each day. Use this information to set up a proportion.

$$\frac{x \text{ tablets}}{7 \text{ days}} = \frac{2 \text{ tablets}}{1 \text{ day}}$$

Then use the means–extremes property of proportions to cross multiply.

$$x \text{ tablets } (1 \text{ day}) = 2 \text{ tablets } (7 \text{ days})$$

$$x = 14 \text{ tablets}$$

Verify your answer by checking that the product of the means equals the product of the extremes.

Dimensional Analysis Method

To begin, you know that 1 tablet contains 200 mg and that the patient will take 1 tablet every 12 hours. You also know that there are 24 hours in a day. Therefore, you can determine the number of tablets the patient will need in a 24-hour period (1 day).

$$\frac{1 \text{ tablet}}{12 \text{ hours}} \times \frac{24 \text{ hours}}{1 \text{ day}} \times \frac{7 \text{ days}}{1} = 14 \text{ tablets}$$

Answer: The pharmacy will dispense 14 tablets for a 7-day supply.

When the quantity to dispense has been determined, you will then select the proper dispensing container. Commonly, amber bottles (ovals) are used for liquids and amber vials for tablets or capsules. Amber bottles are often marked with both fluid ounce (fl oz) and milliliter (mL) lines. Common practice uses the metric system, so the quantity indicated on the prescription drug label will usually be indicated in milliliters. When preparing tablets or capsules to fill a prescription, the tablets or capsules are generally counted out by fives, using a specially designed tray and a plastic or metal spatula, and then placed in amber vials.

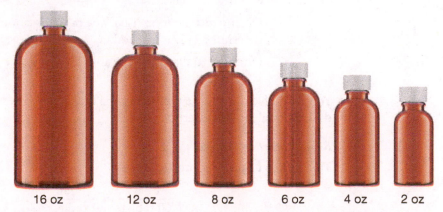

| 16 oz | 12 oz | 8 oz | 6 oz | 4 oz | 2 oz |

Amber medication bottles come in many sizes. As a pharmacy technician, you must select the appropriate size to match the dispensed volume.

Days' Supply

Whether prescriptions are written for a specified number of doses or a specified duration of time, you need to calculate the **days' supply** (the number of days that a prescription medication will last a patient when taken as directed). For example, a prescription that is written for a specified number of doses such as #30 and with a dosing schedule of three times daily will last 10 days. Another prescription may be written for a patient to use a medication *TID* (an abbreviation that means "three times a day") for 10 days, and the physician has indicated the quantity as *QS* (an abbreviation that means "a sufficient quantity"). You would calculate that the patient needs 30 doses to complete the therapy prescribed by the physician.

Days' supply is an important concept in pharmacy practice for two reasons. One reason is that it ensures that the quantity dispensed will meet the needs of the patient according to what the prescriber has indicated. Another reason is that it allows prescription insurance to be billed appropriately. Consider a situation in which you filled a patient's prescription with an order for a 30 days' supply of medication and 6 refills. In one instance, imagine that you correctly calculated and entered the days' supply as 30 and billed the patient's prescription insurance provider. If the patient took the medication as prescribed and requested a refill after the supply was gone (on day 30), the patient's prescription insurance provider should accept the refill claim. On the other hand, imagine that you incorrectly calculated the days' supply as 60 on the first fill and billed the patient's prescription insurance provider. If the patient took the medication as prescribed and requested a refill after the supply was gone (on day 30), the patient's prescription insurance provider would deny the refill claim. This denial is because the insurance provider would think that the patient still had more medication (30 additional days), even though the patient truly needed a refill.

To calculate days' supply, you can use either the ratio-proportion method or the dimensional analysis method. The following examples utilize both these methods.

Example 3.1.6

Calculate the days' supply for the following prescription.

Name Exchange

The generic drug ibuprofen is commonly known as Motrin, one of several brand names for this medication.

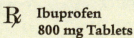

℞ **Ibuprofen**
   800 mg Tablets

   Dosing instructions: Take one tablet by mouth two times daily with food.

   Quantity to dispense: 60 tablets

You can solve this problem by using the ratio-proportion method or by using the dimensional analysis method.

Ratio-Proportion Method

To begin, set up a proportion.

$$\frac{x \text{ days}}{60 \text{ tablets}} = \frac{1 \text{ day}}{2 \text{ tablets}}$$

Then use the means–extremes property of proportions to cross multiply.

$$x \text{ days } (2 \text{ tablets}) = 1 \text{ day } (60 \text{ tablets})$$
$$x = 30 \text{ days}$$

Verify your answer by checking that the product of the means equals the product of the extremes.

Dimensional Analysis Method

$$\frac{60 \text{ tablets}}{1} \times \frac{1 \text{ day}}{2 \text{ tablets}} = 30 \text{ days}$$

Answer: The days' supply for this prescription is 30 days.

Example 3.1.7

Calculate the days' supply for the following prescription.

$R\!\!\!/$ **Ibuprofen**
200 mg Tablets

Dosing instructions: Take 2 po q8h.

Quantity to dispense: 60 tablets

You can solve this problem by using the ratio-proportion method or by using the dimensional analysis method.

Ratio-Proportion Method

To begin, set up an equivalent proportion to determine the number of tablets that are being taken each day. Using information from this label, you know that the patient is taking a dose every 8 hours. Therefore, the patient is taking 3 doses a day.

$$\frac{x \text{ tablets}}{3 \text{ doses}} = \frac{2 \text{ tablets}}{1 \text{ dose}}$$
$$x \text{ tablets } (1 \text{ dose}) = 2 \text{ tablets } (3 \text{ doses})$$
$$x = 6 \text{ tablets}$$

Next, set up a proportion to determine the number of days 60 tablets will last.

$$\frac{x \text{ days}}{60 \text{ tablets}} = \frac{1 \text{ day}}{6 \text{ tablets}}$$
$$x \text{ days } (6 \text{ tablets}) = 1 \text{ day } (60 \text{ tablets})$$
$$x = 10 \text{ days}$$

Dimensional Analysis Multi-Step Method

To begin, determine the number of tablets taken each day.

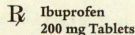

$$\frac{2 \text{ tablets}}{\text{dose}} \times \frac{3 \text{ doses}}{\text{day}} = 6 \text{ tablets per day}$$

Next, determine the number of days 60 tablets will last.

$$\frac{60 \text{ tablets}}{1} \times \frac{\text{day}}{6 \text{ tablets}} = 10 \text{ days}$$

Dimensional Analysis One-Step Method

$$\frac{60 \text{ tablets}}{1} \times \frac{\text{dose}}{2 \text{ tablets}} \times \frac{\text{day}}{3 \text{ doses}} = 10 \text{ days}$$

Answer: The days' supply for this prescription is 10 days.

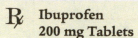 **Example 3.1.8**

Calculate the days' supply for the following prescription.

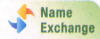 **Name Exchange**

Acetaminophen/codeine elixir is the generic name for the brand name Tylenol-Codeine Elixir.

℞ **Ibuprofen**
200 mg Tablets

Dosing instructions: Take 2 po q12h.

Quantity to dispense: 120 tablets

You can solve this problem by using the ratio-proportion method or by using the dimensional analysis method.

Ratio-Proportion Method

To begin, you know that the patient is taking a dose every 12 hours. Therefore, the patient is taking 2 doses a day. Then set up a proportion to determine the number of tablets that are being taken each day. Finally, solve for the unknown variable x.

$$\frac{x \text{ tablets}}{2 \text{ doses}} = \frac{2 \text{ tablets}}{1 \text{ dose}}$$

$$x \text{ tablets (1 dose)} = 2 \text{ tablets (2 doses)}$$

$$x = 4 \text{ tablets}$$

Next, set up a proportion to determine the number of days 120 tablets will last. Then solve for the unknown variable x.

$$\frac{x \text{ days}}{120 \text{ tablets}} = \frac{1 \text{ day}}{4 \text{ tablets}}$$

$$x \text{ days (4 tablets)} = 1 \text{ day (120 tablets)}$$

$$x = 30 \text{ days}$$

Dimensional Analysis Multi-Step Method

To begin, determine the number of tablets taken each day.

$$\frac{2 \text{ tablets}}{\text{dose}} \times \frac{2 \text{ doses}}{\text{day}} = 4 \text{ tablets per day}$$

Then determine the number of days 120 tablets will last.

$$\frac{120 \text{ tablets}}{1} \times \frac{\text{day}}{4 \text{ tablets}} = 30 \text{ days}$$

Dimensional Analysis One-Step Method

$$\frac{120 \text{ tablets}}{1} \times \frac{\text{dose}}{2 \text{ tablets}} \times \frac{\text{day}}{2 \text{ doses}} = 30 \text{ days}$$

Answer: The days' supply for this prescription is 30 days.

3.1 Problem Set   *odd only*

Determine the validity of the following DEA numbers by verifying the prescriber identifiers and using the check digit verification process. Justify your answers.

1. JC2169870 for
   James Cardillo, MD

2. MG3081659 for
   nurse-midwife Laura Gonzales

3. BH9998070 for
   Blanche McKennon, MD

4. AL6230618 for
   George Lewis, DO

5. AD7638224 for
   Anita Chan, MD

6. BN4412209 for
   Srisha Narayana, DO

7. AK3051492 for
   Satoru Kudaishi, MD

8. MS2864228 for
   clinical nurse specialist Katherine Schultz

9. BK1179870 for
   Jess Kolesar, MD

10. AA2170758 for
    Sara Alvarez, MD

Identify the information indicated for each drug label.

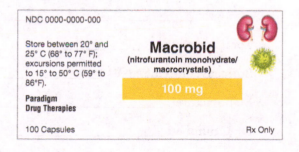

NDC 0000-0000-000

Store between 20° and 25° C (68° to 77° F); excursions permitted to 15° to 50° C (59° to 86°F).

Paradigm Drug Therapies

Macrobid
(nitrofurantoin monohydrate/ macrocrystals)

100 mg

100 Capsules   Rx Only

11. Brand name: _____

    Generic name: _____

    Dosage form: _____

    Strength: _____

    Total quantity: _____

    Storage requirement(s): _____

    Manufacturer: _____

    NDC number: _____

NDC 0000-0000-000

Store between 20° and 25° C (68° to 77° F); excursions permitted to 15° to 50° C (59° to 86° F).

Paradigm Drug Therapies

Prozac
(fluoxetine)

20 mg

100 Capsules   Rx Only

12. Brand name: _____

    Generic name: _____

    Dosage form: _____

    Strength: _____

    Total quantity: _____

    Storage requirement(s): _____

    Manufacturer: _____

    NDC number: _____

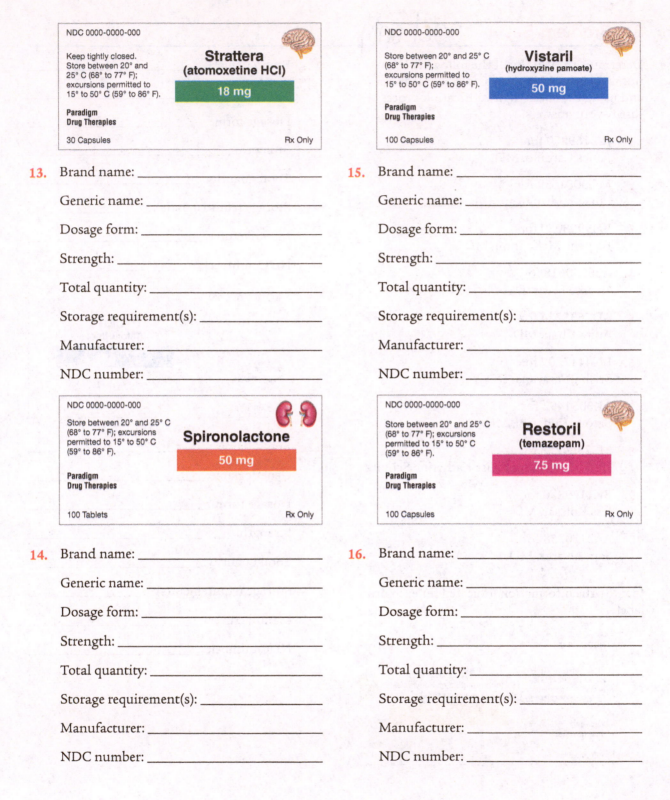

NDC 0000-0000-000

Keep tightly closed.
Store between 20° and
25° C (68° to 77° F);
excursions permitted to
15° to 50° C (59° to 86° F).

**Paradigm
Drug Therapies**

30 Capsules

**Strattera
(atomoxetine HCl)**

18 mg

Rx Only

13. Brand name: _____

Generic name: _____

Dosage form: _____

Strength: _____

Total quantity: _____

Storage requirement(s): _____

Manufacturer: _____

NDC number: _____

NDC 0000-0000-000

Store between 20° and 25° C
(68° to 77° F); excursions
permitted to 15° to 50° C
(59° to 86° F).

**Paradigm
Drug Therapies**

100 Tablets

Spironolactone

50 mg

Rx Only

14. Brand name: _____

Generic name: _____

Dosage form: _____

Strength: _____

Total quantity: _____

Storage requirement(s): _____

Manufacturer: _____

NDC number: _____

NDC 0000-0000-000

Store between 20° and 25° C
(68° to 77° F);
excursions permitted to
15° to 50° C (59° to 86° F).

**Paradigm
Drug Therapies**

100 Capsules

**Vistaril
(hydroxyzine pamoate)**

50 mg

Rx Only

15. Brand name: _____

Generic name: _____

Dosage form: _____

Strength: _____

Total quantity: _____

Storage requirement(s): _____

Manufacturer: _____

NDC number: _____

NDC 0000-0000-000

Store between 20° and 25° C
(68° to 77° F); excursions
permitted to 15° to 50° C
(59° to 86° F).

**Paradigm
Drug Therapies**

100 Capsules

**Restoril
(temazepam)**

7.5 mg

Rx Only

16. Brand name: _____

Generic name: _____

Dosage form: _____

Strength: _____

Total quantity: _____

Storage requirement(s): _____

Manufacturer: _____

NDC number: _____

Applications

How much medication should be dispensed for the following prescriptions?

17.
Rx **Ibuprofen**
400 mg Tablets
#XX

Take one tablet by mouth four times daily with food.

18.
Rx **Amoxicillin**
500 mg Capsules

Take one capsule three times daily for 10 days.

How much medication should be dispensed for the following prescriptions?

19.
Rx **Prednisone**
5 mg Tablets
Take four tablets twice daily for two days;
then three tablets twice daily for two days;
then four tablets once daily for two days;
then three tablets once daily for two days;
then two tablets once daily for two days;
then one tablet once daily for two days.

20.
Rx **Milk of Magnesia**
Take one ounce every night at bedtime for one week.

21.
Rx **Phenytoin**
100 mg Capsules
#CL

Take three capsules every morning.

What is the days' supply for the following prescriptions?

22.
Rx **Cephalexin**
500 mg Capsules
#28

Take one capsule by mouth every 12 hours.

23.
Rx **Bactrim DS**
Tablets
#90

Take one tablet by mouth each morning.

24.
Rx **Norpace**
100 mg Capsules
#120

Take one capsule by mouth every 6 hours.

25.
Rx **Advair HFA 45/21**

Dosing instructions: Use one dose (puff) two times daily.

Quantity to dispense: Dispense one inhaler with 120 doses.

Self-check your work in Appendix A.

3.2 Medication Orders

A **medication order**—also referred to as a *med order*, *medical order*, or *physician order*—is a set of instructions given by a prescriber that specifies medications for an inpatient at a hospital or a resident of a long-term care facility. The prescriber who issues a medication order must have the appropriate credentials and privileges within that institution to relay the order to an on-site pharmacy. Because the hospital or inpatient facility that fills the order typically has the prescriber's address and DEA number on file, this information is generally not required on a medication order.

Understanding Different Types of Medication Orders

Medication orders may be given verbally, written, or transmitted electronically. Written and electronic orders are generally preferred because there is a greater likelihood of medication errors when an order is given verbally. In many facilities, medication orders are entered directly into a computer by a prescriber. These orders communicate patient care directives to all members of the healthcare team. In addition to delivering instructions to the pharmacy, medication orders may provide directions for laboratory, radiology, dietary, physical therapy, and other departments within a healthcare facility. However, some smaller facilities continue to house medication orders within paper medical records.

There are several types of medication orders, including admission orders, daily orders, single orders, stat orders, prn orders, standing orders, and discharge orders. These orders are discussed below.

Admission Orders

An **admission order** is written by a physician upon patient admission to a hospital (see Figure 3.5). The order may be written in an emergency department or in a patient's room. This type of medication order may contain drugs prescribed and taken before admission; suspected diagnoses; requests for laboratory tests or radiology examinations; instructions for the nursing staff; ordered medications, including the notation of drug allergies; activity instructions; and a patient's dietary requirements.

Daily Orders

A **daily order** is an order for a medication to be administered regularly following the same instructions until the prescriber stops the order (see Figure 3.6). Typically, a physician or another healthcare professional examines a patient on a daily basis, but this frequency varies according to patient need. Critically ill patients may be examined several times a day. Patients may also be seen by numerous healthcare practitioners, according to their particular health issues. Every time a practitioner examines a patient, new orders, or changes to existing medication orders, may be written.

Single Orders

A **single order** is a one-time order that is administered at a specified time. For example, an order for medication to be given to a patient before surgery or another medical procedure is considered a single order.

FIGURE 3.5 Admission Order

A physician typically creates an admission order after examining a newly admitted patient.

	IN DOSAGE FORM AND THERAPEUTIC ACTIVITY MAY BE ADMINISTERED UNLESS CHECKED	Patient Information Below

PHARMACY **B 427687**	**START EACH NEW SERIES OF ORDERS BELOW**
	
	 Check one: (FOR NEW PATIENTS OR CHANGE IN STATUS)
	
	 ☐ OBSERVATION: short stay expected ☒ Admit – inpatient; longer stay expected
	
	 Patient name: *Amy Hayashi* ID number: *S1008994566* Room number: *420*
	 DOB: *08/24/1950* Height: *5'3"* Weight: *179 lb*
	 Diagnosis: Ⓛ *Leg DVT, Fe deficiency anemia*
	 Activity: *Bed rest c̄ bedside commode × 24° then ad lib*
	 Diet: *cardiac*
	 Allergies: *NKDA* Reactions:
	 ① *Admit to Medicine – Dr. Galangal*
	 ② *Condition – stable*
	 ③ *Vitals per routine*
	 ④ *Labs – PT/INR q AM – call c̄ results of PT/INR tonight*
	   – *guaiac stools × 3*
	   – *Fe/Ferritin next lab draw*
	 ⑤ *IV – HL flush q shift*
	
	 NURSE'S SIGNATURE DATE TIME
		ID#: S1008994566
		 Name: Hayashi, Amy
		 DOB: 08/24/1950
		 Room: 420
		 Dr.: George Galangal, MD

PHARMACY **B 427687**	**START EACH NEW SERIES OF ORDERS BELOW**
	 ⑥ *Meds – Lovenox 1 mg/kg SQ q 12*
	   – *warfarin 10 mg PO tonight × ī dose*
	   – *Fe-Tinic 150 mg PO bid*
	   – *Vicodin 1–2 PO q6h prn*
	   – *Colace 100 mg PO bid – hold per loose stool*
	   – *LOC prn*
	   – *Benadryl 50 mg PO qHS prn insomnia*
	 ⑦ *Call per acute changes*
	 ⑧ *Nutrition consult re: vitamin K diet*
	
	 SIGNATURE: **George Galangal, MD**
	 NURSE'S SIGNATURE DATE *11/16/2025* TIME *1130*
		ID#: S1008994566
		 Name: Hayashi, Amy
		 DOB: 08/24/1950
		 Room: 420
		 Dr.: George Galangal, MD

	7ØØ781 (2-97) H-NSO781B **MERCY HOSPITAL** **PHYSICIAN'S INITIAL ORDERS SHEET**	

Chapter 3 *Developing Prescription and Medication Order Literacy Skills*   **97**

FIGURE 3.6 Daily Order

A physician creates a daily order after each patient examination, when changing the order, or when submitting a new order.

ID#: J1008912345	MEMORIAL HOSPITAL
Name: Echeverria, Begonia	PHYSICIAN'S MEDICATION ORDER
DOB: 12/01/1939	
Room: 804	
Dr.: Yuka Sun, MD	BEAR DOWN ON HARD SURFACE WITH BALLPOINT PEN

Patient Name: *Begonia Echeverria*	ID number: *J1008912345*	Room number: *804*
DOB: *12/01/1939*	Height: *5'7"*	Weight: *186 lb*

⬇ GENERIC EQUIVALENT IS AUTHORIZED UNLESS CHECKED IN THIS COLUMN

ALLERGY OR SENSITIVITY TO _____ *Ø* _____ NONE KNOWN ☐ SIGNED:	DIAGNOSIS *S/P Hernia Repair*		COMPLETED OR DISCONTINUED

DATE	TIME	ORDERS		NAME	DATE	TIME
6/10/2025	*1600*	*Routine Orders*				
		Height 5'7" Weight 186 lb				
		Condition – stable				
		VS : q4° × 2, then q shift				
		Diet: Regular				
		D5 ½ NS w/ 20 mEq KCl /Liter				
		run at 100 mL/hr, DC when taking PO well				
		Meds:				
		Vistaril 25 mg IM q3h prn pain				
		Halcion 0.25 mg PO q hs prn				
		LOC prn				
		cefazolin 1 gram IVPB q6h				
		Lance wound on foot in am				
		Call H.O. for: T > 101.5				
		BP > 180/100, or < 80/60				

SIGNATURE: *Yuka Sun, MD   06/10/2025*

PHARMACY COPY

Stat Orders

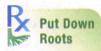

Put Down Roots

The medical term *stat* is a shortened form of the Latin word *statim*, which means "without delay" or "immediately."

A **stat order** is an emergency order that is typically called in or sent electronically to a pharmacy. This type of order must receive priority attention and, consequently, must be immediately input into a pharmacy's database and filled. After a final verification from a pharmacist, the medication is then sent to a patient care unit by a pharmacist or pharmacy technician for patient administration.

Prn Orders

A **prn order** is an order for a specific amount of a medication to be administered on an "as needed" basis rather than at a regularly prescribed interval. Typically, this medication is administered to treat a specific sign or symptom, such as pain, anxiety, fever, or constipation. Whenever an "as needed" dose is administered, healthcare personnel must immediately document the date, the time given, and the reason that the medication was administered.

Standing Orders

A **standing order** is a medication order in which the same set of medications and treatments applies for each patient who receives a similar treatment or surgery (see Figure 3.7). A physician or another prescriber may then sign this preprinted order or slightly modify the standing order by adding or deleting items before signing the form. For example, an orthopedic surgeon who specializes in knee replacement surgery may order the same medications, laboratory tests, and nursing directives for all patients having that procedure. Postoperative (postop) orders written after surgery are another example of standing orders.

Discharge Orders

A **discharge order** is an order that provides take-home instructions for a patient who is being discharged from a hospital. This order includes all prescribed medications and dosages. Prescriptions are commonly written for a seven-day or one-month period, or are designed to last until the patient's follow-up visit with the healthcare practitioner.

Learning the Components of Medication Orders

Regardless of the type, each medication order must contain the same components. Similar to prescriptions, the legal requirements for information necessary on a medication order are regulated by state law and vary among states. Patient information, prescriber information, and medication information must be included on a medication order. You should also be aware that a facility's policy may dictate additional parameters that must be included on a medication order.

Patient Information

Standard patient information on medication orders is highlighted in Figures 3.5, 3.6, and 3.7. This information includes the patient's name, unique identification number, room number, birth date, and physician's name. Patient information must provide sufficient data to uniquely identify the patient, thereby discerning one patient from another.

Other patient information may not be included on a medication order but needs to be accessible to personnel who participate in the management of a patient's medications. This information may be accessed via the electronic health record (EHR) or patient chart. Patient information such as height, weight, allergy information, diagnoses, and current medications should be accessible. Information on pregnancy and lactation status and laboratory results should also be available, when necessary.

Prescriber Information

The signature and authority of the prescriber must be included on a medication order. Because many institutions utilize EHR and medication order entry systems, this signature may be electronic. Prescriber information is shown in Figures 3.5, 3.6, and 3.7.

Medication Information

Although prescriptions require the date, a medication order must include both the date and time of the order. The name of the medication, dosage, route of administration, and time or frequency of administration must also be included. Medication information is highlighted on the medications orders in Figures 3.5, 3.6, and 3.7.

Time of Day

Math Morsel

Computer systems do not always permit the use of a colon when entering time. Consequently, pharmacy technicians may see a time entry as a four-digit entry—for example, 0430 rather than 04:30. Both time entries indicate 4:30 a.m.

Telling time is a skill that you learn as a child. For many individuals, this skill was taught using a clock with movable hands: one hand indicating the hours and one hand indicating the minutes. In addition to these traditional clocks, digital clocks that display the hours and minutes as numbers separated by a colon are also used to tell time. Digital clocks are commonly seen on computer software programs. Both types of clocks typically indicate what is known as **standard time**, or a system of time based on a 12-hour format. Standard time, also known as *civilian time*, uses the designations of *a.m.* and *p.m.*

The healthcare setting, including the pharmacy setting, uses a different time system known as **24-hour time**. As its name indicates, this system is based on a 24-hour format and, consequently, does not use the designations of *a.m.* and *p.m.* In fact, most countries—with the exception of the United States and Canada—have adopted the 24-hour system as their official time standard.

The 24-hour system uses the numbers 0–24 to represent the 24-hour day. To provide consistency and prevent confusion, the 24-hour system uses four digits: The first two digits represent the number of hours past midnight; the last two digits represent the number of minutes past the hour. Times earlier than 10:00 a.m. will often be preceded by one or two leading zeros so that the hour has two digits. To see how 24-hour time compares with standard time, see Table 3.2.

The start of each day is designated as 0000, and midnight is designated as 2400. These two designations are actually the same time, so some computer systems will accept times up to 2400 and then require the first minute after midnight to be entered as 0001, thereby skipping the 0000 time display.

In the healthcare setting, the 24-hour system is used for accuracy. This system prevents ambiguity and provides a simple means of documenting the precise time in a 24-hour day. The 24-hour system may be used to document what time a medication is to be administered, what time an event (such as an adverse reaction) occurs, or what time an intravenous (IV) medication runs out. Precise minutes are also used, so if a medication is to be given at 6:30 a.m., it would be recorded as 0630 to indicate the exact time.

FIGURE 3.7 **Standing Order**

A physician saves time and aids hospital efficiency and communication by using a preprinted standing order form.

ID#: M03822015669
Name: Cruz, Nestor
DOB: 05/11/1955
Room: 400
Dr.: Gary R. Smith, MD – Standing Orders

DR. GARY R. SMITH
STANDING ORDERS FOR POST-OP DISCECTOMY

1. VS q2h × 4, then q4h overnight.

2. Turn q2h.

3. May stand to void.

4. Bathroom privileges with assistance, if tolerated.

5. Ambulate with assistance ~~in A.M.,~~ if tolerated.

6. Heat lamp ~~back~~ 20 minutes QID

7. Reinforce dressing PRN.

8. Diet as tolerated after nausea subsides.

9. Percocet 5 mg/325 mg one or two q3h PRN pain.

10. M.S. 10 mg or 15 mg IM q3h PRN more severe pain.

11. Restoril 15 mg hs PRN sleep. MR × 1.

12. Tylenol 325 mg PO q4h PRN temperature elevation above 101 degrees.

13. Tigan 200 mg IM q6h PRN nausea.

14. Docusate sodium 100 mg PO prn constipation.

15. Laxative of choice.

16. Decadron 4 mg IV or PO q6h × 24 hr. Then start Medrol Dosepak and label for home use.

17. ~~Tagamet 300 mg IV or PO b.i.d.~~

18. Intermittent cath. q 4–6h PRN.

19. R/L 90 cc qh DC after nausea subsides. × 1

20. *Resume home dosage of Prozac post nausea.*

21.

22.

23.

DOB: 05/11/55
5'6"
217#
NKDA
Rm 400

DATE: *August 21ˢᵗ, 2024*

TIME: *0600*

SIGNATURE: *Gary R. Smith, MD*

Dr. Gary R. Smith, MD
711 W. 30th Street, Suite 200
Kalamazoo, MI 49001
Phone 269-555-0423
Fax 269-555-0566

TABLE 3.2 Standard Time and 24-Hour Time Equivalents

Standard Time	24-Hour Time	Standard Time	24-Hour Time
1:00 a.m.	0100 hours	1:00 p.m.	1300 hours
2:00 a.m.	0200 hours	2:00 p.m.	1400 hours
3:00 a.m.	0300 hours	3:00 p.m.	1500 hours
4:00 a.m.	0400 hours	4:00 p.m.	1600 hours
5:00 a.m.	0500 hours	5:00 p.m.	1700 hours
6:00 a.m.	0600 hours	6:00 p.m.	1800 hours
7:00 a.m.	0700 hours	7:00 p.m.	1900 hours
8:00 a.m.	0800 hours	8:00 p.m.	2000 hours
9:00 a.m.	0900 hours	9:00 p.m.	2100 hours
10:00 a.m.	1000 hours	10:00 p.m.	2200 hours
11:00 a.m.	1100 hours	11:00 p.m.	2300 hours
12:00 p.m. (noon)	1200 hours	12:00 a.m. (midnight)	2400 hours

Safety Alert

Because errors in converting standard time to 24-hour time are more common for times after 12:00 p.m. (1200), pharmacy technicians should verify these conversions for accuracy.

Because the healthcare system has adopted the 24-hour system, you need to become familiar with the time equivalents and be able to accurately convert times without looking at a chart. The times that occur in the morning hours are simple and straightforward because they are similar to the display on a typical digital clock. The times that occur in the afternoon and evening (1:00 p.m. to 12:00 a.m.) have numbers that many individuals are not accustomed to seeing when telling time: 1300 to 2400. For these 24-hour times, remember this simple rule: These designations can quickly be converted back to standard time by subtracting 1200. For example, if you subtract 1200 from 1900 hours, you get 7:00—the standard time designation for 7:00 p.m.

Example 3.2.1

Use Table 3.2 to convert the following times from standard time to 24-hour time.

3:45 a.m.	6:13 p.m.	12:10 a.m.
9:20 a.m.	11:56 p.m.	

Answer: In the 24-hour time system, 3:45 a.m. becomes 0345; 9:20 a.m. becomes 0920; 6:13 p.m. becomes 1813; 11:56 p.m. becomes 2356; and 12:10 a.m. becomes 0010.

Example 3.2.2

Use Table 3.2 to convert the following times from 24-hour time to standard time.

0128	1530
0456	2215

Answer: In the standard time system, 0128 becomes 1:28 a.m.; 0456 becomes 4:56 a.m.; 1530 becomes 3:30 p.m.; and 2215 becomes 10:15 p.m.

Example 3.2.3

According to a patient's EHR, the patient received medication at the following times: 0700, 1300, and 1900. Use Table 3.2 to convert these 24-hour times to standard times.

Answer: In the standard time system, 0700 becomes 7:00 a.m.; 1300 becomes 1:00 p.m.; and 1900 becomes 7:00 p.m.

3.2 Problem Set

Match the following medication order type with its description below.

1. ___ admission order
2. ___ daily order
3. ___ single order
4. ___ stat order
5. ___ prn order
6. ___ standing order
7. ___ discharge order

a. emergency order that is typically called in or sent electronically to a pharmacy

b. one-time order that is administered at a specified time

c. order for a medication to be administered regularly following the same instructions until the prescriber stops the order

d. order for a specific amount of a medication to be administered on an "as needed" basis

e. order in which the same set of medications and treatments applies for each patient who receives a similar treatment or surgery

f. order that provides take-home instructions for a patient who is being discharged from a hospital

g. order written upon patient admission to a hospital

Convert the following standard times to 24-hour times.

8. 7:30 a.m.
9. 4:28 p.m.
10. 12:45 a.m.
11. 9:20 p.m.
12. 2:24 a.m.
13. 10:58 p.m.
14. 11:50 p.m.
15. 1:20 a.m.
16. 12:03 a.m.
17. 12:20 p.m.

Convert the following 24-hour times to standard times.

18. 1730

19. 2349

20. 1522

21. 0034

22. 1204

23. 0355

24. 2245

25. 1719

26. 1300

27. 0145

Applications

28. Sun Ng, a patient who arrived in the emergency room around midnight, reported taking pain medication three times during the day: at 8:15 in the morning, at 1:15 in the afternoon with lunch, and at 7:00 in the evening. Using the 24-hour system, what times should be reflected in the patient's health record?

29. A prescription states that Lucy Andrews, a pediatric patient in the intensive care unit, is to take medication three times a day, every eight hours, beginning at 5:00 a.m. Using the 24-hour system, what time should the medication therapy begin?

30. Dr. Dominic Estores has written a prescription for a patient to take a preoperative medication at 2200 on the evening before the patient's scheduled surgery. Using the standard time system, what time should you tell the patient to take the medication?

31. The IV medications prepared each afternoon for overnight administration have to be delivered to the floors between 1800 and 1900. According to the clock in the pharmacy, when should you deliver the medications?

32. Ms. Singh has just been brought to the hospital via ambulance. During admittance, the patient reported placing one nitroglycerin tablet under the tongue at 3:00 p.m. and placing a second tablet under the tongue at 3:05 p.m. Because the chest pain didn't go away, the patient placed a third tablet under the tongue five minutes after the second one. Using 24-hour time, determine the times that the patient placed the three tablets.

Self-check your work in Appendix A.

3.3 Medical Abbreviations, Acronyms, and Symbols

The origin of medical terminology can be traced back to medical treatments developed by the Greek physicians Hippocrates and Galen, as well as ancient practitioners of the Roman Empire. Their discoveries shaped medical science and, as a result, approximately 75% of medical terminology is rooted in the Greek and Latin languages. Medical terminology uses approximately 35,000 abbreviations, acronyms, and symbols as a shorthand method in healthcare communications. It is important for you to become familiar with this specialized healthcare language that is used on prescriptions, medication orders, and medication labels.

Learning Healthcare Abbreviations and Acronyms

Safety Alert

Pharmacy personnel must exercise care when interpreting abbreviations on prescriptions and medication orders to prevent medication errors.

Healthcare abbreviations often use the initial letters of words or phrases as shorthand on prescriptions and medication orders. Many of these abbreviations are derived from the initial letters of Latin words or phrases and refer to common routes of administration, times of administration, or dosage forms. For example, the abbreviation *po* is from the Latin words *per os*, meaning "by mouth" (route of administration); the abbreviation *prn* comes from the Latin words *pro re nata*, meaning "as necessary" (time of administration); and the abbreviation *ung* is from the Latin word *unguentum*, meaning "salve" or "ointment" (dosage form).

Like abbreviations, acronyms are often formed from the initial letters of terms or phrases. However, these letters are frequently capitalized and are pronounced together as one term, not as separate letters. For example, the acronym *AIDS* is a shortened form of "acquired immune deficiency syndrome" and is pronounced as the word "aids." The acronym *SUBCUT* (also expressed as *subcut*) is an abbreviated form of "subcutaneous" and is pronounced "sub-cute." The acronym *NICU* is an abbreviated form of "neonatal intensive care unit" and is pronounced "nick-u."

Work Wise

Pharmacy technicians should ask for clarification for unfamiliar abbreviations. There are also a number of medical dictionaries that technicians can use as resources. One resource is Stedman's Online, which provides access to more than 75,000 medical abbreviations and acronyms. Technicians should check whether their facility has a subscription to this online service.

When abbreviations and acronyms are standardized (have only one meaning) and are clearly written, this medical shorthand saves prescribers and other healthcare practitioners space and time. However, the use of this shorthand can cause serious problems if the medical abbreviations are misinterpreted by others. Sometimes, confusion occurs when the same set of letters has two different meanings. For example, the use of the abbreviation *IVP* on a hospital medication order may mean two different procedures. This abbreviation may mean "IV Push," or the use of a syringe to inject an IV medication into a vein. However, the abbreviation *IVP* may also indicate a request for an "intravenous pyelogram," or an X-ray examination of the urinary tract.

Abbreviations are also problematic when they are not expressed clearly. For example, the abbreviation *qhs* means "nightly at bedtime" but could be misread as *qhr*, meaning "every hour." Consider a situation where a dose was meant to be ordered as 10 units. If the order was written using *U* as an abbreviation for "units," an error could occur. The *U* could be misread for a *0* (zero), and the patient could receive 100 units instead of the intended 10 (a tenfold overdose).

Certain abbreviations are so error-prone that The Joint Commission (TJC)—an independent organization that evaluates and accredits practices in hospital systems— has declared that these abbreviations are absolutely unacceptable for use in accredited institutions. To that end, TJC has published the *Official "Do Not Use" List* containing abbreviations that may lead to confusion among healthcare personnel and, consequently, may result in medication errors. This list can be found at http://PhCalc7e .ParadigmEducation.com/JointCommission.

Another organization, the Institute for Safe Medication Practices (ISMP), has published an extensive list of dangerous abbreviations and symbols to avoid in the healthcare setting. This document, called the ISMP's *List of Error-Prone Abbreviations, Symbols, and Dose Designations*, can be found at http://PhCalc7e.ParadigmEducation.com/ISMP.

You should commit the common abbreviations to memory because they are a part of the pharmacy technician's everyday language. You may want to start by memorizing the abbreviations that indicate how many times per day a patient should take a medication: BID (twice daily), TID (three times daily), and QID (four times daily). The abbreviations are sometimes written in lowercase letters and sometimes written in uppercase letters. The use of periods should be avoided as these punctuation marks can be a source of medication errors. The letter *q* means "every" and is sometimes placed in front of other abbreviations. Common prescription and medication order abbreviations are listed in Table 3.3. For an expanded list, refer to *Appendix B: Common Pharmacy Abbreviations and Acronyms* in this textbook.

need to know

TABLE 3.3 Common Prescription and Medication Order Abbreviations

Abbreviation	Meaning	Abbreviation	Meaning
ac	before meals	NKA	no known allergy
AD	right ear	NKDA	no known drug allergy
AM	morning	npo	nothing by mouth
AS	left ear	OD	right eye
AU	both ears	OS	left eye
bid, BID	twice daily	OU	both eyes
c̄	with	pc	after meals
cap	capsule	po, PO	by mouth
DAW	dispense as written	prn, PRN	as needed
D/C	discontinue	q	every
g	gram	qh	every hour
gr	grain	q2h	every 2 hours
gtt	drop	qhs	every night at bedtime
h, hr	hour	qid, QID	four times daily
hs	bedtime	qs	a sufficient quantity
IM	intramuscular	*stat*	immediately
IV	intravenous	tab	tablet
L	liter	tid, TID	three times daily
mcg	microgram	ud, utd	as directed
mEq	milliequivalent	wk	week
mL	milliliter		

Note: Some prescribers may write abbreviations using capital letters or periods. However, periods should not be used with metric units or medical abbreviations as they can be a source of medication errors.

Recognizing Common Medical Symbols

In addition to knowing medical abbreviations and acronyms commonly seen in pharmacy practice, you must also recognize a number of symbols used on medication orders in particular. Symbols such as ↑ and ↓ are frequently used by prescribers to indicate "increase" and "decrease," respectively. For example, a physician may order a change in an IV flow rate to increase the dose of a medication, such as ↑ *normal saline to 150 mL per hour.* Another common symbol is the Greek delta symbol (Δ), which is used to indicate a desired change. For example, the medication order *famotidine Δ from 20 mg IV to 40 mg PO* communicates that the prescriber wants to change the dose (from 20 mg to 40 mg) and the route of administration (from intravenous [IV] to oral [PO]).

Because symbols are drawn by hand, and handwriting may be poor or at least vary significantly among personnel, symbols can be misinterpreted easily. Therefore, you should take extra care when using or interpreting medical symbols. Computer-generated symbols are preferred over handwritten symbols, whenever possible.

Translating Directions for Patients

Because most patients are not familiar with the abbreviations and acronyms used on prescriptions, directions must be "translated" from the "sig" and written on the medication label placed on the dispensing package or container so that patients can understand the directions. Sometimes, descriptive terms are added, if appropriate. For example, a prescription for a fentanyl transdermal patch may have the sig *i q 3d*. The pharmacy label on the patient's package, however, must state, "Apply one patch every 72 hours." Similarly, a prescription for hydrochlorothiazide 25 mg tablets may bear a sig of *12.5 mg po qam*, but the pharmacy label on the patient's container must state, "Take one-half (¹/₂) tablet by mouth every morning."

It is important that directions for taking a medication be stated in clear terms on the medication label affixed to the dispensing package or container, even if the patient's physician and pharmacist provide verbal instructions to the patient. Written directions on a label provide a necessary reminder to a patient at every dose, which helps to ensure safe medication use.

Even with appropriate translation of prescription instructions, patients may still require additional assistance. For example, patients who are receiving liquid medications typically have their prescribed doses designated in milliliters. Most patients are not familiar with measuring volumes in milliliters. Therefore, special measuring devices—such as dosing syringes, spoons, and cups—are typically dispensed with the medications.

Safety Alert

Instructions to patients on dispensed medications must be clear and should not include medical abbreviations.

3.3 Problem Set

Write out the meanings of these common abbreviations used in prescriptions and medication orders.

1. bid
2. DAW
3. IM
4. IV
5. mL
6. NKA
7. npo
8. q3h
9. qid
10. tid

Applications

Translate the following directions from a prescription order into wording that would be appropriate on a label for the patient's use.

11. ℞ **Diphenhydramine 25 mg Capsules**

ii cap po four times daily prn itching

12. ℞ **Nitroglycerin Transdermal Patch**

i on qhs off qam

13. ℞ **Nitroglycerin 2% Ointment**

Apply ¹/₂ inch (7.5 mg) BID; qam and 6h after first application.

14. ℞ **Nateglinide 60 mg Tablets**

120 mg po tid ac

15. ℞ **Potassium Chloride 20 mEq Tablets**

10 mEq po bid

write out

Self-check your work in Appendix A.

3.4 Interpretation of Prescriptions and Medication Orders

With a good understanding of the types and components of prescriptions and medication orders as well as a familiarity with medical abbreviations, acronyms, and symbols, you are ready to assimilate this information. To do so, you need to practice the correct interpretation of prescriptions and medication orders so that you can perform accurate pharmacy calculations in the pharmacy setting. Honing these skills is an important responsibility of pharmacy technicians and is critical to the safe dispensing of medications to patients.

Interpreting Prescriptions

Whether prescriptions are written, faxed, or communicated via a phone or a digital device, you must be able to accurately interpret the information these orders contain. Patient information, prescriber information, and medication information must be readily identified and transcribed, if necessary. The use of medical abbreviations, acronyms, and symbols must be translated as well. The interpretation of this information may lead to subsequent pharmacy calculations such as days' supply and quantity to dispense. The following example will apply the literacy skills of this chapter into the interpretation of a prescription.

Example 3.4.1

Review the following prescription and answer the associated questions.

Patient Profile

Patient	DENNIS GEORGE	Birth Date	08/13/1953
Address	19 WALNUT STREET PITTSBURGH, PA 15807	Birth Sex	MALE
		Self-Identified Gender Identity	MALE
Phone	555-217-0624		

New Prescription

Rx Number	12597
Drug	ZOLPIDEM 5 MG TABLET
Quantity	60 TABLETS
Sig Code	10 MG PO QHS PRN INSOMNIA
Sig	TAKE 2 TABLETS BY MOUTH EVERY NIGHT AT BEDTIME AS NEEDED FOR INSOMNIA
Refills	0
Date Written	04/15/2025
Rx Expiration	10/15/2025
Rx Origin	ELECTRONIC
Prescriber	STANLEY FRAY
DEA Number	BF3456781
DAW 0, No DAW	NO DAW

Date Written	04/15/2025		
Doctor	Stanley Fray	Doctor	555-636-4200
Address	3333 Burnet Avenue Location A, 8th Floor Pittsburgh, PA 15809	DEA	BF3456781
Patient Name	Dennis George	Phone	555-217-0624
Address	19 Walnut Street Pittsburgh, PA 15807	Birth Date	08/13/1953

℞

	Zolpidem 5 mg tablets
Instructions	10 mg po qhs prn insomnia
Quantity	60
Refills	0
DAW	No

1. **Which type of prescription is pictured?**

   Answer: This screen capture depicts an electronic prescription (e-prescription).

2. **What is the patient's name on this prescription?**

   Answer: The patient's name is Dennis George.

3. **What is the prescriber's name on this prescription?**

   Answer: The prescriber's name is Stanley Fray.

4. **What is the prescriber's DEA number?**

   Answer: The prescriber's DEA number is BF3456781.

5. **Could the prescriber's DEA be valid? Utilize the DEA check digit verification process to support your answer.**

   To begin, review the letters of the DEA number. The first letter matches the prescriber's level of authority (the letters *A*, *B*, or *F* for a primary practitioner). The second letter matches the first initial of the prescriber's last name (the letter *F*).

   Next, utilize the DEA check digit verification process to determine potential validity of the number.

   Step 1. Add the first, third, and fifth digits of the DEA number.

   $$3 + 5 + 7 = 15$$

   Step 2. Add the second, fourth, and sixth digits of the DEA number.

   $$4 + 6 + 8 = 18$$

   Step 3. Multiply the sum obtained in Step 2 by 2.

   $$18 \times 2 = 36$$

   Step 4. Add the results of Steps 1 and 3. The last digit of this sum or the check-sum, should match the check digit, the last digit of the prescriber's DEA number (the number *1*).

   $$15 + 36 = 51$$

   Answer: The prescriber's DEA number could be valid.

6. **What drug, strength, and quantity are listed on the inscription and the subscription?**

   Recall that the inscription is the part of the prescription that lists the medication prescribed. The subscription lists instructions to the pharmacist.

   Answer: The inscription on this e-prescription is for zolpidem tablets. The strength is 5 mg. The quantity to dispense is 60 tablets.

7. **Which label indicates the medication needed to fill the prescription?**

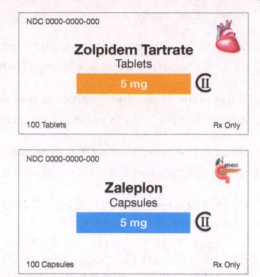

NDC 0000-0000-000

Zolpidem Tartrate
Tablets

5 mg ℃Ⅱ

100 Tablets   Rx Only

NDC 0000-0000-000

Zaleplon
Capsules

5 mg ℃Ⅱ

100 Capsules   Rx Only

Answer: The medication labeled as zolpidem 5 mg (pictured on top) should be selected.

8. **What directions for use are listed in the signa (sig)? Please translate any abbreviations into language that the patient would understand. Then determine the quantity of medication needed for each dose.**

To begin, find the sig on the e-prescription. The sig states *10 mg po qhs prn insomnia*.

Next, translate the sig into language that the patient would understand. The abbreviation *po* means "by mouth," and the abbreviation *qhs* means "every night at bedtime." The abbreviation *prn* means "as needed for." The sig *10 mg po qhs prn insomnia* translates to "10 mg by mouth every night at bedtime as needed for insomnia."

Now, using the dimensional analysis method, set up an equation with the information from the e-prescription: the prescribed drug's strength (5 mg/tablet) and its dose (10 mg/dose). Then cancel like units to determine the number of tablets needed for each dose.

$$\frac{10 \text{ mg}}{\text{dose}} \times \frac{1 \text{ tablet}}{5 \text{ mg}} = 2 \text{ tablets per dose}$$

Answer: The sig states *10 mg po qhs prn insomnia*, which is translated to "10 mg by mouth every night at bedtime as needed for insomnia." The patient will need 2 tablets by mouth for every dose.

9. **If the patient takes the medication every night, what is the days' supply of this prescription?**

Recall that days' supply is the number of days that a prescription medication will last a patient when taken as directed. In this example, two tablets are needed for each dose, and one dose is taken per day. To calculate days' supply, you can solve this problem by using the ratio-proportion method or by using the dimensional analysis method.

Ratio-Proportion Method

$$\frac{x \text{ days}}{60 \text{ tablets}} = \frac{1 \text{ day}}{2 \text{ tablets}}$$

$$x \text{ days } (2 \text{ tablets}) = 1 \text{ day } (60 \text{ tablets})$$

$$x = 30 \text{ days}$$

Dimensional Analysis Method

Set up your dimensional analysis using the information provided. Then cancel like units (in this case, "tablets") and multiply.

$$\frac{60 \text{ tablets}}{1} \times \frac{\text{day}}{2 \text{ tablets}} = 30 \text{ days}$$

Answer: The days' supply of the prescription is 30 days.

10. How many refills are indicated on the prescription?

Answer: The subscription indicates that no refills are allowed.

Interpreting Medication Orders

As discussed earlier, a pharmacy receives different types of medication orders either electronically or in written form. As a pharmacy technician, you must be able to accurately identify and interpret the patient, prescriber, and medication information these orders contain. You must also be able to convert 24-hour time to standard time for patient ease and understanding. The following example will apply the literacy skills of this chapter to the interpretation of a medication order.

Example 3.4.2

Review the medication order and answer the associated questions.

1. Which type of medication order is shown here?

Answer: This order is a daily medication order.

2. What is the patient's name?

Answer: The patient's name is Heidi McCarthy.

3. What allergies or sensitivities does the patient have?

Answer: The patient has no known allergies.

4. What is the patient's weight and height?

Answer: The patient's weight is 186 lb, and the patient's height is 5′7″.

5. What is the prescriber's name?

Answer: The prescriber's name is Yuka Sun.

6. What is the prescriber's authority?

Answer: The prescriber is an MD, or medical doctor.

7. **On what date was the medication order written?**

   Answer: The medication order was written on 06/24/2025.

8. **What time was the medication order written? Please state your answer in 24-hour time and in standard time.**

   Answer: The medication order was written at 1800, which is 24-hour time. To convert the 24-hour time to standard time, subtract 1200 from 1800. The standard time for this order is 6:00 p.m.

ID#: J1008912345 **Name:** McCarthy, Heidi **DOB:** 06/04/82 **Room:** 804 **Dr.:** Yuka Sun, MD	**MEMORIAL HOSPITAL** **PHYSICIAN'S MEDICATION ORDER** BEAR DOWN ON HARD SURFACE WITH BALLPOINT PEN

Patient Name: *Heidi McCarthy*		ID number: *J1008912345*		Room number: *804*
DOB: *06/04/1982*		Height: *5'7"*		Weight: *186 lb*

GENERIC EQUIVALENT IS AUTHORIZED UNLESS CHECKED IN THIS COLUMN

ALLERGY OR SENSITIVITY TO _____ *Ø* _____ NONE KNOWN ☑ SIGNED:	DIAGNOSIS *S/P Hernia* *Repair*		COMPLETED OR DISCONTINUED	

DATE	TIME	ORDERS	PHYSICIAN'S SIG.	NAME	DATE	TIME
6/24/2025	1800	*Routine Orders*				
		Height 5'7" Weight 186 lb				
		Condition – stable				
		VS: q4° × 2, then q shift				
		Diet: Regular				
		Meds:				
		Vistaril 25 mg IM q3h prn pain				
		Halcion 0.25 mg PO q hs prn sleep				
		cefazolin 1 gram IVPB q6h				
		Lance wound on foot in am				
		Call H.O. for: T > 101.5				
		BP > 180/100, or < 80/60				

SIGNATURE: *Yuka Sun, MD,   6/24/2025*

PHARMACY COPY

9. **What drugs, strengths, routes of administration, and frequencies of administration are listed on the medication order? Please translate any abbreviations or acronyms.**

The "Meds" section of the order prescribes the following medications for the patient:

- *Vistaril 25 mg IM q3h prn pain*, which translates to "Vistaril 25 mg intramuscularly every 3 hours as needed for pain"
- *Halcion 0.25 mg PO qhs prn sleep*, which translates to "Halcion 0.25 mg by mouth every night at bedtime as needed for sleep"
- *Cefazolin 1 gram IVPB q6h*, which is translated to "cefazolin 1 gram by intravenous piggyback every 6 hours"

Answer: The prescriber has ordered Vistaril 25 mg intramuscularly every 3 hours as needed for pain, Halcion 0.25 mg by mouth every night at bedtime as needed for sleep, and cefazolin 1 gram by intravenous piggyback every 6 hours.

10. **If the patient's first dose of cefazolin is at 0800, when should the second and third doses be administered? Include 24-hour time and standard time in your answer.**

Answer: If the patient takes the first dose of cefazolin at 0800 (8:00 a.m.) and is to take the medication every 6 hours, the patient will take the second dose at 1400 (2:00 p.m.) and the third dose at 2000 (8:00 p.m.).

3.4 Problem Set

Review the following prescription and answer the associated questions.

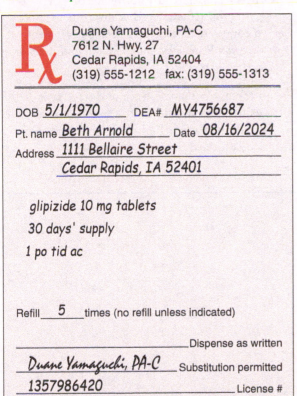

1. Which type of prescription is shown here?

2. What is the patient's name?

3. What is the prescriber's name?

4. What is the prescriber's DEA number?

5. Determine the validity of the DEA number by verifying the prescriber identifiers and using the check digit verification process.

6. What drug, dosage form, and strength are listed on the inscription?

7. Which label indicates the medication needed to fill the prescription?

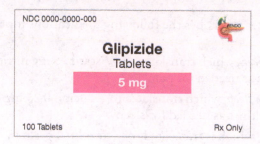

NDC 0000-0000-000

Glipizide
Tablets

5 mg

100 Tablets   Rx Only

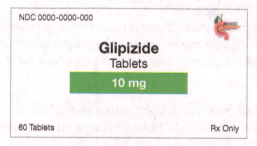

NDC 0000-0000-000

Glipizide
Tablets

10 mg

60 Tablets   Rx Only

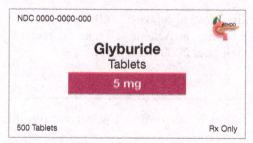

NDC 0000-0000-000

Glyburide
Tablets

5 mg

500 Tablets   Rx Only

8. What directions for use are listed on the signa (sig)? Translate any abbreviations into language that the patient would understand. (If you need additional support to complete this exercise, refer to *Appendix B: Common Pharmacy Abbreviations and Acronyms* in this textbook.)

9. What is the days' supply of this prescription? What is the quantity to dispense?

10. How many refills are indicated on the prescription?

Review the medication order on the following page and answer the associated questions.

11. Which type of medication order is shown here?

12. What is the patient's name?

13. What allergies or sensitivities does the patient have?

14. What is the patient's height and weight?

15. What is the prescriber's name?

16. What is the prescriber's authority?

17. What date was the medication order written?

18. What time was the medication order written? Include both 24-hour time and standard time in your answer.

19. What drugs, strengths, routes of administration, and frequencies of administration are listed on the medication order? Translate any abbreviations or acronyms. (If you need additional support to complete this exercise, refer to *Appendix B: Common Pharmacy Abbreviations and Acronyms* in this textbook.)

20. If the patient's first dose of docusate is at 0800, when should the patient's second dose be administered? Include both 24-hour time and standard time in your answer.

Self-check your work in Appendix A.

| | IN DOSAGE FORM AND THERAPEUTIC ACTIVITY MAY BE ADMINISTERED UNLESS CHECKED | Patient Information Below |

START EACH NEW SERIES OF ORDERS BELOW

Check one: (FOR NEW PATIENTS OR CHANGE IN STATUS)

☐ OBSERVATION: short stay expected   ☒ Admit – inpatient; longer stay expected

Patient name: *Caycie Pasqual*   ID number: *S1008994566*   Room number: *420*

DOB: *02/14/1990*   Height: *5'3"*   Weight: *132 lb*

Diagnosis: Ⓛ *Leg DVT, Fe deficiency anemia*

Activity: *Bed rest c̄ bedside commode × 24° then ad lib*

Diet: *cardiac*

Allergies: *NKDA*   Reactions:

① *Admit to Medicine – Dr. Galangal*
② *Condition – stable*
③ *Vitals per routine*
④ *Labs – PT/INR q AM – call c̄ results of PT/INR tonight*
     – guaiac stools × 3
     – Fe/Ferritin next lab draw
⑤ *IV – HL flush q shift*

NURSE'S SIGNATURE   DATE   TIME

START EACH NEW SERIES OF ORDERS BELOW

⑥ *Meds – Lovenox 1 mg/kg SQ q 12*
     – warfarin 10 mg PO tonight × ī dose
     – docusate 100 mg PO q12h – hold per loose stool
     – Benadryl 50 mg PO qHS prn insomnia
⑦ *Call per acute changes*
⑧ *Nutrition consult re: vitamin K diet*

SIGNATURE: *Greg Galangal, MD*

NURSE'S SIGNATURE   DATE *11/16/2025*   TIME *1430*

700781 (2-97)
H-NSO781B

MERCY HOSPITAL

PHYSICIAN'S INITIAL ORDERS SHEET

PHARMACY   B 427687   PHARMACY   B 427687

ID#: S1008994566   Name: Pasqual, Caycie   DOB: 02/14/1990   Room: 420   Dr.: Greg Galangal, MD

ID#: S1008994566   Name: Pasqual, Caycie   DOB: 02/14/1990   Room: 420   Dr.: Greg Galangal, MD

Review and Assessment

CHAPTER SUMMARY

- A prescription is an order of medication for a patient that is issued by a physician or another licensed healthcare prescriber.

- Prescriptions can be written, faxed, telephoned, or prescribed electronically.

- Controlled substances have specific prescription requirements.

- All prescriptions must include patient information, prescriber information, and medication information.

- The patient's full name and birth date must appear on a prescription.

- In most states, prescribers must include their name, authority, and telephone number on prescriptions.

- A DEA number is a registration code that signifies the authority of the holder to prescribe or handle controlled substances.

- A DEA number comprises two letters followed by seven digits.

- The check digit verification process can be used to determine if a DEA number is fraudulent.

- The date a prescription is written or ordered must be on the document.

- The inscription is the part of the prescription that lists the medication prescribed, including the strength and amount.

- A drug may be identified by its generic name or brand name.

- The signa (commonly referred to as the "sig") is the part of the prescription that communicates the directions for use.

- The subscription is the part of the prescription that lists the instructions to the pharmacist about dispensing the medication, including quantity to dispense, compounding instructions, labeling instructions, information about the appropriateness of dispensing drug equivalents, and refill information.

- Quantity to dispense may be indicated on a prescription, or it may need to be calculated.

- Days' supply is the number of days that a prescription will last a patient when taken as directed by the prescriber.

- Quantity to dispense and days' supply can be calculated by using the ratio-proportion method or by using the dimensional analysis method.

- A medication order is a set of instructions given by a prescriber that specifies medications for an inpatient at a hospital or a resident of a long-term care facility.

- Medication orders may be given verbally, written, or transmitted electronically.

- Admission orders, daily orders, single orders, stat orders, prn orders, standing orders, and discharge orders are all types of medication orders.

- Both the date and time must be included on a medication order.

- Time may be expressed in 24-hour time or in standard time.

- Medical abbreviations, acronyms, and symbols may appear on prescriptions and medication orders.

- Common abbreviations, acronyms, and symbols are shorthand communication methods used by prescribers on prescriptions and medication orders and must be translated for patient understanding.

FORMULAS FOR SUCCESS

DEA Check Digit Verification Process (Section 3.1)

Step 1. Add the first, third, and fifth digits of the DEA number.

Step 2. Add the second, fourth, and sixth digits of the DEA number.

Step 3. Double the sum obtained in Step 2 (i.e., multiply it by 2).

Step 4. Add the results of Steps 1 and 3. The last digit of this checksum should match the check digit, or the last digit of the DEA number.

CHECK YOUR UNDERSTANDING

Take a moment to review what you have learned in this chapter and answer the following questions.

1. The number of refills on a prescription
   a. should be filled in by the patient.
   b. is zero if left blank by the prescriber.
   c. is always one unless otherwise indicated.
   d. may be altered if the dose is not appropriate for the patient's weight.

2. A DEA number is issued to
   a. prescribers who are known to have abused controlled substances.
   b. prescribers who have authority to prescribe controlled substances.
   c. all physicians and nurses.
   d. emergency room physicians who need special privileges.

3. The quantity to dispense is
   a. determined only by calling or verifying the amount dispensed with the prescriber or the prescriber's staff.
   b. calculated from information on the prescription that describes the daily dose and the duration of therapy.
   c. based on what the patient received on the previous prescription refill.
   d. calculated by what the insurance company will permit as the maximum number of doses.

4. The directions for patients on a prescription are called the
   a. "dispense as written" instructions.
   b. signa.
   c. metric conversions.
   d. route of administration.

5. Days' supply is calculated to verify that
   a. the patient will have an adequate supply of medication to take for the duration of therapy.
   b. the prescriber's dosage form selection is appropriate.
   c. the prescriber has selected drug therapy from the available supply in inventory.
   d. the prescription complies with the guidelines of TJC.

6. Which DEA number could be valid for a midwife?
   a. AJ3456781
   b. BM3456781
   c. FL3456781
   d. MM3456781

7. A prescription for cefaclor 250 mg capsules contains the following sig: *1 capsule TID for 14 days*. How many capsules should be dispensed?

a. 14
b. 21
c. 28
d. 42

8. A prescription has a sig that instructs the patient to do the following: *Place ii gtts OD BID*. Where will the patient instill this medication?

a. left ear
b. right eye
c. left eye
d. both eyes

9. A prescription has the following sig: *2 caps po TID ac*. What patient instructions should appear on the label of the medication container?

a. Take 2 capsules twice daily with food.
b. Take 2 capsules three times daily as needed.
c. Take 2 capsules by mouth three times daily before meals.
d. Take 2 capsules after each meal.

10. A prescription has the following sig: *Take 1 cap qhs*. How many days will this prescription last if 45 capsules are dispensed?

a. 11 days
b. 14 days
c. 22 days
d. 45 days

FIND SOLUTIONS

Take a moment to consider what you have learned in this chapter and respond thoughtfully to the prompts.

Note: *To indicate your answers for Scenario C, Questions 9 and 10, ask your instructor for the handout depicting a dosing spoon and an oral syringe and the handout depicting a dosing spoon and a medicine cup.*

Scenario A: A prescription for a large quantity of narcotic pain medication has come into a community pharmacy. Although the prescription is written on a hospital prescription form, you are suspicious that the prescription may not be valid. The written directive is oddly worded, and the dose is not what is typically associated with the medication prescribed. A DEA number is handwritten at the bottom of the prescription.

1. Perform a check digit verification process on the DEA number: AB4423921. Could this DEA number be valid?

2. The sig of this prescription states the following: *Take 3 tabs qid or prn*. How would you translate this sig for patient understanding?

3. The drug name written is NORCO (hydrocodone/acetaminophen). What part of the drug name indicates the brand name, and what part indicates the generic name?

Scenario B: An older adult patient with significant vision loss requires large-print instructions for taking medications. Translate the following sigs for patient understanding.

4. Lasix 20 mg; take 1 tab po QDay in AM for edema

5. cimetidine 800 mg; take 1 tab po BID for GERD

6. acyclovir 800 mg; take 1 tab po QID for 5 days for shingles

7. verapamil 80 mg; take 1 tab po TID for angina

8. diazepam 2 mg; take 1 tab po HS for sleep

Scenario C: Mrs. Zapata has three children with chicken pox, and the pediatrician's office has advised the purchase of OTC Benadryl for itching. The oldest child can take capsules, but the other two children need a liquid formulation.

9. On the handout that you obtained from your instructor, select the most accurate measuring device (either the dosing spoon or the oral syringe) to administer a ½ tsp dose to a child. Fill in the correct volume on the measuring device.

10. On the handout that you obtained from your instructor, select the most accurate measuring device (either the dosing spoon or the medicine cup) to administer a 2 tsp dose to a child. Fill in the correct volume on the measuring device.

 Scenario D: Nany Romez brings this prescription to the pharmacy. Use the prescription to answer the following questions.

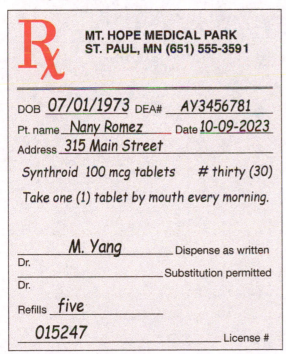

R̶x̶
MT. HOPE MEDICAL PARK
ST. PAUL, MN (651) 555-3591

DOB __07/01/1973__ DEA# __AY3456781__
Pt. name __Nany Romez__ Date __10-09-2023__
Address __315 Main Street__

Synthroid 100 mcg tablets   # thirty (30)

Take one (1) tablet by mouth every morning.

__M. Yang__ _____ Dispense as written
Dr.
_____ Substitution permitted
Dr.

Refills __five__

__015247__ _____ License #

11. Perform a check digit verification process on the DEA number. Could this DEA number be valid?

12. How would you abbreviate the signa?

13. What is the days' supply for this prescription?

14. If the patient wanted a 90 days' supply of this medication, how many tablets would need to be dispensed?

15. How many refills are permitted on this prescription?

Scenario E: Use the prescription below to answer the following questions.

R̶x̶ **Azithromycin 500 mg**
ii tab PO × 1 *stat*

16. Translate the sig from the prescription into wording that would be appropriate on the medication label for a patient.

17. If the instructions included the abbreviation *ac*, how would that change your translation?

 The online course includes additional review and assessment resources.

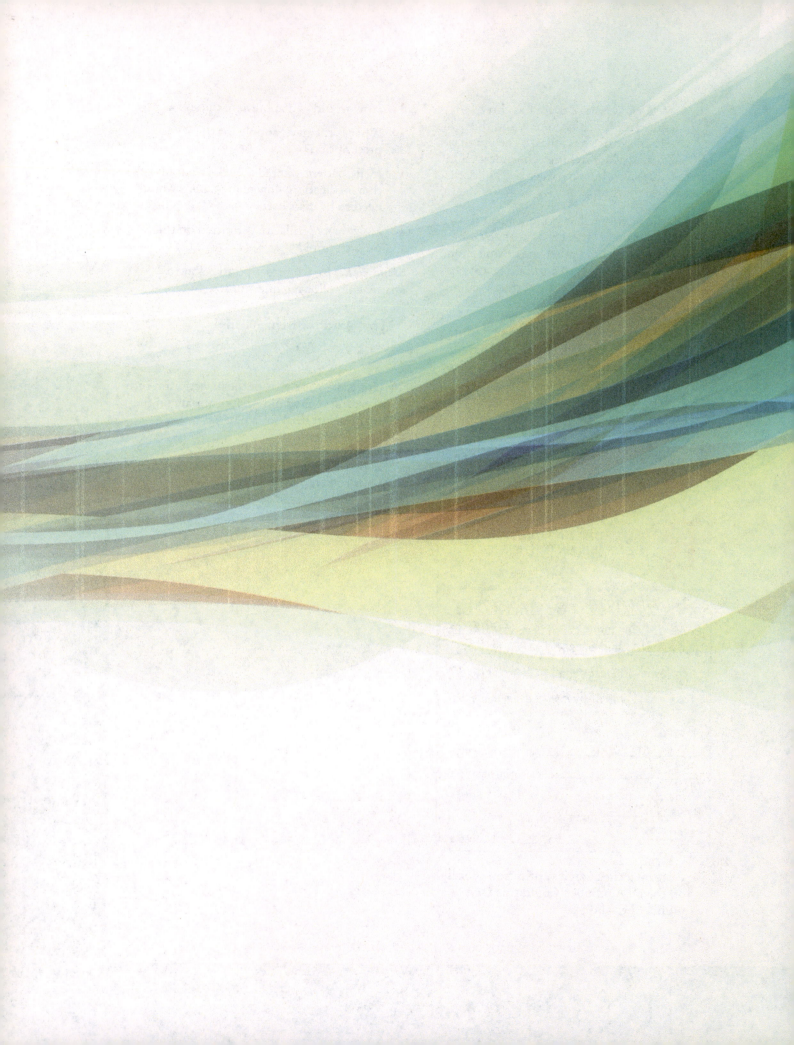

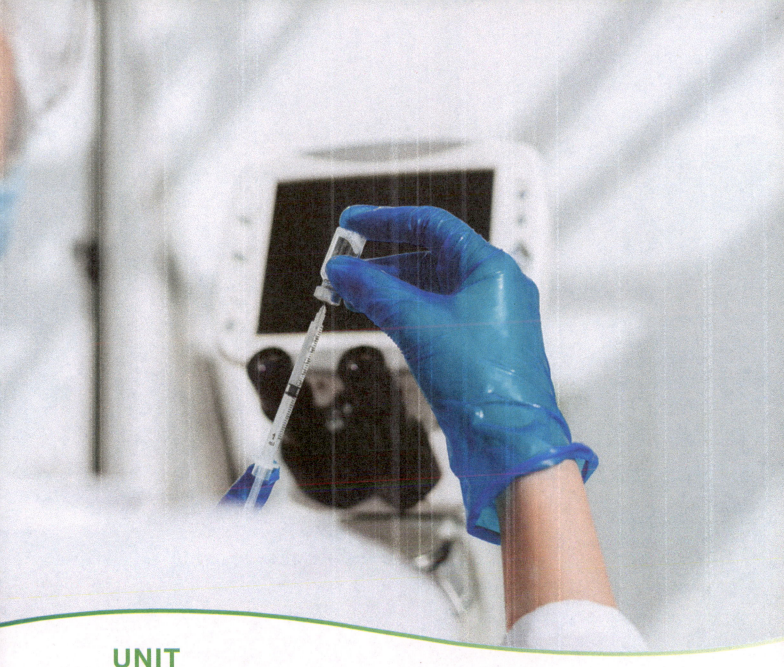

UNIT 2 Common Pharmacy Calculations

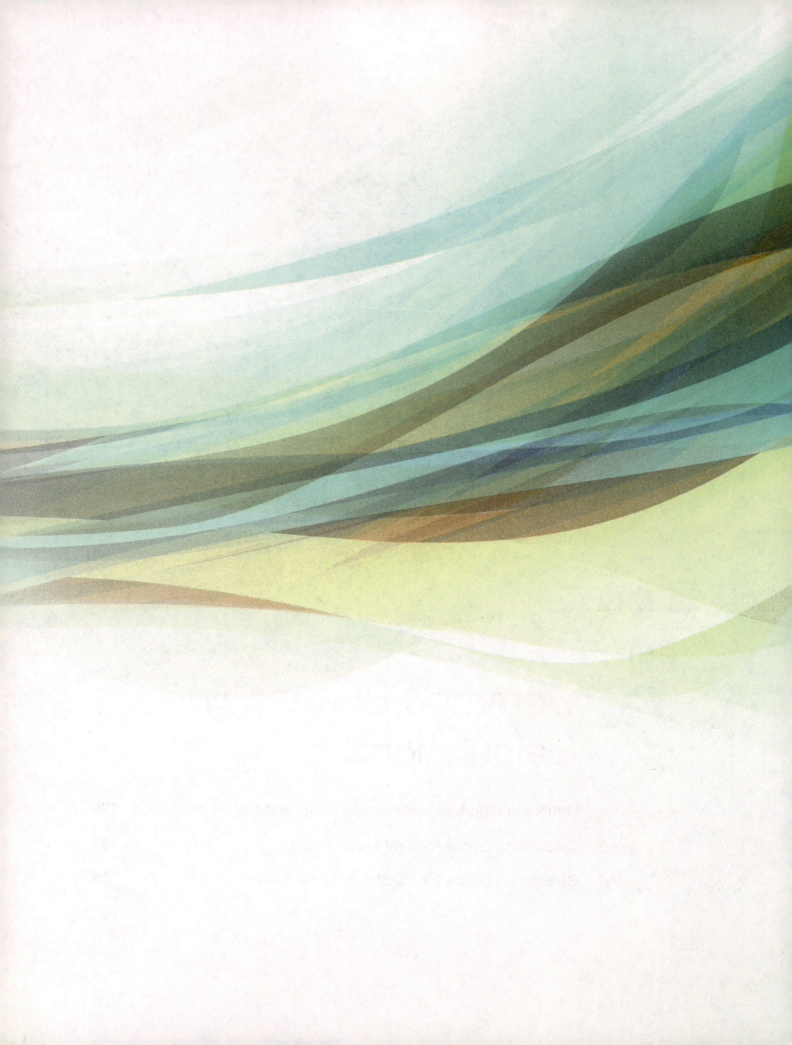

Understanding Measurement Systems and Conversions

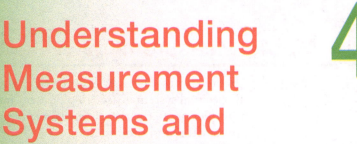

4

Learning Objectives

1 Identify the metric system units of measurement. (Section 4.1)

2 Recognize metric system prefixes and abbreviations and understand their meanings. (Section 4.1)

3 Understand how to write parts of a unit as a decimal. (Section 4.1)

4 Perform conversions within the metric system by multiplying, dividing, and moving the decimal point. (Section 4.2)

5 Convert metric units of measurement by using the ratio-proportion and dimensional analysis methods. (Section 4.2)

6 Identify household system units of measurement. (Section 4.3)

7 Recognize household system abbreviations and their meanings. (Section 4.3)

8 Perform conversions within the household system by using the ratio-proportion and dimensional analysis methods. (Section 4.4)

9 Perform conversions between the metric and household measurement systems using the ratio-proportion and dimensional analysis methods. (Section 4.5)

10 Understand the Celsius and Fahrenheit temperature systems and perform conversions between these systems. (Section 4.6)

For a key to the body system icons that appear in each chapter of this textbook, refer to the Preface.

ASHP/ACPE Accreditation Standards
To view the *ASHP/ACPE Accreditation Standards* addressed in this chapter, refer to Appendix D.

There are two main measurement systems you will encounter in pharmacy practice: the metric measurement system and the household measurement system. Although there is a growing trend toward the use of the metric system, both measurement systems are used by patients, prescribers, and drug manufacturers. For this reason, you must know these measurement systems as well as how to perform conversions both within and between these systems.

4.1 Metric Measurement System

Chapter 1 presented a brief overview of the decimal system. Because of its accuracy, the decimal system is used in pharmacy measurements. Based on subdivisions and multiples of 10, the **metric measurement system** uses decimals to indicate tenths, hundredths, and thousandths.

Identifying Metric System Units of Measurement

The metric system has three basic units of measurement: *meter*, *gram*, and *liter* (see Table 4.1). The **meter**, the unit for measuring length, has limited use in a pharmacy. A patient's height is often measured in feet and inches but may be measured in meters or centimeters. One meter (1 m) is approximately three feet (3 ft), or 39.37 in. The **gram**, the unit for measuring weight (mass), is used in a pharmacy for measuring the amount of medication in a solid dosage form and for indicating the amount of solid medication in a solution. One gram (1 g) is the weight of one cubic centimeter (1 cc) of water at 4° C. The **liter** is the unit used for measuring the volume of liquid medications and liquids for solutions. One liter (1 L) equals 1,000 milliliters (1,000 mL), and one milliliter (1 mL) is approximately the volume of one cubic centimeter (1 cc).

TABLE 4.1 Metric Units of Measurement

Metric Unit	Measurement
meter (m)	length
gram (g)	weight (mass)*
liter (L)	volume

*Mass is a measurement of how much matter is in an object; weight is a measurement of how hard gravity is pulling on that object. Your mass is the same no matter where you are (Earth, the moon, another planet), but your weight differs based on where you are. To prevent confusion, the gram is used as the unit of measurement for weight.

Using Metric System Prefixes and Abbreviations

Metric system prefixes, such as the ones shown in Table 4.2, are added to the names of the basic units to designate larger or smaller values of these units. These prefixes indicate a power of 10 by which the basic units are multiplied or divided. For that reason, metric system prefixes have the same meanings for all basic units. For example, the basic unit *gram* can be multiplied by 1,000 to create the smaller unit *milligram* and can be divided by 1,000 to create the larger unit *kilogram*. The three prefixes most commonly used in pharmacy calculations are *kilo-*, *milli-*, and *micro-*.

All metric system units also have corresponding abbreviations, as shown in Table 4.3. These abbreviations are commonly used in pharmacy practice. Medication labels, prescriptions, medication orders, and measuring devices are examples of items that contain metric system abbreviations. Therefore, you need to be familiar with these abbreviations. However, as mentioned in Chapter 3, you also need to be cautious in your interpretation of these abbreviations. For example, the misinterpretation of the abbreviation *mcg* as *mg* leads to a 1,000-fold increase in a dose.

TABLE 4.2 Metric System Prefixes

Prefix	Value
nano (n)	$\frac{1}{1,000,000,000}$ (one-billionth of the basic unit, or 0.000000001 or 10^{-9})
micro (mc)	$\frac{1}{1,000,000}$ (one-millionth of the basic unit, or 0.000001 or 10^{-6})
milli (m)	$\frac{1}{1,000}$ (one-thousandth of the basic unit, or 0.001 or 10^{-3})
centi (c)	$\frac{1}{100}$ (one-hundredth of the basic unit, or 0.01 or 10^{-2})
deci (d)	$\frac{1}{10}$ (one-tenth of the basic unit, or 0.1 or 10^{-1})
kilo (k)	1,000 (one thousand times the basic unit or 10^3)

TABLE 4.3 Metric System Unit Abbreviations

Measurement	Metric Unit	Abbreviation
weight	kilogram	kg
	gram	g
	milligram	mg
	microgram	mcg
volume	kiloliter	kL
	liter	L
	milliliter	mL*
	microliter	mcL
length	kilometer	km
	meter	m
	millimeter	mm
	micrometer	mcm†

*The abbreviation *mL* is equivalent to the abbreviation *cc*, which signifies cubic centimeters. The use of the abbreviation *cc* is considered a dangerous practice because it can be mistaken for "u."

†Micrometer is sometimes abbreviated as μm. However, the use of the abbreviation μ*m* is considered a dangerous practice because it can be mistaken for the abbreviation *mg*.

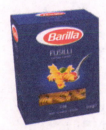 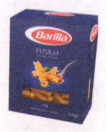

One kilogram (1 kg) is equivalent to a little more than two one-pound (1 lb) boxes of pasta.

A single, large paper clip weighs approximately one gram (1 g).

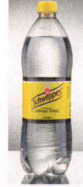

Remembering the amount of liquid that is contained in a standard, one-liter (1 L) bottle will help you visualize the amount of liquid in one liter.

Most people can visualize an object that weighs a kilogram or a gram, and many individuals can create a mental picture of a container that can hold a liter or a milliliter of a liquid. However, it is more difficult to see something that weighs only a microgram. Medications that contain micrograms (mcg), or even milligrams (mg), of an active ingredient almost always contain an inactive filler so that the dosage form becomes measurable. For example, a tablet with a weight of 3 mcg would be hard to see and too small to handle. The tablets shown in Figure 4.1 contain different amounts of levothyroxine, but they are all the same size. Even though levothyroxine is available in a variety of strengths, the tablet sizes remain the same. The colors of the tablets and the package labeling differentiate the amount of active ingredient.

FIGURE 4.1 Levothyroxine Tablet Strengths and Colors

| 25 mcg orange | 50 mcg white | 75 mcg violet | 88 mcg olive | 100 mcg yellow | 112 mcg rose | 125 mcg brown | 137 mcg turquoise | 150 mcg blue | 175 mcg lilac | 200 mcg pink | 300 mcg green |

Writing Parts of a Unit

Safety Alert

For a decimal value less than 1, pharmacy technicians should use a leading zero to prevent medication errors.

Parts of a unit are written as a decimal number. For example, two-and-a-half milligrams is written as 2.5 mg, not 2½ mg. A leading zero is used if there is no whole number preceding the decimal point. For example, one-half liter is written as 0.5 L (not .5 L), and one-quarter gram is written as 0.25 g (not .25 g). These leading zeros help prevent medication errors.

When writing dosage strengths, trailing zeros (unnecessary zeros after the decimal point) are generally left off to reduce the chance of misreading the values. For example, 0.25 mL, 5 L, and 15.6 mL should not be written as 0.250 mL, 5.0 L, and 15.60 mL.

4.1 Problem Set   1-10

State the abbreviation for each of the following metric units.

1. microgram
2. milligram
3. liter
4. gram
5. kilogram
6. meter
7. centimeter
8. milliliter
9. microliter
10. deciliter

Write the following numbers using an Arabic number with a decimal value and the appropriate unit abbreviation.

11. six-tenths of a gram
12. fifty kilograms
13. four-tenths of a milligram
14. four-hundredths of a liter
15. four and two-tenths of a gram
16. five-thousandths of a gram
17. six-hundredths of a gram
18. two and six-tenths of a liter
19. three-hundredths of a liter
20. two-hundredths of a milliliter

Self-check your work in Appendix A.

4.2 Conversions within the Metric Measurement System

To convert units within the metric measurement system, you have three options: multiplying or dividing (moving the decimal point), using the ratio-proportion method, or using the dimensional analysis method. Once you learn the three methods of conversion, you may want to select the most comfortable method and use only that method when making conversions.

Multiplying or Dividing (Moving the Decimal Point)

To change the metric units of a number to smaller or larger units, you can multiply or divide by an appropriate multiple of 1,000 (see Table 4.4). You use multiplication to convert a larger metric unit of measurement to a smaller metric unit of measurement. For example, to convert 5 g to milligrams (mg), you need to know the following metric conversion: 1 g equals 1,000 mg. Therefore, you multiply 5 by 1,000 to get 5,000 mg. You can also multiply by 1,000 by moving the decimal point three places to the right: 5.0 becomes 5000, or 5,000. To convert 17 L to microliters (mcL), you need to know the following metric conversion: 1 L equals 1,000,000 mcL. Therefore, you multiply 17 by 1,000,000 to get 17,000,000 mcL. You can also multiply by 1,000,000 by moving the decimal point six places to the right: 17.0 becomes 17000000, or 17,000,000.

TABLE 4.4 Metric Unit Equivalents

Kilo	Base	Milli	Micro
0.001 kg	1 g	1,000 mg	1,000,000 mcg
0.001 kL	1 L	1,000 mL	1,000,000 mcL
0.001 km	1 m	1,000 mm	1,000,000 mcm

Math Morsel

Moving the decimal point three places to the right is the same as multiplying by 1,000. Moving the decimal point three places to the left is the same as dividing by 1,000.

Conversely, you use division to convert a smaller metric unit of measurement to a larger metric unit of measurement. For example, to convert 3 grams (g) to kilograms (kg), you need to know the following metric conversion: 1,000 g equals 1 kg. Therefore, you divide 3 by 1,000 to get 0.003 kg. You can also divide by 1,000 by moving the decimal point three places to the left: 3.0 becomes 0.003. To convert 22 mL to liters (L), you need to know the following metric conversion: 1,000 mL equals 1 L. Therefore, you divide 22 by 1,000 to get 0.022 L. You can also divide by 1,000 by moving the decimal point three places to the left: 22.0 becomes 0.022.

The key to understanding the relationships of the prefixes *kilo–*, *milli –*, and *micro–* to a base unit in the metric system is to remember that the decimal point must be moved three places when converting from one unit to the next. Moving the decimal point three places is a quick way to multiply or divide the number by 1,000. The three places are representative of the three zeros in 1,000. Table 4.5 summarizes the conversions of common metric units using multiplication, division, and movement of the decimal point.

TABLE 4.5 Common Metric Conversions

Conversion	Instruction	Example
kilograms (kg) to grams (g)	multiply by 1,000 (move decimal point three places to the right)	6.25 kg = 6,250 g
grams (g) to milligrams (mg)	multiply by 1,000 (move decimal point three places to the right)	3.56 g = 3,560 mg
milligrams (mg) to grams (g)	divide by 1,000 (move decimal point three places to the left)	120 mg = 0.120 g
liters (L) to milliliters (mL)	multiply by 1,000 (move decimal point three places to the right)	2.5 L = 2,500 mL
milliliters (mL) to liters (L)	divide by 1,000 (move decimal point three places to the left)	238 mL = 0.238 L

The following examples show the conversion of a smaller metric unit of measurement to a larger metric unit of measurement. Remember that this type of conversion requires you to move the decimal point three places to the left.

Example 4.2.1

Convert 4,500 mL to liters.

$$4,500 \text{ mL} = 4.500 \text{ L} = 4.5 \text{ L}$$

Answer: A volume of 4,500 mL is equal to 4.5 L.

Example 4.2.2

Convert 1,287 mg to grams.

$$1,287 \text{ mg} = 1.287 \text{ g}$$

Answer: A weight of 1,287 mg is equal to 1.287 g.

Example 4.2.3

Convert 480 mL to liters.

$$480 \text{ mL} = 0.480 \text{ L} = 0.48 \text{ L}$$

Answer: A volume of 480 mL is equal to 0.48 L.

The following examples show the conversion of a larger metric unit of measurement to a smaller metric unit of measurement. Remember that this type of conversion requires you to move the decimal point three places to the right.

Example 4.2.4

Convert 0.954 g to milligrams.

$$0.954 \text{ g} = 954 \text{ mg}$$

Answer: A weight of 0.954 g is equal to 954 mg.

Example 4.2.5

Convert 1.5 g to milligrams.

$$1.5 \text{ g} = 1500 \text{ mg}$$

Answer: A weight of 1.5 g is equal to 1,500 mg.

Example 4.2.6

Convert 0.621 mg to micrograms.

$$0.621 \text{ mg} = 621 \text{ mcg}$$

Answer: A weight of 0.621 mg is equal to 621 mcg.

 ## WORKPLACE WISDOM

At first, it may be difficult to visualize conversions from smaller to larger units. It can be helpful to think about this concept in terms of more familiar units. Suppose you have $1,000,000 all in one-dollar bills (a smaller unit). In other words, you have 1,000,000 one-dollar bills. Suppose you wanted larger units and exchanged your dollar bills for $100 bills. You would then have 10,000 one-hundred-dollar bills (move the decimal point two places to the left). Now suppose you exchange all your $100 bills for $1,000 dollar bills (assume that one-thousand-dollar bills are still printed). You would have 1,000 one-thousand-dollar bills (move the decimal point one place to the left). In the end, you have the same amount of total dollars ($1,000,000), but you changed the units from smaller (one-dollar bills) to larger (one-hundred-dollar bills and then one-thousand-dollar bills).

Using the Ratio-Proportion Method

If you have difficulty remembering which way to move the decimal point when converting between units of measurement in the metric system, the **ratio-proportion method** introduced in Chapter 2 is an effective alternative. This method is a foolproof way to convert metric units. Set up the conversion by placing the unknown variable x and the value to be converted on the left side of the equation and the conversion factor (the ratio of the desired unit to the given unit) on the right side of the equation.

Math Morsel

When setting up proportions, units in the numerators must match, and units in the denominators must match.

Math Morsel

Pharmacy technicians who use the ratio-proportion method can verify their answer by multiplying the means and the extremes in the ratio. The products of the means and of the extremes must be equal.

When setting up a proportion to solve for the unknown variable *x*, remember that the units in the numerators must match and the units in the denominators must match. Checking to make sure that the units match before completing the calculation will ensure accuracy in the conversion. The next examples demonstrate conversions by moving the decimal point, followed by the same conversions using the ratio-proportion method.

Example 4.2.7

Convert 2,300 mg to grams.

To perform this conversion, you can use two methods: multiplying or dividing (moving the decimal point) or using the ratio-proportion method.

Multiplying or Dividing (Moving the Decimal Point)

To begin, recognize that you are converting a smaller unit (milligrams) to a larger unit (grams). Then you can either divide by 1,000 or move the decimal point three places to the left, as shown below.

$$2,300 \text{ mg} = 2.300 \text{ g} = 2.3 \text{ g}$$

Ratio-Proportion Method

To begin, set up a proportion by placing the unknown variable *x* over the value to be converted (2,300 mg) on the left side of the equation. Then place the conversion factor (1 g equals 1,000 mg) on the right side of the equation. Note that the units in the numerators and the units in the denominators match.

$$\frac{x \text{ g}}{2,300 \text{ mg}} = \frac{1 \text{ g}}{1,000 \text{ mg}}$$

Now, cross multiply, cancel similar units (like terms), and divide to solve for the unknown variable *x*.

$$x \text{ g } (1,000 \text{ mg}) = 1 \text{ g } (2,300 \text{ mg})$$

$$x = 2.3 \text{ g}$$

Answer: The conversion indicates that 2,300 mg is equal to 2.3 g.

Example 4.2.8

Convert 3.2 mg to micrograms.

To perform this conversion, you can use two methods: multiplying or dividing (moving the decimal point) or using the ratio-proportion method.

Multiplying or Dividing (Moving the Decimal Point)

To begin, recognize that you are converting a larger unit (milligrams) to a smaller unit (micrograms). Then multiply by 1,000 or move the decimal point three places to the right, as shown below.

$$3.2 \text{ mg} = 3200. \text{ mcg} = 3,200 \text{ mcg}$$

Ratio-Proportion Method

To begin, set up a proportion by placing the unknown variable x over the value to be converted (3.2 mg) on the left side of the equation. Then place the conversion factor (1,000 mcg equals 1 mg) on the right side of the equation. Note that the units in the numerators and the units in the denominators match.

$$\frac{x \text{ mcg}}{3.2 \text{ mg}} = \frac{1,000 \text{ mcg}}{1 \text{ mg}}$$

Now, cross multiply, cancel similar units (like terms), and divide to solve for the unknown variable x.

$$x \text{ mcg } (1 \text{ mg}) = 1,000 \text{ mcg } (3.2 \text{ mg})$$

$$x = 3,200 \text{ mcg}$$

Answer: The conversion indicates that 3.2 mg is equal to 3,200 mcg.

Example 4.2.9

Convert 3.785 L to milliliters.

To perform this conversion, you can use two methods: multiplying or dividing (moving the decimal point) or using the ratio-proportion method.

Multiplying or Dividing (Moving the Decimal Point)

To begin, recognize that you are converting a larger unit (liters) to a smaller unit (milliliters). Then multiply by 1,000 or move the decimal point three places to the right, as shown below.

$$3.785 \text{ L} = 3785. \text{ mL} = 3,785 \text{ mL}$$

Ratio-Proportion Method

To begin, set up a proportion by placing the unknown variable x over the value to be converted (3.785 L) on the left side of the equation. Then place the conversion factor (1,000 mL equals 1 L) on the right side of the equation. Note that the units in the numerators and the units in the denominators match.

$$\frac{x \text{ mL}}{3.785 \text{ L}} = \frac{1,000 \text{ mL}}{1 \text{ L}}$$

Now, cross multiply, cancel similar units (like terms), and divide to solve for the unknown variable x.

$$x \text{ mL } (1 \text{ L}) = 1,000 \text{ mL } (3.785 \text{ L})$$

$$x = 3,785 \text{ mL}$$

Answer: The conversion indicates that 3.785 L is equal to 3,785 mL.

Example 4.2.10

Convert 454 g to kilograms.

To perform this conversion, you can use two methods: multiplying or dividing (moving the decimal point) or using the ratio-proportion method.

Multiplying or Dividing (Moving the Decimal Point)

To begin, recognize that you are converting a smaller unit (grams) to a larger unit (kilograms). Then divide by 1,000 or move the decimal point three places to the left, as shown below.

$$454 \text{ g} = 0.454 \text{ kg} = 0.454 \text{ kg}$$

Ratio-Proportion Method

To begin, set up a proportion by placing the unknown variable x over the value to be converted (454 g) on the left side of the equation. Then place the conversion factor (1 kg equals 1,000 g) on the right side of the equation. Note that the units in the numerators and the units in the denominators match.

$$\frac{x \text{ kg}}{454 \text{ g}} = \frac{1 \text{ kg}}{1,000 \text{ g}}$$

Now, cross multiply, cancel similar units (like terms), and divide to solve for the unknown variable x.

$$x \text{ kg } (1,000 \text{ g}) = 1 \text{ kg } (454 \text{ g})$$

$$x = 0.454 \text{ kg}$$

Answer: The conversion indicates that 454 g is equal to 0.454 kg.

Using the Dimensional Analysis Method

As you learned in earlier chapters, the **dimensional analysis method** is a problem-solving method that uses the math principle that any number or expression can be multiplied by one without changing its value. As a reminder, you can set up the problems so that the starting units cancel one another and, consequently, you are left with the desired units.

$$\text{starting units} \times \frac{\text{desired units}}{\text{starting units}} = \text{desired units}$$

Example 4.2.11

Convert 486 mg to grams.

To begin, you know that the starting units are milligrams (486 mg). You also know that the desired units are grams and that 1 g equals 1,000 mg.

Then use this information to set up your equation. Cancel similar units (like terms) to determine the desired units.

$$\frac{486 \text{ mg}}{1} \times \frac{1 \text{ g}}{1,000 \text{ mg}} = 0.486 \text{ g}$$

Answer: The conversion indicates that 486 mg is equal to 0.486 g.

Example 4.2.12

Convert 4.5 L to milliliters.

To begin, you know that the starting units are liters (4.5 L). You also know that the desired units are milliliters and that 1,000 mL equals 1 L.

Then use this information to set up your equation. Cancel similar units (like terms) to determine the desired units.

$$\frac{4.5 \text{ L}}{1} \times \frac{1,000 \text{ mL}}{1 \text{ L}} = 4,500 \text{ mL}$$

Answer: The conversion indicates that 4.5 L is equal to 4,500 mL.

Example 4.2.13

Convert 240 mL to liters.

To begin, you know that the starting units are milliliters (240 mL). You also know that the desired units are liters and that 1 L equals 1,000 mL.

Then use this information to set up your equation. Cancel similar units (like terms) to determine the desired units.

$$\frac{240 \text{ mL}}{1} \times \frac{1 \text{ L}}{1,000 \text{ mL}} = 0.24 \text{ L}$$

Answer: The conversion indicates that 240 mL is equal to 0.24 L.

Example 4.2.14

Convert 0.725 mg to micrograms.

To begin, you know that the starting units are milligrams (0.725 mg). You also know that the desired units are micrograms and that 1,000 mcg equals 1 mg.

Then use this information to set up your equation. Cancel similar units (like terms) to determine the desired units.

$$\frac{0.725 \text{ mg}}{1} \times \frac{1,000 \text{ mcg}}{1 \text{ mg}} = 725 \text{ mcg}$$

Answer: The conversion indicates that 0.725 mg is equal to 725 mcg.

Example 4.2.15

Convert 0.519 g to micrograms.

To begin, you know that the starting units are grams (0.519 g). You also know that the desired units are micrograms. Therefore, you must perform two conversions.

For the first conversion, you need to change grams to milligrams. You know that 1,000 mg equals 1 g. For the second conversion, you need to change milligrams to micrograms. You know that 1,000 mcg equals 1 mg.

Then use this information to set up your equation. Cancel similar units (like terms) to determine the desired units.

$$\frac{0.519 \text{ g}}{1} \times \frac{1,000 \text{ mg}}{1 \text{ g}} \times \frac{1,000 \text{ mcg}}{1 \text{ mg}} = 519,000 \text{ mcg}$$

Answer: The conversion indicates that 0.519 g is equal to 519,000 mcg.

4.2 Problem Set odd 1-40

Convert the following units within the metric system by using the ratio-proportion method. Retain all significant figures and do not round your answers.

1. 1,964 mcg = _____ mg

2. 418 mg = _____ g

3. 651 mg = _____ mcg

4. 0.84 mg = _____ mcg

5. 0.012 g = _____ mcg

6. 9,213,406 mcg = _____ g

7. 284 mg = _____ g

8. 9,382.5 mcg = _____ mg

9. 12,321 mcg = _____ g

10. 184 g = _____ kg

Convert the following units within the metric system by using the dimensional analysis method. Retain all significant figures and do not round your answers.

11. 52 mL = _____ L

12. 2.06 g = _____ mg

13. 16 mg = _____ mcg

14. 256 mg = _____ g

15. 2,703,000 mcg = _____ g

16. 6.9 L = _____ mL

17. 62.5 mg = _____ g

18. 15 kg = _____ g

19. 2,785,000 mcg = _____ g

20. 8.234 mg = _____ mcg

Convert the following units by moving the decimal point, or by using the method that you prefer. Show all work. Retain all significant figures and do not round your answers.

21. 2 kg = _____ mg

22. 21 L = _____ mL

23. 576 mL = _____ L

24. 823 kg = _____ mg

25. 27 mcg = _____ mg

26. 5,000 mcg = _____ mg

27. 20 mcg = _____ mg

28. 4.624 mg = _____ mcg

29. 3.19 g = _____ mg

30. 8,736 mcg = _____ mg

31. 830 mL = _____ L

32. 0.94 L = _____ mL

33. 1.84 g = _____ mg

34. 560 mg = _____ g

35. 1,200 mcg = _____ mg

36. 125 mcg = _____ mg

37. 0.275 mg = _____ mcg

38. 480 mL = _____ L

39. 239 mg = _____ g

40. 1,500 mg = _____ g

Applications

41. The following prescription has come into your pharmacy. *Note:* One teaspoon (1 tsp) is equivalent to five milliliters (5 mL).

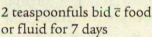

℞ **Clarithromycin Granules
125 mg/5 mL**

2 teaspoonfuls bid c̄ food
or fluid for 7 days

a. How many milliliters will the patient take daily?

b. How many milliliters should be dispensed to the patient?

c. How many grams will the patient take daily?

d. Using the following drug label, how many bottles of clarithromycin will be needed to fill this prescription?.

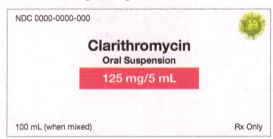

NDC 0000-0000-000

Clarithromycin
Oral Suspension
125 mg/5 mL

100 mL (when mixed)   Rx Only

42. A patient is to take 1.5 g of amoxicillin before a dental procedure. The capsules available are shown in the following label. How many capsules will be dispensed to this patient?

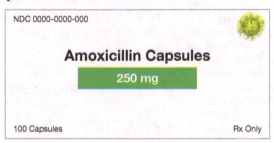

NDC 0000-0000-000

Amoxicillin Capsules
250 mg

100 Capsules   Rx Only

43. A patient is to receive 1,000 mg of vancomycin two times daily, diluted in IV solution. The following label shows the stock available.

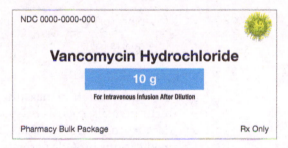

NDC 0000-0000-000

Vancomycin Hydrochloride
10 g
For Intravenous Infusion After Dilution

Pharmacy Bulk Package   Rx Only

a. How many doses are available in one vial?

b. How many days will one unopened vial last? Assume that the patient is the only one using vancomycin from this vial.

Self-check your work in Appendix A.

4.3 Household Measurement System

The **household measurement system** is a system used in homes, particularly in kitchens, in the United States. The units of household measurement for volume are *drop, teaspoon, tablespoon, cup, pint, quart,* and *gallon.* The units of household measurement for weight are *ounces* and *pounds.* Table 4.6 lists the household measurement equivalents and their abbreviations. Figure 4.2 illustrates household measurement equivalents.

TABLE 4.6 Household Measurement System Equivalents

Volume		Weight
3 teaspoonfuls (tsp)	= 1 tablespoonful (tbsp)	1 pound (lb) = 16 ounces (oz)
2 tablespoonfuls (tbsp)	= 1 fluid ounce (fl oz)	
8 fluid ounces (fl oz)	= 1 cup	
2 cups	= 1 pint (pt)	
2 pints (pt)	= 1 quart (qt)	
4 quarts (qt)	= 1 gallon (gal)	

In addition to measuring volumes for cooking and baking, household measurement utensils, such as teaspoons and tablespoons, have been used by patients for decades to administer liquid medications at home. Consequently, labels on these medications provide patient instructions in household measurement units.

However, using household measurement utensils to measure medication volumes can be less accurate than using standard measurement devices that have graduation marks. For that reason, there is a growing trend among prescribers and pharmacies to use the preferred metric measurement system for medication doses. To that end, pharmacies often provide dosing spoons, droppers, and dosing cups marked with both metric and household measurement units.

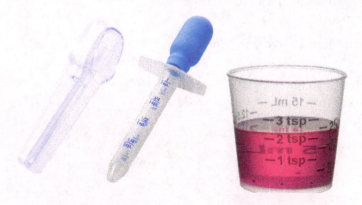

Dosing spoons, droppers, and dosing cups are frequently marked with both metric and household measurement units.

FIGURE 4.2 Household Units for Volume and Their Equivalents

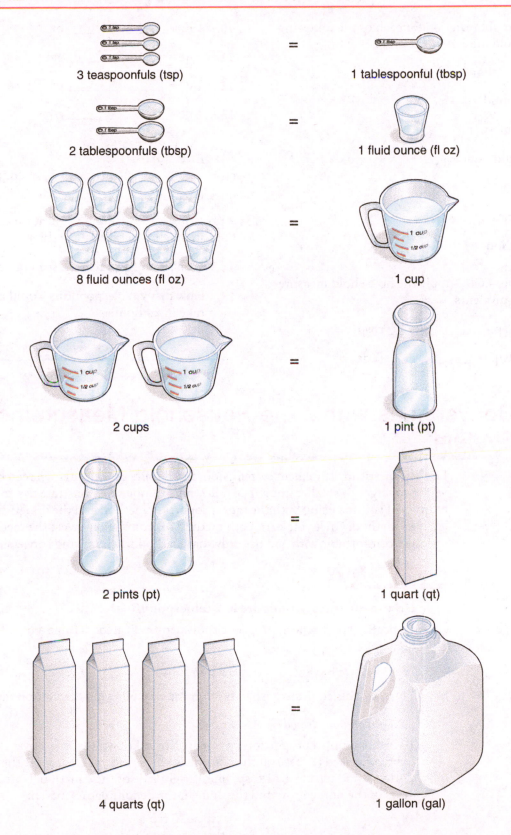

3 teaspoonfuls (tsp) = 1 tablespoonful (tbsp)

2 tablespoonfuls (tbsp) = 1 fluid ounce (fl oz)

8 fluid ounces (fl oz) = 1 cup

2 cups = 1 pint (pt)

2 pints (pt) = 1 quart (qt)

4 quarts (qt) = 1 gallon (gal)

4.3 Problem Set   ALL 1-13

State the abbreviation for each of the following household measurement units.

1. teaspoon

2. pound

3. tablespoon

4. fluid ounce

5. pint

6. quart

7. gallon

Use Table 4.6 to supply the household measurement equivalents.

8. 3 tsp = _____ tbsp

9. 1 cup = _____ fl oz

10. 1 lb = _____ oz

11. 4 qt = _____ gal

12. 1 qt = _____ pt

13. 1 pt = _____ cups

Applications

Use the scenario below to answer the following questions.

A prescription for a liquid medication states that the patient should take 1 fl oz three times daily.

14. What is an equivalent dose in tablespoons?

15. How many tablespoonfuls would a patient take in 24 hours?

Self-check your work in Appendix A.

4.4 Conversions within the Household Measurement System

Like the metric measurement system, household units of measurement can be converted to larger or smaller units. The following examples demonstrate the conversion of units of volume using both the ratio-proportion method and the dimensional analysis method. Once you learn both methods of conversion, select the method you are most comfortable with and use only that method when making conversions.

Example 4.4.1

How many teaspoonfuls are in 2 tablespoonfuls?

To begin, refer to the appropriate equivalent indicated in Table 4.6 and Figure 4.2.

$$3 \text{ tsp} = 1 \text{ tbsp}$$

Then use this equivalent when performing the following calculation methods.

Ratio-Proportion Method

To begin, set up a proportion by placing the unknown variable x over the value to be converted (2 tbsp) on the left side of the equation. Then place the conversion factor (3 tsp equals 1 tbsp) on the right side of the equation. Note that the units in the numerators and the units in the denominators match.

$$\frac{x \text{ tsp}}{2 \text{ tbsp}} = \frac{3 \text{ tsp}}{1 \text{ tbsp}}$$

Now, cross multiply, cancel similar units (like terms), and divide to solve for the unknown variable x.

$$x \text{ tsp (1 tbsp)} = 3 \text{ tsp (2 tbsp)}$$
$$x = 6 \text{ tsp}$$

Dimensional Analysis Method

$$\frac{2 \text{ tbsp}}{1} \times \frac{3 \text{ tsp}}{1 \text{ tbsp}} = 6 \text{ tsp}$$

Answer: There are 6 teaspoonfuls in 2 tablespoonfuls.

Example 4.4.2

How many tablespoonfuls are in 2 cups of medication?

To begin, refer to the appropriate equivalents indicated in Table 4.6 and Figure 4.2.

$$2 \text{ tbsp} = 1 \text{ fl oz}$$
$$1 \text{ cup} = 8 \text{ fl oz}$$

Then use these equivalents when performing the following calculation methods.

Ratio-Proportion Method

To begin, determine the number of fluid ounces in 2 cups by setting up a proportion. Place the unknown variable x over the value to be converted (2 cups) on the left side of the equation. Then place the conversion factor (8 fl oz equals 1 cup) on the right side of the equation. Note that the units in the numerators and the units in the denominators match.

$$\frac{x \text{ fl oz}}{2 \text{ cups}} = \frac{8 \text{ fl oz}}{1 \text{ cup}}$$

Next, cross multiply, cancel similar units (like terms), and divide to solve for the unknown variable x.

$$x \text{ fl oz (1 cup)} = 8 \text{ fl oz (2 cups)}$$
$$x = 16 \text{ fl oz}$$

Now, determine the number of tablespoonfuls in 16 fl oz by setting up another proportion. Place the unknown variable x over the value to be converted (16 fl oz) on the left side of the equation. Then place the conversion factor you cited at the beginning of this example (2 tbsp equals 1 fl oz) on the right side of the equation.

$$\frac{x \text{ tbsp}}{16 \text{ fl oz}} = \frac{2 \text{ tbsp}}{1 \text{ fl oz}}$$

Finally, cross multiply, cancel similar units (like terms), and divide to solve for the unknown variable x.

$$x \text{ tbsp (1 fl oz)} = 2 \text{ tbsp (16 fl oz)}$$
$$x = 32 \text{ tbsp}$$

Dimensional Analysis Method

$$\frac{2 \text{ cups}}{1} \times \frac{8 \text{ fl oz}}{1 \text{ cup}} \times \frac{2 \text{ tbsp}}{1 \text{ fl oz}} = 32 \text{ tbsp}$$

Answer: There are 32 tablespoonfuls in 2 cups of medication.

Example 4.4.3

How many 1 tsp doses are in 3 cups of liquid medication?

To begin, refer to the appropriate equivalents indicated in Table 4.6 and Figure 4.2.

$$3 \text{ tsp} = 1 \text{ tbsp}$$
$$2 \text{ tbsp} = 1 \text{ fl oz}$$
$$8 \text{ fl oz} = 1 \text{ cup}$$

Then use these equivalents when performing the following calculation methods.

Ratio-Proportion Method

To begin, determine the number of fluid ounces in 3 cups by setting up a proportion. Place the unknown variable x over the value to be converted (3 cups) on the left side of the equation. Then place the conversion factor (8 fl oz equals 1 cup) on the right side of the equation. Note that the units in the numerators and the units in the denominators match.

$$\frac{x \text{ fl oz}}{3 \text{ cups}} = \frac{8 \text{ fl oz}}{1 \text{ cup}}$$

Next, cross multiply, cancel similar units (like terms), and divide to solve for the unknown variable x.

$$x \text{ fl oz } (1 \text{ cup}) = 8 \text{ fl oz } (3 \text{ cups})$$
$$x = 24 \text{ fl oz}$$

Now, determine the number of tablespoonfuls in 24 fl oz by setting up another proportion. Place the unknown variable x over the value to be converted (24 fl oz) on the left side of the equation. Then place the conversion factor you cited at the beginning of this example (2 tbsp equals 1 fl oz) on the right side of the equation.

$$\frac{x \text{ tbsp}}{24 \text{ fl oz}} = \frac{2 \text{ tbsp}}{1 \text{ fl oz}}$$

Next, cross multiply, cancel similar units (like terms), and divide to solve for the unknown variable x.

$$x \text{ tbsp } (1 \text{ fl oz}) = 2 \text{ tbsp } (24 \text{ fl oz})$$
$$x = 48 \text{ tbsp}$$

Then determine the number of teaspoonfuls in 48 tablespoonfuls by setting up another proportion. Place the unknown variable x over the value to be converted (48 tbsp) on the left side of the equation. Then place the conversion factor you cited at the beginning of this example (3 tsp equals 1 tbsp) on the right side of the equation.

$$\frac{x \text{ tsp}}{48 \text{ tbsp}} = \frac{3 \text{ tsp}}{1 \text{ tbsp}}$$

Finally, cross multiply, cancel similar units (like terms), and divide to solve for the unknown variable x.

$$x \text{ tsp } (1 \text{ tbsp}) = 3 \text{ tsp } (48 \text{ tbsp})$$
$$x = 144 \text{ tsp}$$

Dimensional Analysis Method

$$\frac{3 \cancel{\text{cups}}}{1} \times \frac{8 \cancel{\text{fl oz}}}{1 \cancel{\text{cup}}} \times \frac{2 \cancel{\text{tbsp}}}{1 \cancel{\text{fl oz}}} \times \frac{3 \text{ tsp}}{1 \cancel{\text{tbsp}}} = 144 \text{ tsp}$$

Answer: There are 144 teaspoonfuls in 3 cups of liquid medication.

Example 4.4.4

How many 1 fl oz doses are in 3 pt of liquid medication?

To begin, refer to the appropriate equivalents indicated in Table 4.6 and Figure 4.2.

$$8 \text{ fl oz} = 1 \text{ cup}$$

$$2 \text{ cups} = 1 \text{ pt}$$

Then use these equivalents when performing the following calculation methods.

Ratio-Proportion Method

To begin, determine the number of cups in 3 pt by setting up a proportion. Place the unknown variable x over the value to be converted (3 pt) on the left side of the equation. Then place the conversion factor (2 cups equal 1 pt) on the right side of the equation. Note that the units in the numerators and the units in the denominators match.

$$\frac{x \text{ cups}}{3 \text{ pt}} = \frac{2 \text{ cups}}{1 \text{ pt}}$$

Next, cross multiply, cancel similar units (like terms), and divide to solve for the unknown variable x.

$$x \text{ cups } (1 \text{ pt}) = 2 \text{ cups } (3 \text{ pt})$$

$$x = 6 \text{ cups}$$

Now, determine the number of fluid ounces in 6 cups by setting up another proportion. Place the unknown variable x over the value to be converted (6 cups) on the left side of the equation. Then place the conversion factor you cited at the beginning of this example (8 fl oz equals 1 cup) on the right side of the equation.

$$\frac{x \text{ fl oz}}{6 \text{ cups}} = \frac{8 \text{ fl oz}}{1 \text{ cup}}$$

Finally, cross multiply, cancel similar units (like terms), and divide to solve for the unknown variable x.

$$x \text{ fl oz } (1 \text{ cup}) = 8 \text{ fl oz } (6 \text{ cups})$$

$$x = 48 \text{ fl oz}$$

Dimensional Analysis Method

$$\frac{3 \cancel{\text{pt}}}{1} \times \frac{2 \cancel{\text{cups}}}{1 \cancel{\text{pt}}} \times \frac{8 \text{ fl oz}}{1 \cancel{\text{cup}}} = 48 \text{ fl oz}$$

Answer: There are 48 fl oz doses in 3 pt of liquid medication.

Example 4.4.5

How many 1 fl oz doses are in 2 qt of liquid medication?

To begin, refer to the appropriate equivalents indicated in Table 4.6 and Figure 4.2.

$$8 \text{ fl oz} = 1 \text{ cup}$$
$$2 \text{ cups} = 1 \text{ pt}$$
$$2 \text{ pt} = 1 \text{ qt}$$

Then use these equivalents when performing the following calculation methods.

Ratio-Proportion Method

To begin, determine the number of pints in 2 qt by setting up a proportion. Place the unknown variable x over the value to be converted (2 qt) on the left side of the equation. Then place the conversion factor (2 pt equal 1 qt) on the right side of the equation. Note that the units in the numerators and the units in the denominators match.

$$\frac{x \text{ pt}}{2 \text{ qt}} = \frac{2 \text{ pt}}{1 \text{ qt}}$$

Next, cross multiply, cancel similar units (like terms), and divide to solve for the unknown variable x.

$$x \text{ pt} (1 \text{ qt}) = 2 \text{ pt} (2 \text{ qt})$$
$$x = 4 \text{ pt}$$

Now, determine the number of cups in 4 pt by setting up another proportion. Place the unknown variable x over the value to be converted (4 pt) on the left side of the equation. Then place the conversion factor you cited at the beginning of this example (2 cups equal 1 pt) on the right side of the equation.

$$\frac{x \text{ cups}}{4 \text{ pt}} = \frac{2 \text{ cups}}{1 \text{ pt}}$$

Then cross multiply, cancel similar units (like terms), and divide to solve for the unknown variable x.

$$x \text{ cups} (1 \text{ pt}) = 2 \text{ cups} (4 \text{ pt})$$
$$x = 8 \text{ cups}$$

Next, determine the number of fluid ounces in 8 cups.

$$\frac{x \text{ fl oz}}{8 \text{ cups}} = \frac{8 \text{ fl oz}}{1 \text{ cup}}$$

Finally, cross multiply, cancel similar units (like terms), and divide to solve for the unknown variable x.

$$x \text{ fl oz} (1 \text{ cup}) = 8 \text{ fl oz} (8 \text{ cups})$$
$$x = 64 \text{ fl oz}$$

Dimensional Analysis Method

$$\frac{2 \text{ qt}}{1} \times \frac{2 \text{ pt}}{1 \text{ qt}} \times \frac{2 \text{ cups}}{1 \text{ pt}} \times \frac{8 \text{ fl oz}}{1 \text{ cup}} = 64 \text{ fl oz}$$

Answer: There are 64 fl oz doses in 2 qt of liquid medication.

4.4 Problem Set

Convert the given volumes within the household measurement system. Round your answers to the nearest tenth when necessary.

1. 8 cups = _____ pt

2. 3 pt = _____ fl oz

3. 1 pt = _____ tbsp

4. 3 qt = _____ fl oz

5. 28 tsp = _____ fl oz

6. 1 pt = _____ qt

7. 6 cups = _____ tsp

Applications

Complete the following conversions. Round your answers to the nearest tenth when necessary.

8. How many 1 tsp doses are in 2 pt, 6 fl oz?

9. How many 2 tsp doses are in 3 cups?

10. How many 1 tbsp doses are in 12 bottles containing 16 fl oz each?

4.5 Conversions between the Metric and Household Measurement Systems

Because metric system units are more accurate than household system units, it is preferable that you work with metric units in your pharmacy calculations. In addition, some pharmacy software programs accept only amounts given in metric units. With that in mind, you need to be adept at performing conversions between these two measurement systems.

When working in an institutional or a long-term care facility, you will see medication orders that are written using both metric and household units of measurement. Typically, computerized provider order entry (CPOE) software is set up to accept metric units. However, in the event household units are used by a prescriber, you must convert the quantity ordered into metric units.

In a community pharmacy, you may also receive prescriptions written in both metric and household units of measurement. For prescriptions written in household units, you should convert any quantity measurements to metric units and then enter the information into the computerized patient's profile. Typically, the computer software is set up to accept milliliters for liquid medications and grams for solid medications, such as creams or ointments. When a prescription is written for a liquid, the volume to be dispensed and the quantity to be given at each dose is used to calculate the days' supply. Calculating the volume to be dispensed and the days' supply are important steps in the processing of each prescription. These calculations provide the pharmacist and you with the information needed to accurately fill the prescription, thereby ensuring that the patient is getting the prescribed therapy.

Although some references list exact values for conversions between the household measurement system and the metric measurement system, the equivalents shown in Table 4.7 and Figure 4.3 on the following page are generally accepted for use for these conversions in daily pharmacy practice. You should commit these conversion values to memory.

Quick Study

A pharmacy technician should memorize the approximate equivalent measurements for common units such as the following:

- 1 m = 3 ft
- 1 kg = 2.2 lb
- 1 lb = 454 g
- 1 oz = 30 mL

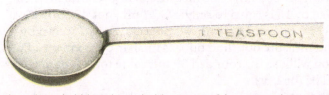

The volume held by a household teaspoonful may vary, but a true teaspoonful equals 5 mL.

TABLE 4.7 Household Unit and Metric Unit Equivalents

Volume		Weight	
1 tsp	= 5 mL	1 oz	= 30 g†
1 tbsp	= 15 mL	1 lb	= 454 g
1 fl oz	= 30 mL*	2.2 lb	= 1 kg
1 cup	= 240 mL		
1 pt	= 480 mL*		
1 qt	= 960 mL		
1 gal	= 3,840 mL*		

*There are actually 29.57 mL in 1 fl oz, but 30 mL is usually used. When packaging a pint, companies will typically include 473 mL, rather than the full 480 mL. Additionally, 1 gal is actually equivalent to 3,785 mL.

†There are actually 28.34952 g in a household ounce; however, pharmacy personnel often round up to 30 g.

FIGURE 4.3 Household Units for Volume and Their Metric Equivalents

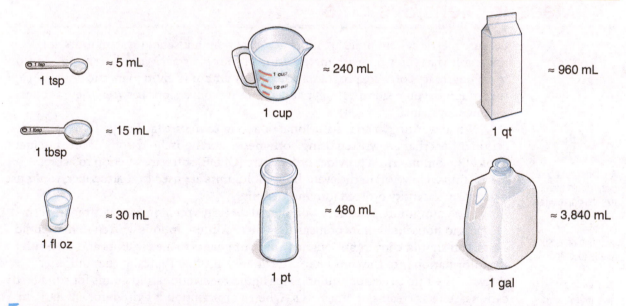

≈ 5 mL
1 tsp

≈ 240 mL
1 cup

≈ 960 mL
1 qt

≈ 15 mL
1 tbsp

≈ 30 mL
1 fl oz

≈ 480 mL
1 pt

≈ 3,840 mL
1 gal

For Good Measure

Using the household measurement equivalents given in this chapter, 1 pt equals 480 mL. However, pharmacy technicians should be aware that some pharmacies consider 473 mL to be equivalent to 1 pt.

As indicated in Table 4.7 and Figure 4.3, it is common practice to round a household fluid ounce from 29.57 mL to 30 mL. When measuring this amount, this estimation is often appropriate because the volume differs by such a small amount. When measuring multiple fluid ounces that have been rounded up to 30 mL, however, the discrepancy becomes far more apparent. For example, if asked to measure a pint (16 fl oz), you would measure roughly 480 mL. This measurement becomes problematic because 29.57 mL multiplied by 16 is equal to only 473.12 mL, not 480 mL. Most pint stock medication containers are labeled 473 mL, yet pharmacies bill according to the estimation of 480 mL and measure out fluid ounces in 30 mL increments. For the purposes of this chapter, you will use the rounded 30 mL value for 1 fl oz and the rounded 480 mL value for 16 fl oz (or 1 pt).

The following examples show some typical conversion problems you must be able to solve when working in a pharmacy.

Example 4.5.1

You are to dispense 300 mL of morphine sulfate 100 mg/5 mL solution. The prescription states that the patient is to take 2 tsp two times daily. How many doses will the dispensed volume contain?

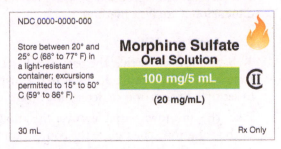

You can solve this problem by using the ratio-proportion method or by using the dimensional analysis method.

Ratio-Proportion Method

To begin, convert the household measurement unit (2 tsp) to a metric measurement unit by using the conversion values in Table 4.7 and Figure 4.3. Place the unknown variable *x* over the known value (2 tsp) on the left side of the equation. Then place the conversion factor (1 tsp equals 5 mL) on the right side of the equation. Note that the units in the numerators and the units in the denominators match.

$$\frac{x \text{ mL}}{2 \text{ tsp}} = \frac{5 \text{ mL}}{1 \text{ tsp}}$$

Then cross multiply, cancel similar units (like terms), and divide to solve for the unknown variable *x*.

$$x \text{ mL (1 tsp)} = 5 \text{ mL (2 tsp)}$$

$$x = 10 \text{ mL}$$

Next, determine the number of doses needed by setting up a proportion. Place the unknown variable *x* over the known value (300 mL) on the left side of the equation. Then place the conversion factor (1 dose equals 10 mL) on the right side of the equation. Note that the units in the numerators and the units in the denominators match.

$$\frac{x \text{ doses}}{300 \text{ mL}} = \frac{1 \text{ dose}}{10 \text{ mL}}$$

Then cross multiply, cancel similar units (like terms), and divide to solve for the unknown variable *x*.

$$x \text{ doses (10 mL)} = 1 \text{ dose (300 mL)}$$

$$x = 30 \text{ doses}$$

Dimensional Analysis Method

$$\frac{300 \ \cancel{\text{mL}}}{1} \times \frac{\text{dose}}{2 \ \cancel{\text{tsp}}} \times \frac{1 \ \cancel{\text{tsp}}}{5 \ \cancel{\text{mL}}} = 30 \text{ doses}$$

Answer: The dispensed volume will contain 30 doses.

Example 4.5.2

Using the medication and dosing instructions in Example 4.5.1, how many days will the 300 mL of morphine sulfate last?

You can solve this problem by using the ratio-proportion method or by using the dimensional analysis method.

Ratio-Proportion Method

To begin, you know that the patient takes 1 dose twice daily and, as calculated in Example 4.5.1, there are 30 doses in the dispensed volume. Use this information to set up a proportion to determine how many days the 300 mL will last.

Place the unknown variable x over the known value (30 doses) on the left side of the equation. Then place the conversion factor (1 day equals 2 doses) on the right side of the equation. Note that the units in the numerators and the units in the denominators match.

$$\frac{x \text{ days}}{30 \text{ doses}} = \frac{1 \text{ day}}{2 \text{ doses}}$$

Then cross multiply, cancel similar units (like terms), and divide to solve for the unknown variable x.

$$x \text{ days } (2 \text{ doses}) = 1 \text{ day } (30 \text{ doses})$$
$$x = 15 \text{ days}$$

Dimensional Analysis Method

$$30 \text{ doses} \times \frac{1 \text{ day}}{2 \text{ doses}} = 15 \text{ days}$$

Answer: The 300 mL of morphine sulfate will last 15 days.

Example 4.5.3

A patient is to purchase a 12 fl oz bottle of antacid. The patient is to take 15 mL before each meal and at bedtime. How many doses does the bottle contain?

You can solve this problem by using the ratio-proportion method or by using the dimensional analysis method.

Ratio-Proportion Method

To begin, convert the household measurement unit (12 fl oz) using the conversion values in Table 4.7 and Figure 4.3.

$$1 \text{ fl oz} = 30 \text{ mL}$$

Now, place the unknown variable x over the known value (12 fl oz) on the left side of the equation. Then place the conversion factor (1 fl oz equals 30 mL) on the right side of the equation. Note that the units in the numerators and in the denominators match.

$$\frac{x \text{ mL}}{12 \text{ fl oz}} = \frac{30 \text{ mL}}{1 \text{ fl oz}}$$

Then cross multiply, cancel similar units (like terms), and divide to solve for the unknown variable x.

$$x \text{ mL } (1 \text{ fl oz}) = 30 \text{ mL } (12 \text{ fl oz})$$
$$x = 360 \text{ mL}$$

Next, determine the number of doses needed by setting up a proportion. Place the unknown variable x over the known value (360 mL) on the left side of the equation. Then place the conversion factor (1 dose equals 15 mL) on the right side of the equation. Note that the units in the numerators and the units in the denominators match.

$$\frac{x \text{ doses}}{360 \text{ mL}} = \frac{1 \text{ dose}}{15 \text{ mL}}$$

Then cross multiply, cancel similar units (like terms), and divide to solve for the unknown variable x.

$$x \text{ doses } (15 \text{ mL}) = 1 \text{ dose } (360 \text{ mL})$$

$$x = 24 \text{ doses}$$

Dimensional Analysis Method

$$\frac{12 \text{ fl oz}}{1} \times \frac{30 \text{ mL}}{1 \text{ fl oz}} \times \frac{1 \text{ dose}}{15 \text{ mL}} = 24 \text{ doses}$$

Answer: The bottle of antacid contains 24 doses.

Example 4.5.4

Use the medication and dosing instructions in Example 4.5.3 to solve the following problem. If the patient eats three times a day, how many days will the 12 fl oz bottle of antacid last?

To begin, you know that the patient is to take 1 dose with every meal and at bedtime. You also know that the patient eats three meals a day. Therefore, the patient will take four doses per day (one for each of three meals plus the bedtime dose).

$$\left(\frac{1 \text{ dose}}{\text{meal}} \times \frac{3 \text{ meals}}{\text{day}} \right) + 1 \text{ dose at bedtime} = \frac{4 \text{ doses}}{\text{day}}$$

Then use your answer in Example 4.5.3 (24 doses) to determine how many days the bottle will last.

$$24 \text{ doses} \times \frac{1 \text{ day}}{4 \text{ doses}} = 6 \text{ days}$$

Answer: The 12 fl oz bottle of antacid will last 6 days.

Example 4.5.5

How many 2 tbsp doses are in 480 mL?

You can solve this problem by using the ratio-proportion method or by using the dimensional analysis method.

Ratio-Proportion Method

To begin, convert the household measurement unit (2 tbsp) using the conversion values in Table 4.7 and Figure 4.3.

$$1 \text{ tbsp} = 15 \text{ mL}$$

Place the unknown variable x over the known value (2 tbsp) on the left side of the equation. Then place the conversion factor (1 tbsp equals 15 mL) on the right side of the equation. Note that the units in the numerators and the units in the denominators match.

$$\frac{x \text{ mL}}{2 \text{ tbsp}} = \frac{15 \text{ mL}}{1 \text{ tbsp}}$$

Then cross multiply, cancel similar units (like terms), and divide to solve for the unknown variable x.

$$x \text{ mL } (1 \text{ tbsp}) = 15 \text{ mL } (2 \text{ tbsp})$$
$$x = 30 \text{ mL}$$

Next, determine the number of doses needed by setting up a proportion. Place the unknown variable x over the known value (480 mL) on the left side of the equation. Then place the conversion factor (1 dose equals 30 mL) on the right side of the equation. Note that the units in the numerators and the units in the denominators match.

$$\frac{x \text{ doses}}{480 \text{ mL}} = \frac{1 \text{ dose}}{30 \text{ mL}}$$

Then cross multiply, cancel similar units (like terms), and divide to solve for the unknown variable x.

$$x \text{ doses } (30 \text{ mL}) = 1 \text{ dose } (480 \text{ mL})$$
$$x = 16 \text{ doses}$$

Dimensional Analysis Method

$$\frac{480 \text{ mL}}{1} \times \frac{1 \text{ tbsp}}{15 \text{ mL}} \times \frac{1 \text{ dose}}{2 \text{ tbsp}} = 16 \text{ doses}$$

Answer: There are 16 doses (2 tbsp/dose) in 480 mL.

Example 4.5.6

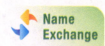

Name Exchange

Theophylline elixir is also known by the brand name *Elixophyllin*, a combination of the words *elixir* and *theophylline*.

A medication order indicates that a patient should take theophylline elixir. Theophylline elixir contains 80 mg/15 mL. One dose is 2 tbsp. How many milligrams are in one dose of the theophylline elixir?

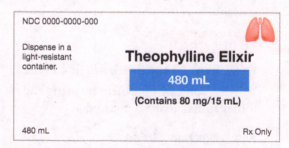

NDC 0000-0000-000

Dispense in a light-resistant container.

Theophylline Elixir

480 mL

(Contains 80 mg/15 mL)

480 mL   Rx Only

You can solve this problem by using the ratio-proportion method or by using the dimensional analysis method.

Ratio-Proportion Method

To begin, convert the household measurement unit (2 tbsp) to a metric measurement unit by using the conversion values in Table 4.7 and Figure 4.3.

$$1 \text{ tbsp} = 15 \text{ mL}$$

Place the unknown variable x over the known value (2 tbsp) on the left side of the equation. Then place the conversion factor (1 tbsp equals 15 mL) on the right side of the equation. Note that the units in the numerators and the units in the denominators match.

$$\frac{x \text{ mL}}{2 \text{ tbsp}} = \frac{15 \text{ mL}}{1 \text{ tbsp}}$$

Then cross multiply, cancel similar units (like terms), and divide to solve for the unknown variable x.

$$x \text{ mL } (1 \text{ tbsp}) = 15 \text{ mL } (2 \text{ tbsp})$$

$$x = 30 \text{ mL}$$

Next, determine the number of milligrams in one dose by setting up a proportion. Place the unknown variable x over the conversion value (30 mL) on the left side of the equation. Then place the concentration of the medication (80 mg/15 mL) on the right side of the equation. Note that the units in the numerators and the units in the denominators match.

$$\frac{x \text{ mg}}{30 \text{ mL}} = \frac{80 \text{ mg}}{15 \text{ mL}}$$

Then cross multiply, cancel similar units (like terms), and divide to solve for the unknown variable x.

$$x \text{ mg } (15 \text{ mL}) = 80 \text{ mg } (30 \text{ mL})$$

$$x = 160 \text{ mg}$$

Dimensional Analysis Method

$$\frac{2 \text{ tbsp}}{1} \times \frac{15 \text{ mL}}{1 \text{ tbsp}} \times \frac{80 \text{ mg}}{15 \text{ mL}} = 160 \text{ mg}$$

Answer: There are 160 mg in one dose of the theophylline elixir.

Like volumes, weights can be converted between household measurement units and metric measurement units. The most common conversions are between the household measurements of pounds and ounces and the metric measurements of kilograms and grams. These conversions are shown in Table 4.7.

Example 4.5.7

A medication order was received by the pharmacy for a 1.5 oz tube of ointment. How many grams of ointment are needed?

You can solve this problem by using the ratio-proportion method or by using the dimensional analysis method.

Ratio-Proportion Method

To begin, convert the household measurement unit (1 oz) to a metric measurement unit by using the conversion value in Table 4.7.

$$1 \text{ oz} = 30 \text{ g}$$

Next, determine the number of grams by setting up a proportion. Place the unknown variable x over the known value (1.5 oz) on the left side of the equation. Then place the conversion factor (30 g/1 oz) on the right side of the equation. Note that the units in the numerators and the units in the denominators match.

$$\frac{x \text{ g}}{1.5 \text{ oz}} = \frac{30 \text{ g}}{1 \text{ oz}}$$

Then cross multiply, cancel similar units (like terms), and divide to solve for the unknown variable x.

$$x \text{ g} (1 \text{ oz}) = 30 \text{ g} (1.5 \text{ oz})$$
$$x = 45 \text{ g}$$

Dimensional Analysis Method

$$\frac{1.5 \text{ \cancel{oz}}}{1} \times \frac{30 \text{ g}}{1 \text{ \cancel{oz}}} = 45 \text{ g}$$

Answer: There are 45 g in a 1.5 oz tube of ointment.

Example 4.5.8

You have a 1 lb jar of ointment available. You are instructed to use this stock medication to fill smaller jars with 20 g of ointment each. How many jars can you fill?

You can solve this problem by using the ratio-proportion method or by using the dimensional analysis method.

Ratio-Proportion Method

To begin, convert the household measurement unit (1 lb) to a metric measurement unit by using the conversion value in Table 4.7.

$$1 \text{ lb} = 454 \text{ g}$$

Next, determine the number of grams by setting up a proportion. Place the unknown variable x over the conversion factor (454 g) on the left side of the equation. Then place the known value (1 jar equals 20 g) on the right side of the equation. Note that the units in the numerators and the units in the denominators match.

$$\frac{x \text{ jars}}{454 \text{ g}} = \frac{1 \text{ jar}}{20 \text{ g}}$$

Then cross multiply, cancel similar units (like terms), and divide to solve for the unknown variable x.

$$x \text{ jars} (20 \text{ g}) = 1 \text{ jar} (454 \text{ g})$$
$$x = 22.7 \text{ jars, or 22 full jars}$$

Dimensional Analysis Method

$$\frac{454 \text{ \cancel{g}}}{1} \times \frac{1 \text{ jar}}{20 \text{ \cancel{g}}} = 22.7 \text{ jars, or 22 full jars}$$

Answer: You can fill 22 full jars, with each jar containing 20 g of ointment.

In both solutions, there is 0.7 g of ointment remaining. You can determine how many grams of ointment are left over with the following calculation:

$$\frac{20 \text{ g}}{\text{jar}} \times 0.7 \text{ jar leftover ointment} = 14 \text{ g leftover ointment}$$

Converting Body Weight

Medications are sometimes dosed based on the weight of a patient. Increasingly, drug manufacturers are providing a recommended dose based on a specific dose in milligrams per kilogram (mg/kg) of a patient's weight. Because most medications are dosed based on kilograms, you may need to convert a patient's weight from pounds to kilograms before calculating the appropriate dose.

Example 4.5.9

A patient weighs 134 lb. What is this patient's weight in kilograms?

You can solve this problem by using the ratio-proportion method or by using the dimensional analysis method.

Ratio-Proportion Method

To begin, use the conversion value in Table 4.7.

$$1 \text{ kg} = 2.2 \text{ lb}$$

Next, determine the number of kilograms by setting up a proportion. Place the unknown variable x over the known value (134 lb) on the left side of the equation. Then place the conversion factor (1 kg equals 2.2 lb) on the right side of the equation. Note that the units in the numerators and the units in the denominators match.

$$\frac{x \text{ kg}}{134 \text{ lb}} = \frac{1 \text{ kg}}{2.2 \text{ lb}}$$

Then cross multiply, cancel similara units (like terms), and divide to solve for the unknown variable x.

$$x \text{ kg } (2.2 \text{ lb}) = 1 \text{ kg } (134 \text{ lb})$$
$$x = 60.909 \text{ kg, rounded to } 60.9 \text{ kg}$$

Dimensional Analysis Method

$$\frac{134 \text{ lb}}{1} \times \frac{1 \text{ kg}}{2.2 \text{ lb}} = 60.909 \text{ kg, rounded to } 60.9 \text{ kg}$$

Answer: The patient's weight is 60.909 kg, rounded to 60.9 kg.

Example 4.5.10

A patient weighs 76 lb. What is this patient's weight in kilograms?

You can solve this problem by using the ratio-proportion method or by using the dimensional analysis method.

Ratio-Proportion Method

To begin, use the conversion value in Table 4.7.

$$1 \text{ kg} = 2.2 \text{ lb}$$

Next, determine the number of kilograms by setting up a proportion. Place the unknown variable x over the known value (76 lb) on the left side of the equation. Then place the conversion factor (1 kg equals 2.2 lb) on the right side of the equation. Note that the units in the numerators and the units in the denominators match.

$$\frac{x \text{ kg}}{76 \text{ lb}} = \frac{1 \text{ kg}}{2.2 \text{ lb}}$$

Then cross multiply, cancel similar units (like terms), and divide to solve for the unknown variable x.

$$x \text{ kg} (2.2 \text{ lb}) = 1 \text{ kg} (76 \text{ lb})$$

$$x = 34.545 \text{ kg, rounded to } 34.5 \text{ kg}$$

Dimensional Analysis Method

$$\frac{76 \text{ lb}}{1} \times \frac{1 \text{ kg}}{2.2 \text{ lb}} = 34.545 \text{ kg, rounded to } 34.5 \text{ kg}$$

Answer: The patient's weight is 34.545 kg, rounded to 34.5 kg.

Although it is important to understand the conversion using both the ratio-proportion and the dimensional analysis methods, a shorthand method for converting a patient's weight from pounds to kilograms is to divide the patient's weight by 2.2 lb/1 kg. Similarly, you can convert a patient's weight from kilograms to pounds by multiplying the patient's weight by 2.2 lb/1 kg.

Example 4.5.11

A patient weighs 58 kg. What is this patient's weight in pounds?

$$58 \text{ kg} \times \frac{2.2 \text{ lb}}{1 \text{ kg}} = 127.6 \text{ lb}$$

Answer: The patient's weight is 127.6 lb.

To verify your answer, convert it from pounds back to kilograms.

$$127.6 \text{ lb} \times \frac{1 \text{ kg}}{2.2 \text{ lb}} = 58 \text{ kg}$$

Example 4.5.12

A patient in the neonatal intensive care unit weighs 1,250 g. What is the patient's weight in pounds?

To begin, convert grams to kilograms.

$$1,250 \text{ g} = 1.25 \text{ kg}$$

Then convert kilograms to pounds.

$$1.25 \text{ kg} \times \frac{2.2 \text{ lb}}{1 \text{ kg}} = 2.75 \text{ lb}$$

Answer: The patient's weight is 2.75 lb.

To verify your answer, convert it from pounds back to kilograms.

$$2.75 \text{ lb} \times \frac{1 \text{ kg}}{2.2 \text{ lb}} = 1.25 \text{ kg}$$

Example 4.5.13

A patient's weight is recorded as 150 and does not include units. If the weight was reported in kilograms, how many pounds does the patient weigh?

$$150 \text{ kg} \times \frac{2.2 \text{ lb}}{1 \text{ kg}} = 330 \text{ lb}$$

Answer: The patient's weight is 330 lb.

WORKPLACE WISDOM

Many medications are dosed by weight (typically, milligrams per kilogram [mg/kg]). However, you may find a patient's weight recorded without a unit of measurement, either by the patient, by the patient's caregiver, or by a healthcare practitioner. You may also find the patient's weight without a unit of measurement in the patient's profile. If the unit of measurement is missing, it is imperative that you do not make assumptions regarding the unit and that you verify the patient's weight *and* units. Mistaking pounds for kilograms can result in a patient receiving more than double the intended dose of medication. With some medications, a dose increase of that magnitude could result in harm or, possibly, death.

4.5 Problem Set

Convert the following volumes from the household measurement system to the metric measurement system. Round your answers to the nearest tenth when necessary.

1. 3 tbsp = _____ mL

2. 1 fl oz = _____ mL

3. 2 fl oz = _____ mL

4. 3 fl oz = _____ mL

5. 4 fl oz = _____ mL

6. 5 fl oz = _____ mL

7. 6 fl oz = _____ mL

8. 7 fl oz = _____ mL

9. 8 fl oz = _____ mL

10. 12 fl oz = _____ mL

11. 16 fl oz = _____ mL

Convert the given volumes between the household measurement and metric measurement systems. Round your answers to the nearest tenth when necessary.

12. 80 mL = _____ tbsp

13. 6 fl oz = _____ mL

14. 90 mL = _____ fl oz

15. 800 mL = _____ pt

16. 53 mL = _____ tsp

17. 35 mL = _____ tsp

18. 10 L = _____ gal

19. 4 tbsp = _____ mL

20. 15 mL = _____ tsp

21. 720 mL = _____ pt

22. 30 tsp = _____ mL

23. 120 mL = _____ fl oz

24. ½ gal = _____ mL

25. 2 L = _____ pt

Convert the following patient weights from pounds to kilograms. Round your answers to the nearest tenth when necessary.

26. 3.5 lb = _____ kg

27. 14 lb = _____ kg

28. 42 lb = _____ kg

29. 97 lb = _____ kg

30. 112 lb = _____ kg

31. 165 lb = _____ kg

32. 178 lb = _____ kg

33. 247 lb = _____ kg

Convert the following weights between the household and metric measurement systems. Round your answers to the nearest tenth when necessary.

34. 2 oz = _____ g

35. 1.5 oz = _____ g

36. 8 oz = _____ g

37. 906 g = _____ lb

38. 30 g = _____ lb

39. 0.8 oz = _____ g

Applications

In solving these problems, convert all quantities to the metric system. Round your answers to the nearest tenth when necessary.

40. How many 5 mL doses are in a 5 fl oz bottle?

41. How many 3 tsp doses are in 1 pt?

42. A dose of 1.5 fl oz is to be given three times daily. How many milliliters will be given in one day?

43. How many $1\frac{1}{2}$ tsp doses are in an 8 fl oz bottle of cough syrup?

Use the following label to answer questions 44 and 45. Round your answers to the nearest tenth when necessary.

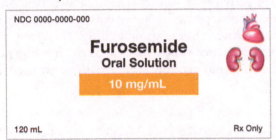

44. A prescription states that a patient is to take ½ tsp of furosemide oral solution daily. Using the furosemide label shown above, how many milligrams are in a dose?

45. Using the furosemide label shown above, how many days will a 4 fl oz bottle last a patient who is taking 20 mg daily?

Use the following label to answer questions 46–50. Round your answers to the nearest tenth when necessary.

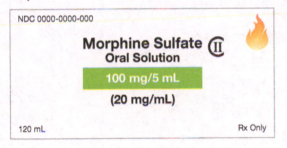

46. A prescription states that a patient is to take 2.5 mL morphine sulfate oral solution four times daily as needed for pain. Using the provided label, calculate the equivalent dose measured in teaspoonfuls.

47. How many days will 320 mL of morphine sulfate oral solution last if a patient is taking 3 tsp daily?

48. A physician prescribes the following dose of medication for an adult patient: 2 tsp/68 kg/dose. How many doses would a 300 mL bottle contain for a patient who weighs 180 lb?

49. A physician prescribes the following dose of medication for a pediatric patient: 1 tsp/20 kg/dose. How many doses will a 4 fl oz bottle provide for a 52 lb patient?

50. A nurse practitioner writes the following prescription for a laxative: 2 tbsp/50 kg/dose. How many doses will a 12 fl oz bottle last for a patient who weighs 172 lb?

Self-check your work in Appendix A.

4.6 Temperature Measurement Systems

As a pharmacy technician, you may be asked to monitor the refrigerator and freezer temperatures of stored medications. For that reason, you need to have a good understanding of the two temperature scales used in pharmacy practice: the Fahrenheit temperature scale and the Celsius temperature scale. You must also be able to convert temperature readings between these two scales.

Understanding Temperature Measurement Systems

Daniel Fahrenheit, a German physicist, invented a temperature scale in 1724. The **Fahrenheit temperature scale** was based on ice water and salt as a low point (0° F) and the human body temperature as the high point (100° F). Fahrenheit used his own

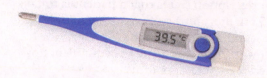

Pharmacy technicians may be asked to help patients convert between temperature readings in degrees Celsius and degrees Fahrenheit. As with all conversions, this calculation must be done accurately.

body temperature as the standard but, in the years that followed, scientists learned that body temperature varied. Therefore, the Fahrenheit scale was keyed to water for both the low point and the high point. The freezing point of water at sea level was set at 32° F, and the boiling point of water at sea level was set at 212° F.

In the early 1740s, Anders Celsius, a Swedish astronomer, developed a thermometer with a difference of 100 degrees between freezing and boiling. Therefore, the **Celsius temperature scale** uses 0° C as the freezing point and 100° C as the boiling point. The Celsius temperature scale is commonly used in science as well as in healthcare settings.

Converting Celsius and Fahrenheit Temperatures

As mentioned earlier, you need to understand the conversions between Fahrenheit and Celsius temperature scales. The formulas for these conversions are based on the fact that each Celsius degree equals 1.8 or $^9/_5$ of each Fahrenheit degree. Below are the conversion formulas. Note that temperatures are rounded to the nearest tenth.

Degrees Celsius to Degrees Fahrenheit

$$° F = \left(\frac{9 \times ° C}{5} \right) + 32°$$

or

$$° F = (1.8 \times ° C) + 32°$$

Degrees Fahrenheit to Degrees Celsius

$$° C = (° F - 32°) \times \frac{5}{9}$$

or

$$° C = \frac{° F - 32°}{1.8}$$

Example 4.6.1

Convert 40° C to its equivalent on the Fahrenheit temperature scale.

Solution 1

$$° F = \left(\frac{9 \times ° C}{5} \right) + 32°$$

$$= \left(\frac{9 \times 40°}{5} \right) + 32°$$

$$= \frac{360°}{5} + 32°$$

$$= 72° + 32°$$

$$= 104° F$$

Solution 2

$$°F = (1.8 \times °C) + 32°$$

$$= (1.8 \times 40°) + 32°$$

$$= 72° + 32°$$

$$= 104° F$$

Answer: A temperature of 40° C is equivalent to 104° F.

Example 4.6.2

Convert 82° F to its equivalent on the Celsius temperature scale.

Solution 1

$$°C = (°F - 32°) \times \frac{5}{9}$$

$$= (82° - 32°) \times \frac{5}{9}$$

$$= 50° \times \frac{5}{9}$$

$$= 27.777° \text{ C, rounded to } 27.8° \text{ C}$$

Solution 2

$$°C = \frac{(°F - 32°)}{1.8}$$

$$= \frac{(82° - 32°)}{1.8}$$

$$= \frac{50°}{1.8}$$

$$= 27.777° \text{ C, rounded to } 27.8° \text{ C}$$

Answer: A temperature of 82° F is equivalent to 27.8° C.

Monitoring Temperature in Pharmacy Practice

Medications are required to be stored under specific temperature conditions. Some medications must be stored in refrigerated conditions, which are defined as being between 2° C and 5° C (35.6° F and 41° F). Other medications must be stored in frozen conditions. Freezers for medication storage should be maintained at temperatures between –25° C and –10° C (–13° F and 14° F). The storage of drugs outside of these recommended temperature parameters compromises the quality and safety of the medications.

As mentioned earlier, you may be asked to monitor the pharmacy refrigerators and freezers for medication storage and to record these temperatures daily. Many pharmacies use specific charts for recording temperatures of refrigerators and freezers used for drug storage. See Figure 4.4 and Figure 4.5 for examples of the Celsius and Fahrenheit refrigerator temperature charts. To view examples of the freezer temperature charts for these two scales, see Figure 4.6 and Figure 4.7.

FIGURE 4.4 **Drug Storage Refrigerator Temperature Chart (Celsius)**

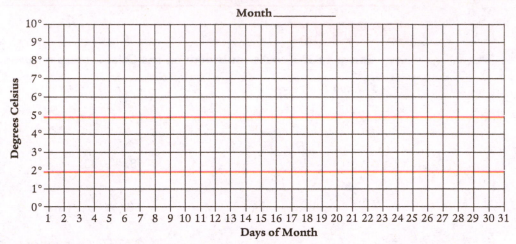

Graph freezer temperature on chart once daily. If temperature is less than **2 degrees** or greater than **5 degrees,** check the thermostat setting and correct as necessary. Recheck temperature in one hour, and, if temperature is out of stated range, contact maintenance for evaluation and repair. Contact the appropriate area for storage of supplies.

Documentation of Repairs: _____   Documentation of Cleaning: _____
_____   _____
_____   _____
_____   _____

FIGURE 4.5 **Drug Storage Refrigerator Temperature Chart (Fahrenheit)**

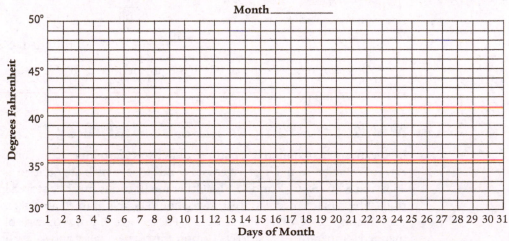

Graph refrigerator temperature on chart once daily. If temperature is less than **35.6 degrees** or greater than **41 degrees,** check the thermostat setting and correct as necessary. Recheck temperature in one hour, and, if temperature is out of stated range, contact maintenance for evaluation and repair. Contact the appropriate area for storage of supplies.

Documentation of Repairs: _____   Documentation of Cleaning: _____
_____   _____
_____   _____
_____   _____

FIGURE 4.6 Drug Storage Freezer Temperature Chart (Celsius)

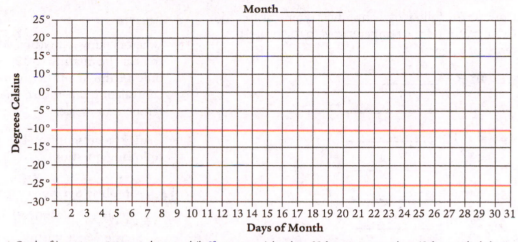

Graph refrigerator temperature on chart once daily. If temperature is less than **–25 degrees** or greater than **–10 degrees,** check the thermostat setting and correct as necessary. Recheck temperature in one hour, and, if temperature is out of stated range, contact maintenance for evaluation and repair. Contact the appropriate area for storage of supplies.

Documentation of Repairs: _____   Documentation of Cleaning: _____

_____   _____

_____   _____

_____   _____

FIGURE 4.7 Drug Storage Freezer Temperature Chart (Fahrenheit)

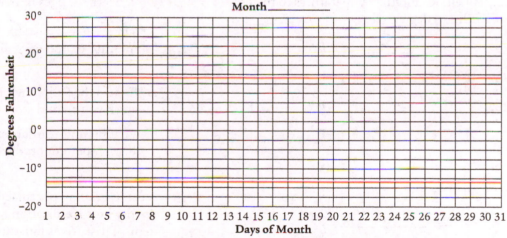

Graph freezer temperature on chart once daily. If temperature is less than **–13 degrees** or greater than **14 degrees,** check the thermostat setting and correct as necessary. Recheck temperature in one hour, and, if temperature is out of stated range, contact maintenance for evaluation and repair. Contact the appropriate area for storage of supplies.

Documentation of Repairs: _____   Documentation of Cleaning: _____

_____   _____

_____   _____

4.6 Problem Set

Convert the following Fahrenheit temperatures to Celsius. Round the temperatures to the nearest tenth of a degree.

1. 0° F = _____ ° C

2. 23° F = _____ ° C

3. 36° F = _____ ° C

4. 40° F = _____ ° C

5. 64° F = _____ ° C

6. 72° F = _____ ° C

7. 98.6° F = _____ ° C

8. 100.5° F = _____ ° C

9. 102.8° F = _____ ° C

10. 105° F = _____ ° C

Convert the following Celsius temperatures to Fahrenheit. Round the temperatures to the nearest tenth of a degree.

11. −15° C = ___5___ ° F

12. 18° C = _____ ° F

13. 27° C = _____ ° F

14. 31° C = _____ ° F

15. 38° C = _____ ° F

16. 40° C = _____ ° F

17. 49° C = _____ ° F

18. 63° C = _____ ° F

19. 99.8° C = _____ ° F

20. 101.4° C = _____ ° F

Applications

21. When making a mixture, you are instructed to heat the mixture to 130° C. You have only a Fahrenheit thermometer. What is the equivalent temperature on the Fahrenheit temperature scale?

22. Using the prescription below, answer the following questions.

> ℞ **Alteplase Syringes**
>
> Alteplase 2 mg/mL 50 mg
>
> Sterile Water for Injection (SWFI)
>   25 mL
>
> 1. Reconstitute the alteplase with SWFI.
>
> 2. Draw up 5 mL in 10 mL syringes.
>
> 3. Label syringes with contents, concentration, and date of preparation.
>
> 4. Place syringes in freezer.
>
> The syringes are stable for six months, or 180 days, at −20° C.

a. What is the Fahrenheit temperature at which you should store this product?

b. What beyond-use date should you put on this compound if today is February 1, 2025?

23. A compounding pharmacy is required to use dry heat sterilization for certain supply items. These items must undergo sterilization in a 300° F oven for 12 hours. At what Celsius temperature should the oven be set? Round the temperature to the nearest tenth of a degree.

24. Convert the following refrigerator temperatures and log them on the Celsius chart. Round the temperatures to the nearest tenth degree, and note any temperatures that fall outside the safe range.

Date	Degrees F	Degrees C
5/5	36.1°	a. _____
5/6	37.7°	b. _____
5/7	39.0°	c. _____
5/8	35.7°	d. _____
5/9	36.9°	e. _____
5/10	34.9°	f. _____
5/11	36.4°	g. _____
5/12	36.8°	h. _____
5/13	35.5°	i. _____
5/14	38.8°	j. _____

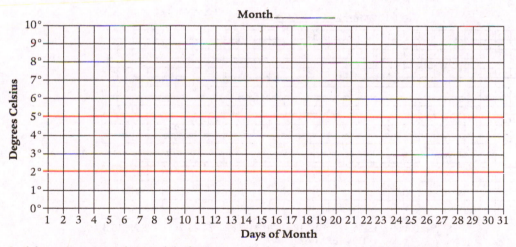

Month _____

Days of Month

Graph freezer temperature on chart once daily. If temperature is less than **2 degrees** or greater than **5 degrees,** check the thermostat setting and correct as necessary. Recheck temperature in one hour, and, if temperature is out of stated range, contact maintenance for evaluation and repair. Contact the appropriate area for storage of supplies.

Documentation of Repairs: _____   Documentation of Cleaning: _____

25. Convert the following refrigerator temperatures and log them on the Fahrenheit chart. Round the temperatures to the nearest tenth degree, and note any temperatures that fall outside the safe range.

Date	Degrees C	Degrees F
7/12	1.8°	a. _____
7/13	3.1°	b. _____
7/14	2.8°	c. _____
7/15	3.0°	d. _____
7/16	4.5°	e. _____
7/17	3.2°	f. _____
7/18	3.9°	g. _____
7/19	2.5°	h. _____
7/20	4.1°	i. _____
7/21	4.7°	j. _____

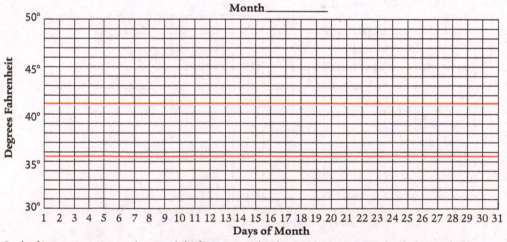

Month_____

Graph refrigerator temperature on chart once daily. If temperature is less than **35.6 degrees** or greater than **41 degrees,** check the thermostat setting and correct as necessary. Recheck temperature in one hour, and, if temperature is out of stated range, contact maintenance for evaluation and repair. Contact the appropriate area for storage of supplies.

Documentation of Repairs: _____   Documentation of Cleaning: _____

Review and Assessment

 ## CHAPTER SUMMARY

- The basic units of measurement in the metric system are meter (length), gram (weight), and liter (volume).

- The metric system uses prefixes that describe the values of the units, which are multiples of 10, 100, or 1,000.

- The *meter* and the *centimeter* are the two most common units of measurement used to describe lengths and heights in a healthcare setting.

- A meter is about the same length as 1 yard, or 3 feet.

- The *milligram* and the *microgram* are the two most common units of measurement for weight in a pharmacy.

- A gram weighs about the same as a large paper clip.

- The *liter* and the *milliliter* are the two most common units of measurement for volume in a pharmacy.

- Converting units in the metric system often requires multiplying or dividing by 1,000, or moving the decimal point three places when changing the unit of measurement.

- Use the ratio-proportion method to convert the unit if you need a foolproof way to perform the conversion—especially if you get confused as to which direction you should move the decimal point.

- The dimensional analysis method can be used to convert units of measurement.

- Patients are more familiar with household units of measurement such as teaspoonfuls and cups rather than metric units of measurement.

- Household measuring devices are often less accurate than the measuring devices used in a pharmacy.

- Household units of measurement may be easily converted to metric units of measurement using either the ratio-proportion method or the dimensional analysis method.

- Some drugs are dosed based on a patient's weight in kilograms.

- Weights measured in pounds may be converted to kilograms by dividing the number of pounds by 2.2.

- Teaspoonful and fluid ounce conversions should be memorized: 1 tsp equals 5 mL and 1 fl oz equals 30 mL.

- The Celsius temperature scale uses 0° as the freezing point and 100° as the boiling point.

- The Fahrenheit temperature scale uses 32° as the freezing point and 212° as the boiling point.

- Temperatures in pharmacy refrigerators and freezers must be checked daily to ensure that medications are being stored within the appropriate temperature ranges.

FORMULAS FOR SUCCESS

Metric Unit Equivalents (Section 4.2)

Kilo	Base	Milli	Micro
0.001 kg	1 g	1,000 mg	1,000,000 mcg
0.001 kL	1 L	1,000 mL	1,000,000 mcL
0.001 km	1 m	1,000 mm	1,000,000 mcm

Household Unit Equivalents (Section 4.3)

3 teaspoonfuls (tsp) = 1 tablespoon (tbsp)	2 cups = 1 pint (pt)
2 tablespoonfuls (tbsp) = 1 fluid ounce (fl oz)	2 pints (pt) = 1 quart (qt)
8 fluid ounces (fl oz) = 1 cup	4 quarts (qt) = 1 gallon (gal)

Degrees Celsius to Degrees Fahrenheit (Section 4.6)

$$°\,F = \left(\frac{9 \times °\,C}{5} \right) + 32°$$

or

$$°\,F = (1.8 \times °\,C) + 32°$$

Degrees Fahrenheit to Degrees Celsius (Section 4.6)

$$°\,C = (°\,F - 32°) \times \frac{5}{9}$$

or

$$°\,C = \frac{°\,F - 32°}{1.8}$$

CHECK YOUR UNDERSTANDING

Take a moment to review what you have learned in this chapter and answer the following questions.

1. The metric system unit of measurement for length is a(n)
   a. inch.
   b. foot.
   c. meter.
   d. mile.

2. The metric system unit of measurement for volume is a
   a. cup.
   b. gallon.
   c. liter.
   d. quart.

3. When converting from a larger unit (liter) to a smaller unit (milliliter), move the decimal point
   a. two places to the left.
   b. two places to the right.
   c. three places to the left.
   d. three places to the right.

4. Which amount indicates the correct conversion of 125 mcg to milligrams?
   a. 0.125 mg
   b. 1.25 mg
   c. 12.5 mg
   d. 125,000 mg

5. Which equivalent is correct?
   a. 3 tsp = 1 tbsp
   b. 3 tsp = 1 fl oz
   c. 3 tsp = ½ cup
   d. 3 tsp = 1 cup

6. Most medications that are dosed based on a patient's weight use _____ as the unit of measurement for the patient's weight.
   a. pounds
   b. pounds and ounces
   c. kilograms
   d. grams

7. Which mathematical operation can be used to convert pounds to kilograms?
   a. add 2.2
   b. divide by 2.2
   c. multiply by 2.2
   d. subtract 2.2

8. Convert 1 pt of Bactrim Suspension to fluid ounces.
   a. 64 fl oz
   b. 32 fl oz
   c. 16 fl oz
   d. 4 fl oz

9. If a patient takes 1 tsp TID, how many milliliters will be needed for a 7-day course of therapy?
   a. 90 mL
   b. 100 mL
   c. 105 mL
   d. 125 mL

10. How many tablespoonful doses are in 1 pt?
    a. 64 tbsp
    b. 32 tbsp
    c. 16 tbsp
    d. 4 tbsp

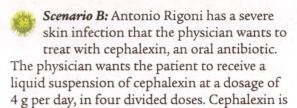

FIND SOLUTIONS

Take a moment to consider what you have learned in this chapter and respond thoughtfully to the prompts.

Note: To indicate your answer for Scenario B, Question 7, ask your instructor for the handout depicting a medicine cup.

Scenario A: You are working at a community pharmacy and receive a prescription for diphenhydramine elixir (2.5 mg/mL) with instructions for the patient to take 1 tsp po q8h as needed for itching. You check the pharmacy stock medication and find that you have two unopened bottles of diphenhydramine elixir (12.5 mg/5 mL) and each container is 1 pt.

1. Is the prescribed diphenhydramine concentration the same as the pharmacy stock concentration?

2. How many milliliters is the ordered dose?

3. How many milliliters is the daily dose?

4. What is the daily dose in tablespoonfuls?

5. Using the household measurement system equivalencies provided in this chapter, determine how many milliliters are in each unopened bottle of diphenhydramine.

6. How many total milliliters does the pharmacy have of diphenhydramine elixir?

Scenario B: Antonio Rigoni has a severe skin infection that the physician wants to treat with cephalexin, an oral antibiotic. The physician wants the patient to receive a liquid suspension of cephalexin at a dosage of 4 g per day, in four divided doses. Cephalexin is available in a 250 mg/5 mL suspension.

7. How many milliliters will be given at each dose? On the handout that you obtained from your instructor, indicate on the measuring device the amount of medication that should be administered to the patient.

8. How many teaspoonfuls are in each dose?

9. How many milliliters will the patient need to complete a 10-day course of therapy?

10. The physician would like to be notified if Antonio's temperature is greater than 39° C. What is this temperature in degrees Fahrenheit?

The online course includes additional review and assessment resources.

Calculating Doses for Oral Medications

Learning Objectives

1 Calculate drug doses in word problems that use the ratio-proportion and dimensional analysis methods. (Section 5.1)

2 Determine quantity to dispense for oral solid dosage forms. (Section 5.2)

3 Determine volumes for liquid oral dosage forms. (Section 5.2)

4 Calculate quantity to dispense and days' supply for liquid oral dosage forms. (Section 5.2)

5 Utilize dosing tables to identify pediatric doses. (Section 5.2)

6 Calculate a patient-specific dose based on weight. (Section 5.3)

7 Calculate a patient-specific dose based on body surface area. (Section 5.3)

For a key to the body system icons that appear in each chapter of this textbook, refer to the Preface.

ASHP/ACPE Accreditation Standards

To view the *ASHP/ACPE Accreditation Standards* addressed in this chapter, refer to Appendix D.

Whether you are a pharmacy technician in a community pharmacy or in an institutional pharmacy, you are expected to accurately perform medication dose calculations. This chapter provides a solid foundation for specific types of dose calculations, with an emphasis on the ratio-proportion and dimensional analysis methods. Oral dose calculations for commonly prescribed dosage forms such as capsules, tablets, and liquids are addressed. In addition, patient-specific dosing factors, including body weight and body surface area, are discussed.

5.1 Ratio-Proportion and Dimensional Analysis Dose Calculations

As a pharmacy technician, you will face situations every day that require you to solve mathematical problems presented as scenarios. These situational problems, also known as *word problems*, require good critical-thinking skills and a methodical approach to finding the solutions. When faced with a word problem or another problem in which the calculation needed is not absolutely clear, you may find it helpful to ask yourself the following question: *What am I looking for to solve the problem?* Asking this question before performing dose calculations in a pharmacy setting can also help you determine the best approach to solving the problem. For dose calculations, the answer to this question is typically a weight, expressed in milligrams (mg), or a volume, expressed in milliliters (mL).

Using the Ratio-Proportion Method to Calculate a Medication Dose

In Chapter 2, you learned some basic calculations using the ratio-proportion method and applied that method to converting between metric units of measurement in Chapter 4. Now you will apply the mathematical concepts of ratios and proportions to compare a readily available medication with a particular strength, consisting of a vehicle and an active ingredient, to a desired (prescribed) dose. A **vehicle** is an inert (chemically inactive) medium, such as a syrup, in which a medication is administered. An **active ingredient** is the biologically active component of a medication. The equation below represents this proportional relationship.

Math Morsel

When setting up ratios, the active ingredients or the vehicles may appear in either the numerators or in the denominators as long as the units are in the same positions on both sides of the equation.

$$\frac{\text{active ingredient (desired)}}{\text{vehicle (desired)}} = \frac{\text{active ingredient (on hand)}}{\text{vehicle (on hand)}}$$

Keep in mind that the ratios on the two sides of the equation may be inverted. For example, the vehicle may be in the numerator and the active ingredient may be in the denominator. However, the same units must appear in both the numerators and the denominators.

You can follow the steps outlined in Table 5.1 to solve dose calculation word problems using the ratio-proportion method.

TABLE 5.1 **Steps for Using the Ratio-Proportion Method for Solving Word Problems**

Step 1. Read through the entire problem and identify what the problem is asking you to find. This unknown amount is designated by the variable *x*, labeled with the unit you are looking for such as *x* mg or *x* mL.

Step 2. Identify the prescriber's order. Circle the dose ordered by the prescriber.

Step 3. Identify the appropriate stock medication in the pharmacy. The ratio, dosage strength, or concentration of the pharmacy stock medication, such as 1 mg/tablet or 125 mg/5 mL, is typically shown on the label of the drug used in the pharmacy. Underline this information.

Step 4. Identify any extraneous information, or information that is not needed to solve the problem. Then draw a single line through this information to prevent you from using it in the setup of your ratio.

Step 5. Estimate what your answer should be by comparing the ordered dose to the stock medication ratio. Will the ordered dose be larger or smaller than the stock medication ratio?

Step 6. Use the ratio-proportion method to solve for the unknown variable *x*. When using the ratio-proportion method to solve the problem, place the prescriber-ordered dose on the left side of the equation and the pharmacy stock medication ratio on the right side of the equation.

Step 7. Round your answer appropriately. Follow the rounding rules specific to your practice setting. In this textbook, weights are typically rounded to the nearest whole milligram, and volumes are typically rounded to the nearest tenth of a milliliter.

Example 5.1.1

A physician has ordered 370 mg of a medication, and you have on hand a 10 mL vial of solution containing 250 mg/3 mL. How many milliliters will you measure out?

Step 1. Identify the question being asked. You need to find the number of milliliters, so *x* mL is the unknown amount.

Step 2. Identify the prescribed amount and circle it. In this problem, the physician has ordered 370 mg.

Step 3. Identify the product available in the pharmacy and underline it. In this problem, the pharmacy has 250 mg/3 mL of the medication.

Step 4. Identify extraneous information and draw a line through it. In this problem, it is not important to know that the medication is available in a 10 mL vial.

Step 5. Estimate the answer. The ordered dose of 370 mg is greater than the dose of the available product, which is 250 mg. Therefore, the dose volume should be greater than 3 mL.

Step 6. Use the ratio-proportion method to solve for *x*.

$$\frac{x \text{ mL}}{370 \text{ mg}} = \frac{3 \text{ mL}}{250 \text{ mg}}$$

$$x \text{ mL } (250 \text{ mg}) = 3 \text{ mL } (370 \text{ mg})$$

$$x = 4.44 \text{ mL}$$

Step 7. Because the amount is a volume, you will round your answer to the nearest tenth: 4.4 mL.

Answer: You will measure out 4.4 mL of medication.

Example 5.1.2

A physician has ordered 100 mg of amoxicillin to be given to a child three times a day for 10 days. Amoxicillin is available in a 150 mL bottle with a dosage strength (concentration) of 125 mg/5 mL. How many milliliters will the child need at each dose?

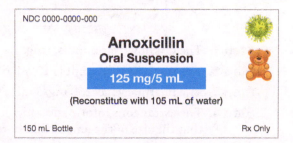

NDC 0000-0000-000

Amoxicillin
Oral Suspension
125 mg/5 mL
(Reconstitute with 105 mL of water)
150 mL Bottle   Rx Only

Step 1. Identify the question being asked. You need to find the number of milliliters, so *x* mL is the unknown amount.

Step 2. Identify the prescribed amount and circle it. In this problem, the physician has ordered 100 mg at each dose.

Step 3. Identify the product available in the pharmacy and underline it. In this problem, the pharmacy has 125 mg/5 mL of amoxicillin.

Step 4. Identify extraneous information and draw a line through it. In this problem, it is not important to know "three times a day for 10 days" and that the size of the amoxicillin bottle is 150 mL.

Step 5. Estimate the answer. The ordered dose of 100 mg is less than the dose strength of 125 mg, so the dose volume should be less than 5 mL.

Step 6. Use the ratio-proportion method to solve for x.

$$\frac{x \text{ mL}}{100 \text{ mg}} = \frac{5 \text{ mL}}{125 \text{ mg}}$$

$$x \text{ mL} (125 \text{ mg}) = 5 \text{ mL} (100 \text{ mg})$$

$$x = 4 \text{ mL}$$

Step 7. No rounding is needed because this volume does not extend beyond a tenth of a milliliter.

Answer: The child will need 4 mL of amoxicillin at each dose.

Some medications are ordered by a certain volume (typically milliliters) rather than by milligrams or other units of weight. For example, a cough syrup may be ordered as 10 mL every 4 hours, and it may be necessary to calculate how much of the active ingredient is in this dose. The steps presented in Table 5.1 can also be used to solve this type of problem. In this case, however, the unknown amount will be the amount of the active ingredient instead of the overall volume.

Example 5.1.3

A physician has ordered 10 mL of amoxicillin to be given to a child three times a day for 7 days. Amoxicillin is available in a 150 mL bottle with a dosage strength (concentration) of 250 mg/5 mL. How many milligrams will the child receive at each dose?

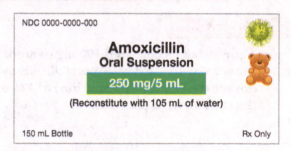

NDC 0000-0000-000

Amoxicillin
Oral Suspension

250 mg/5 mL

(Reconstitute with 105 mL of water)

150 mL Bottle   Rx Only

Step 1. The unknown amount is x mg.

Step 2. The prescribed amount is 10 mL of amoxicillin.

Step 3. The pharmacy has 250 mg/5 mL of amoxicillin.

Step 4. The extraneous information includes "three times a day for 7 days" and that the size of the amoxicillin bottle is 150 mL.

Step 5. The answer will be greater than 250 mg because 10 mL is greater than 5 mL.

Step 6. Use the ratio-proportion method to solve for x.

$$\frac{x \text{ mg}}{10 \text{ mL}} = \frac{250 \text{ mg}}{5 \text{ mL}}$$

$$x \text{ mg} (5 \text{ mL}) = 250 \text{ mg} (10 \text{ mL})$$

$$x = 500 \text{ mg}$$

Step 7. No rounding is needed because this weight does not have a decimal point, and the significant figures are correct.

Answer: The child will receive 500 mg of amoxicillin at each dose.

Example 5.1.4

A physician has ordered cefaclor 375 mg/5 mL oral suspension for a patient. A 100 mL bottle is prepared and is labeled to administer 7.5 mL twice daily for 5 days. How many milligrams is the patient receiving at each dose?

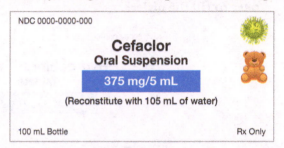

NDC 0000-0000-000

Cefaclor
Oral Suspension

375 mg/5 mL

(Reconstitute with 105 mL of water)

100 mL Bottle   Rx Only

Step 1. The unknown amount is x mg.

Step 2. The prescribed amount is 7.5 mL of oral suspension.

Step 3. Once the oral suspension is prepared, it contains 375 mg of cefaclor/5 mL of oral suspension.

Step 4. The extraneous information includes "twice daily for 5 days" and that the size of the cefaclor bottle is 100 mL.

Step 5. The answer will be greater than 375 mg because 7.5 mL is greater than 5 mL.

Step 6. Use the ratio-proportion method to solve for x.

$$\frac{x \text{ mg}}{7.5 \text{ mL}} = \frac{375 \text{ mg}}{5 \text{ mL}}$$

$$x \text{ mg } (5 \text{ mL}) = 375 \text{ mg } (7.5 \text{ mL})$$

$$x = 562.5 \text{ mg, rounded to } 563 \text{ mg}$$

Step 7. The weight of 562.5 mg is rounded to the nearest whole milligram, or 563 mg.

Answer: The patient is receiving 563 mg at each dose.

Using Dimensional Analysis to Calculate a Medication Dose

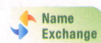

Name Exchange

The terms *concentration* and *strength* are often used interchangeably in pharmacy practice. Both terms refer to the amount of medication per volume (such as 5 mg/125 mL).

Just as you used the dimensional analysis method to convert metric units of measurement in Chapter 4, you can now use this method to solve medication dose problems by "converting" a dose from milligrams to tablets, or from milligrams to milliliters. You accomplish this task by multiplying the dose ordered by the prescriber by the dosage strength or concentration of the pharmacy stock medication. As in the metric conversions practiced in Chapter 4, you set up the ratio so that the units of the ordered dose and the units in the denominator cancel out. When using the dimensional analysis method to solve drug dosage problems, you can still use the steps in Table 5.1 to analyze the information. The only difference is in the setup of the calculation in Step 6.

The dimensional analysis method tends to be used most frequently for simple dosage calculations such as the number of tablets. For example, if a physician has prescribed 100 mg of a medication, and you have that medication on hand in 50 mg tablets, you can quickly determine that the patient will need two 50 mg tablets for the prescribed 100 mg dose. Although you may be able to perform mental calculations in the following exercises, it is important to work through the steps to ensure your understanding of the calculations process.

Example 5.1.5

A physician has ordered a 25 mg dose of hydrochlorothiazide. You have a 100-count bottle of 50 mg tablets. How many tablets will you need to prepare to fill the order?

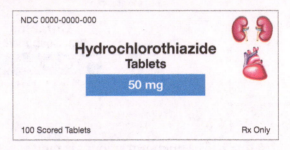

NDC 0000-0000-000

Hydrochlorothiazide
Tablets

50 mg

100 Scored Tablets   Rx Only

Step 1. The unknown is *x* tablets.

Step 2. The prescribed amount is 25 mg.

Step 3. The pharmacy has 50 mg tablets.

Step 4. The extraneous information includes "100-count bottle."

Step 5. The answer will be less than 1 tablet, as the requested dose is less than the number of milligrams in 1 tablet.

Step 6. Use the dimensional analysis method to convert the units.

$$\frac{25 \text{ mg}}{1} \times \frac{1 \text{ tablet}}{50 \text{ mg}} = 0.5 \text{ tablet}$$

Step 7. No rounding is required.

Answer: You will prepare 0.5 tablet to fill the order.

Example 5.1.6

A physician has ordered a 750 mg dose of amoxicillin. You have 150 mL of a 250 mg/5 mL oral suspension. How many milliliters will you prepare to fill the order?

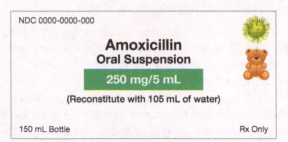

NDC 0000-0000-000

Amoxicillin
Oral Suspension

250 mg/5 mL

(Reconstitute with 105 mL of water)

150 mL Bottle   Rx Only

Step 1. The unknown amount is *x* mL.

Step 2. The prescribed amount is 750 mg of amoxicillin.

Step 3. The pharmacy has 250 mg/5 mL.

Step 4. The extraneous information includes "150 mL" and "oral suspension."

Step 5. The answer will be approximately three times as large as the unit given.

Step 6. Use dimensional analysis to convert the units.

$$\frac{750 \text{ mg}}{1} \times \frac{5 \text{ mL}}{250 \text{ mg}} = 15 \text{ mL}$$

Step 7. No rounding is required.

Answer: You will prepare 15 mL to fill the order.

Example 5.1.7

A prescriber has ordered that a patient take 250 mg of amoxicillin twice daily for 10 days. You have 150 mL of 250 mg/5 mL amoxicillin oral suspension in stock. How many milliliters are needed for a 1-day supply?

Step 1. The unknown amount is x mL.

Step 2. The prescriber ordered 250 mg twice daily.

Step 3. The pharmacy has 250 mg/5 mL of amoxicillin.

Step 4. The extraneous information includes "10 days" and "150 mL."

Step 5. The answer will be greater than 5 mL (the volume of 250 mg of amoxicillin).

Step 6. Use dimensional analysis to convert the units.

$$\frac{250 \text{ mg}}{\text{dose}} \times \frac{2 \text{ doses}}{\text{day}} \times \frac{5 \text{ mL}}{250 \text{ mg}} = \frac{10 \text{ mL}}{\text{day}}$$

Step 7. No rounding is required.

Answer: You will need 10 mL of the amoxicillin oral suspension for a 1-day supply.

Example 5.1.8

Using the same prescription and amoxicillin oral suspension from Example 5.1.7, calculate how many milliliters of amoxicillin 250 mg/5 mL oral suspension are needed for a 10 days' supply. The patient weighs 25 kg.

Dimensional Analysis Multi-Step Method

Step 1. The unknown amount is x mL.

Step 2. The prescriber ordered 250 mg twice daily for 10 days.

Step 3. The pharmacy has amoxicillin 250 mg/5 mL oral suspension.

Step 4. The extraneous information includes the patient's weight.

Step 5. The answer will be greater than 10 mL.

Step 6. Use dimensional analysis to convert the units.

$$\frac{10 \text{ days}}{1} \times \frac{10 \text{ mL}}{\text{day}} = 100 \text{ mL}$$

Step 7. No rounding is required.

You solved for a 10 days' supply using two separate calculations. First, you converted milligrams/dose to milliliters/day in Example 5.1.7. Then you converted milliliters/day to milliliters for a 10 days' supply. You can alternately solve this problem using a one-step method.

Dimensional Analysis One-Step Method

$$\frac{10 \text{ days}}{1} \times \frac{2 \text{ doses}}{\text{day}} \times \frac{250 \text{ mg}}{\text{dose}} \times \frac{5 \text{ mL}}{250 \text{ mg}} = 100 \text{ mL}$$

Answer: You will need 100 mL of the amoxicillin oral suspension for a 10 days' supply.

5.1 Problem Set

Calculate the following doses using the ratio-proportion method.

1. A patient has a prescription order for 30 mg of a medication. The pharmacy has a partial container of 7.5 mg tablets. How many tablets will the patient need?

2. A prescription order is written for 20 mg of medication. The pharmacy has on hand a 10 mL vial of 25 mg/2 mL solution. How many milliliters will be prepared for this patient?

3. A patient is prescribed 125 mg of carbamazepine suspension. The label provided shows the medication that the pharmacy has in stock. How many milliliters will be prepared for this patient?

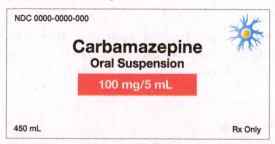

4. A patient is to receive 4 mg of haloperidol. The pharmacy has on hand a 1 mL vial of 5 mg/1 mL solution. How many milliliters are needed to fill this prescription?

5. A loading dose of 1,750 mg is needed. The pharmacy has on hand a 500-count bottle of 250 mg capsules. How many capsules will be needed to fill this prescription?

6. A patient is to receive 40 mg of morphine sulfate. The pharmacy has the following medication available. How many milliliters will be prepared for this patient?

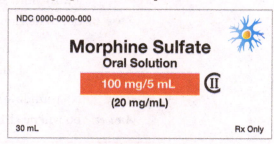

7. A patient is to receive 400 mg of erythromycin ethylsuccinate three times daily. The label provided shows the available medication. How many milliliters will be prepared for the morning dose?

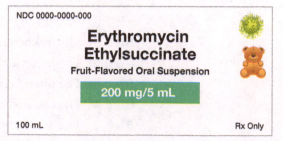

8. The pharmacy receives the following order.

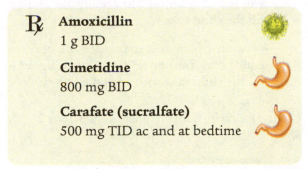

Rx **Amoxicillin**
1 g BID

Cimetidine
800 mg BID

Carafate (sucralfate)
500 mg TID ac and at bedtime

a. Amoxicillin is available as a 250 mg/5 mL suspension. How many milliliters of medication would you draw up in each oral syringe for the patient?

b. Cimetidine is available as 300 mg/5 mL. How many milliliters will you draw up in each oral syringe for the patient?

c. Carafate is available as 1 g tablets. How many tablets will be needed for one day?

9. A total regimen of therapy calls for 10 mg of a medication to be given to a patient over several days. In the pharmacy, a solution is available with 40 mcg/mL. How many milliliters must be dispensed to complete the regimen?

10. A patient was given 2 mL of gentamicin, shown in the label below. How many milligrams were given to the patient?

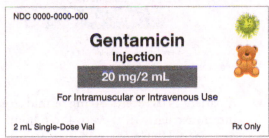

NDC 0000-0000-000

Gentamicin
Injection

20 mg/2 mL

For Intramuscular or Intravenous Use

2 mL Single-Dose Vial   Rx Only

11. A patient receives 1 mg of atropine, shown in the label below. How many milliliters did the patient receive?

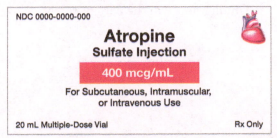

NDC 0000-0000-000

Atropine
Sulfate Injection

400 mcg/mL

For Subcutaneous, Intramuscular, or Intravenous Use

20 mL Multiple-Dose Vial   Rx Only

12. A patient receives 1.2 mL of the atropine solution shown in the preceding problem. How many micrograms did the patient receive?

13. A prescriber orders a 0.63 mL dose of medication. The pharmacy stock solution contains 80 mg/15 mL. How many micrograms are in the dose?

14. A capsule contains 35 mg of an active ingredient. How many capsules would you need to accumulate 1.05 kg of the active ingredient?

15. A total regimen of therapy calls for 880 mg of a medication to be given. If two doses provide 80 mg, how many doses will have to be given?

16. You have 560 mL of a solution that contains 1,600 mg. How many micrograms are in 4 mL of solution? Round your answer to the nearest microgram.

17. A total regimen of therapy calls for 10 mg of a medication to be given to a patient over several days. In the pharmacy, a solution is available with 40 mcg/mL. How many milliliters must be dispensed to complete the regimen?

18. A patient is to receive 2,000 units of heparin. Use the following label to determine how many milliliters of heparin you will prepare.

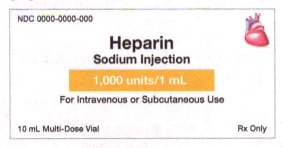

NDC 0000-0000-000

Heparin
Sodium Injection

1,000 units/1 mL

For Intravenous or Subcutaneous Use

10 mL Multi-Dose Vial   Rx Only

Use the following label to answer questions 19 and 20.

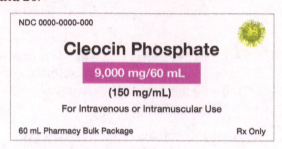

NDC 0000-0000-000

Cleocin Phosphate

9,000 mg/60 mL

(150 mg/mL)

For Intravenous or Intramuscular Use

60 mL Pharmacy Bulk Package   Rx Only

19. A medication order states that the patient is to take 900 mg of Cleocin. How many milliliters are in this dose?

20. A patient receives 4 mL of Cleocin. How many milligrams are in this dose?

Use the following label to answer questions 21 and 22.

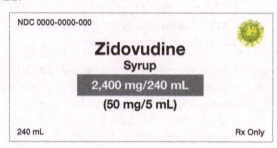

NDC 0000-0000-000

Zidovudine
Syrup

2,400 mg/240 mL

(50 mg/5 mL)

240 mL   Rx Only

21. A patient is to take 12.5 mL of zidovudine syrup as shown. How many milligrams are in this dose?

22. A patient is prescribed 100 mg of zidovudine syrup as shown. How many milliliters are in this dose?

Use the following label to answer questions 23 and 24.

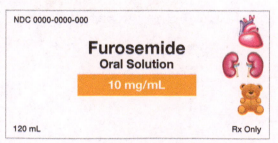

NDC 0000-0000-000

Furosemide
Oral Solution

10 mg/mL

120 mL   Rx Only

23. A pediatric patient is to take 0.5 mL of furosemide oral solution. How many milligrams will the child take with each dose?

24. A pediatric patient is to take 0.8 mL of furosemide oral solution. How many milligrams will the child take with each dose?

Use the following label to answer questions 25 and 26.

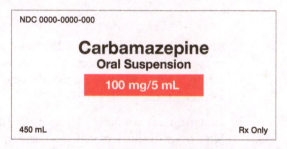

NDC 0000-0000-000

Carbamazepine
Oral Suspension

100 mg/5 mL

450 mL   Rx Only

25. A patient is to take 150 mg of carbamazepine every 12 hours. How many milliliters will the patient take at each dose?

26. A patient is to take 0.5 g of carbamazepine. How many milliliters will be prepared?

Use the following label to answer questions 27 and 28.

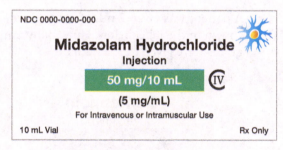

NDC 0000-0000-000

Midazolam Hydrochloride
Injection

50 mg/10 mL   Ⓒ IV

(5 mg/mL)

For Intravenous or Intramuscular Use

10 mL Vial   Rx Only

27. A patient is to receive 50 mg of midazolam intramuscularly (IM) every 4 to 6 hours as needed. How many milliliters will the patient need for one dose?

28. A patient is to receive 0.8 mL of midazolam solution IM stat (immediately). How many milligrams will the patient receive?

Use the following label to answer questions 29 and 30.

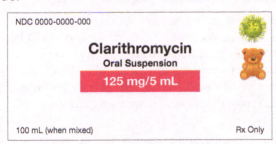

NDC 0000-0000-000

Clarithromycin
Oral Suspension

125 mg/5 mL

100 mL (when mixed)   Rx Only

29. A patient is to take 100 mg of clarithromycin. How many milliliters will the patient receive?

30. A patient is to take 7.5 mL of clarithromycin. How many milligrams will the patient receive?

Use the following label to answer questions 31 and 32.

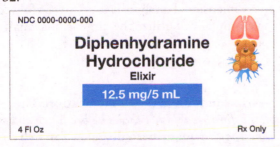

NDC 0000-0000-000

Diphenhydramine Hydrochloride
Elixir

12.5 mg/5 mL

4 Fl Oz   Rx Only

31. A pediatric patient is to receive 20 mg of diphenhydramine hydrochloride. How many milliliters of elixir will the patient receive?

32. An adult patient who has been stung by a wasp is to receive 50 mg of diphenhydramine hydrochloride stat (immediately). How many milliliters of elixir will be administered?

33. A patient is to take 150 mg of nortriptyline per day. The pharmacy has on hand 25 mg, 50 mg, and 75 mg capsules.

a. Select the product that will result in the patient taking the fewest number of capsules daily.

b. How many capsules will need to be dispensed for a 7 days' supply?

34. The pharmacy receives the following order.

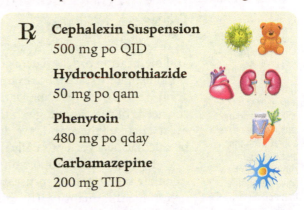

Rx **Cephalexin Suspension**
500 mg po QID

Hydrochlorothiazide
50 mg po qam

Phenytoin
480 mg po qday

Carbamazepine
200 mg TID

a. Cephalexin is available in a 250 mL bottle of 250 mg/5 mL suspension. How many milliliters will the patient need for the first day?

b. Hydrochlorothiazide is available from the pharmacy in a 1,000-count bottle of 25 mg tablets. How many tablets will be needed for the first day of hospitalization?

c. Phenytoin is available as 125 mg/5 mL. How many milliliters will be measured out for the patient's daily dose?

d. The pharmacy has a 450 mL bottle of 100 mg/5 mL carbamazepine solution. How many milliliters will be prepared for this patient for the first day?

Self-check your work in Appendix A

5.2 Oral Dose Calculations

As a pharmacy technician, you will often fill prescriptions for oral dosage forms such as tablets, capsules, and liquids. Oral medications are commonly ordered by prescribers because these drugs are typically safe, well-tolerated, and cost-effective for patients. In light of that, you must be able to perform oral dose calculations accurately and efficiently. These calculations involve conversions from the metric system to the household system and the determination of dosing and dispensing amounts.

Determining Quantity to Dispense for Solid Oral Dosage Forms

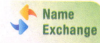
Name Exchange

The abbreviation *QS* may appear on prescriptions and medication orders. This abbreviation means that the pharmacy should dispense a "quantity sufficient" to meet the patient's needs, given the dosing instructions.

As discussed in Chapter 3, prescribers indicate quantity to dispense on prescriptions and medication orders. There are instances, however, where the amount to dispense is not explicitly stated. For example, a prescription or a medication order may use the abbreviation *QS*. This abbreviation means to dispense a "quantity sufficient" to meet the needs of the patient, given the dosing instructions. For this type of order, you must calculate the amount to dispense. The quantity to dispense can be determined by calculating a patient's daily need over the duration of therapy.

Both the ratio-proportion and dimensional analysis methods can be used to calculate quantity to dispense. However, dimensional analysis is used more often to determine this quantity. The following examples will utilize the dimensional analysis method to determine quantity to dispense.

Example 5.2.1

A patient has brought in a prescription for a diabetes medication. The prescription states, *Take 2 tablets before breakfast, 1 tablet before lunch and dinner, and 1 tablet at bedtime.* **Determine the quantity to dispense for a 30 days' supply.**

To begin, determine the number of tablets required for one day.

2 tablets before breakfast + 1 tablet before lunch + 1 tablet before dinner + 1 tablet at bedtime = 5 tablets

Then determine a 30 days' supply if the patient takes 5 tablets/day.

$$\frac{5 \text{ tablets}}{\text{day}} \times 30 \text{ days} = 150 \text{ tablets}$$

Answer: The pharmacy should dispense 150 tablets for a 30 days' supply.

Example 5.2.2

A patient has been prescribed prednisone and is to follow a tapered dosing schedule. Determine the quantity of 5 mg tablets to dispense.

℞ **Prednisone 5 mg Tablets**

Take 40 mg for 2 days.

Take 35 mg for 1 day.

Take 30 mg for 2 days.

Then decrease by 5 mg each day for 5 days.

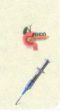

To begin, you need to recognize that the number of tablets taken each day changes. Therefore, the most straightforward approach to determining the quantity to dispense is to perform a series of dimensional analysis calculations.

Then set up your calculations by showing the number of tablets that the patient will take for each day of treatment.

$$\text{Day 1: } 40 \text{ mg} \times \frac{1 \text{ tablet}}{5 \text{ mg}} = 8 \text{ tablets}$$

$$\text{Day 2: } 40 \text{ mg} \times \frac{1 \text{ tablet}}{5 \text{ mg}} = 8 \text{ tablets}$$

$$\text{Day 3: } 35 \text{ mg} \times \frac{1 \text{ tablet}}{5 \text{ mg}} = 7 \text{ tablets}$$

$$\text{Day 4: } 30 \text{ mg} \times \frac{1 \text{ tablet}}{5 \text{ mg}} = 6 \text{ tablets}$$

$$\text{Day 5: } 30 \text{ mg} \times \frac{1 \text{ tablet}}{5 \text{ mg}} = 6 \text{ tablets}$$

$$\text{Day 6: } 25 \text{ mg} \times \frac{1 \text{ tablet}}{5 \text{ mg}} = 5 \text{ tablets}$$

$$\text{Day 7: } 20 \text{ mg} \times \frac{1 \text{ tablet}}{5 \text{ mg}} = 4 \text{ tablets}$$

$$\text{Day 8: } 15 \text{ mg} \times \frac{1 \text{ tablet}}{5 \text{ mg}} = 3 \text{ tablets}$$

$$\text{Day 9: } 10 \text{ mg} \times \frac{1 \text{ tablet}}{5 \text{ mg}} = 2 \text{ tablets}$$

$$\text{Day 10: } 5 \text{ mg} \times \frac{1 \text{ tablet}}{5 \text{ mg}} = 1 \text{ tablet}$$

Finally, add the daily totals of the tablets:

$$8 + 8 + 7 + 6 + 6 + 5 + 4 + 3 + 2 + 1 = 50$$

Answer: The pharmacy should dispense 50 tablets to fill this prescription.

Determining Volumes for Liquid Oral Dosage Forms

Many oral liquid medications are solutions or suspensions. A **solution** is a liquid dosage form that is a mixture of one or more solutes dissolved in a solvent. A **solvent** is the substance in which a solute dissolves. A **solute** is the substance that dissolves in a solvent. Consider the solution created by combining table salt (NaCl) to a glass of hot water. In this example, the solvent is the hot water and the solutes are sodium (Na^+) and chloride (Cl^-). A suspension, like a solution, is a liquid. A **suspension** is a liquid dosage form that contains insoluble (incapable of being dissolved) materials suspended in a liquid. Many liquid antibiotics, for example, are available as suspensions.

Both solutions and suspensions are typically indicated by the weight of active drug per volume of solution or suspension. Metric units for a solution or a suspension are typically expressed as the number of milligrams of active drug per milliliters of solution or suspension. For example, the antibiotic amoxicillin is available as a suspension in the concentration of 125 mg/5 mL. In other words, 5 mL of the suspension contains 125 mg of amoxicillin.

Oral liquid medications may be dosed in household units of measurement such as teaspoonfuls, tablespoonfuls, or fluid ounces and in metric units of measurement such as milliliters. If patient instructions indicate household units, you should convert these units to milliliters if the dose is not easily measured using the household system. Dispensing an oral syringe (shown in Figure 5.1) with the prescription allows patients to measure oral liquids using either the household or metric units of measurement.

Usually, a prescription for an oral liquid medication includes a specific volume to be given at each dose, as well as the total volume to be dispensed. It is important to have a working knowledge of the volumes of oral liquid medications that are commonly prescribed. Most frequently, the dosage amount is between 2 mL and 60 mL, or roughly 1/2 tsp to 2 fl oz.

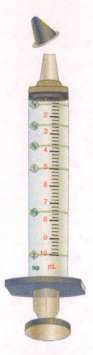

FIGURE 5.1
Oral Syringe

This oral syringe is marked with both household and metric units of measurement.

Example 5.2.3

If a 12 fl oz bottle of mouthwash contains 0.75 g of the active ingredient, how many milligrams will be in a 1 tbsp dose?

You can solve this problem by using the ratio-proportion method or by using the dimensional analysis method.

Ratio-Proportion Method

To begin, convert the household units of measurement to metric units of measurement.

$$12 \text{ fl oz} = 360 \text{ mL}$$
$$1 \text{ tbsp} = 15 \text{ mL}$$

Then convert the metric unit of measurement from grams to milligrams.

$$0.75 \text{ g} = 750 \text{ mg}$$

Next, set up a proportion of the unknown quantity (x mg) over the ordered dose (15 mL) on the left side of the equation, and the milligrams per milliliter of the available stock medication on the right side of the equation. Remember that the units of measurement in the numerators and in the denominators must match. Then solve for x.

$$\frac{x \text{ mg}}{15 \text{ mL}} = \frac{750 \text{ mg}}{360 \text{ mL}}$$

$$x \text{ mg } (360 \text{ mL}) = 750 \text{ mg } (15 \text{ mL})$$

$$x = 31.25 \text{ mg}$$

Dimensional Analysis Method

$$\frac{1 \text{ tbsp}}{1} \times \frac{1 \text{ fl oz}}{2 \text{ tbsp}} \times \frac{0.75 \text{ g}}{12 \text{ fl oz}} \times \frac{1{,}000 \text{ mg}}{\text{g}} = 31.25 \text{ mg}$$

Answer: There are 31.25 mg in a 1 tbsp dose.

Example 5.2.4

The pharmacy receives a prescription for amoxicillin oral suspension 1 g BID. The pharmacy has a supply of amoxicillin 250 mg/5 mL. How many milliliters are in one dose? What will the patient's dosing instructions on the bottle label indicate?

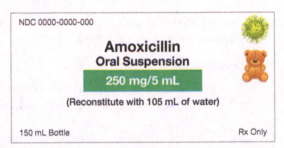

You can solve this problem by using the ratio-proportion method or by using the dimensional analysis method.

Ratio-Proportion Method

To begin, convert the metric unit of measurement from grams to milligrams. That way, you know how many milligrams are needed for one dose.

$$1 \text{ g} = 1{,}000 \text{ mg}$$

Next, set up a proportion of the unknown quantity (x mL) over your conversion (1,000 mg) on the left side of the equation, and the milligrams per milliliter of the available stock medication on the right side of the equation. Remember that the units of measurement in the numerators and in the denominators must match. Then solve for x.

$$\frac{x \text{ mL}}{1{,}000 \text{ mg}} = \frac{5 \text{ mL}}{250 \text{ mg}}$$

$$x \text{ mL} (250 \text{ mg}) = 5 \text{ mL} (1{,}000 \text{ mg})$$

$$x = 20 \text{ mL}$$

Dimensional Analysis Method

$$\frac{1 \text{ g}}{\text{dose}} \times \frac{1{,}000 \text{ mg}}{1 \text{ g}} \times \frac{5 \text{ mL}}{250 \text{ mg}} = 20 \text{ mL}$$

Answer: There are 20 mL of amoxicillin 250 mg/5 mL oral suspension in one dose. The patient's instructions will state, *Take 20 mL (or 4 teaspoonfuls) two times daily.*

Example 5.2.5

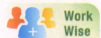

Work Wise

Pharmacy technicians who are comfortable performing oral liquid medication dose calculations may enjoy working in a healthcare setting that specializes in the treatment of pediatric patients. This patient population commonly uses liquid dosage forms.

A patient is to take 7 mL of amoxicillin oral suspension 250 mg/5 mL. How many milligrams of amoxicillin are present in one dose?

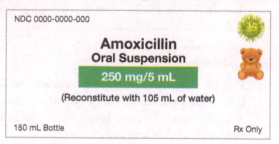

You can solve this problem by using the ratio-proportion method or by using the dimensional analysis method.

Ratio-Proportion Method

To begin, set up a proportion of the unknown quantity (*x* mg) over the known value (7 mL) on the left side of the equation, and the milligrams per milliliter of the available stock medication on the right side of the equation. Remember that the units of measurement in the numerators and in the denominators must match. Then solve for *x*.

$$\frac{x \text{ mg}}{7 \text{ mL}} = \frac{250 \text{ mg}}{5 \text{ mL}}$$

$$x \text{ mg} (5 \text{ mL}) = 250 \text{ mg} (7 \text{ mL})$$

$$x = 350 \text{ mg}$$

Dimensional Analysis Method

$$\frac{7 \text{ mL}}{1} \times \frac{250 \text{ mg}}{5 \text{ mL}} = 350 \text{ mg}$$

Answer: There are 350 mg of amoxicillin present in one dose.

Example 5.2.6

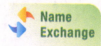

Name Exchange

Diphenhydramine hydrochloride elixir is commonly known by the brand name Benadryl.

A hospitalized patient is taking 4 tsp of diphenhydramine hydrochloride elixir at bedtime. The patient is now able to swallow solids and is being switched to diphenhydramine capsules. The 12.5 mg/5 mL elixir comes in a 4 fl oz bottle and is 14% alcohol. The pharmacy has 25 mg capsules in stock. How many capsules will the patient need to take to equal the dose in the 4 tsp of elixir?

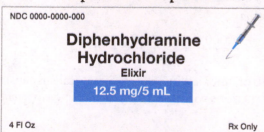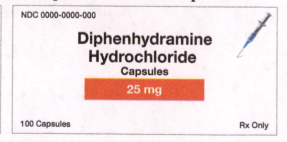

You can solve this problem by using the ratio-proportion method or by using the dimensional analysis method.

Ratio-Proportion Method

To begin, convert the household unit of measurement to a metric unit of measurement.

$$4 \text{ tsp} = 20 \text{ mL}$$

Then set up a proportion of the unknown quantity over the conversion (20 mL) on the left side of the equation, and the milligrams per milliliter of the available stock medication on the right side of the equation. Remember that the units of measurement in the numerators and in the denominators must match. Then solve for x.

$$\frac{x \text{ mg}}{20 \text{ mL}} = \frac{12.5 \text{ mg}}{5 \text{ mL}}$$

$$x \text{ mg } (5 \text{ mL}) = 12.5 \text{ mg } (20 \text{ mL})$$

$$x = 50 \text{ mg}$$

Now, set up a proportion that compares the number of milligrams in the elixir dosage form (50 mg) to the number of milligrams in the capsule dosage form. Remember that the units of measurement in the numerators and in the denominators must match. Then solve for x.

$$\frac{x \text{ capsules}}{50 \text{ mg}} = \frac{1 \text{ capsule}}{25 \text{ mg}}$$

$$x \text{ capsules } (25 \text{ mg}) = 1 \text{ capsule } (50 \text{ mg})$$

$$x = 2 \text{ capsules}$$

Dimensional Analysis Method

$$\frac{4 \text{ tsp}}{1} \times \frac{5 \text{ mL}}{1 \text{ tsp}} \times \frac{12.5 \text{ mg}}{5 \text{ mL}} \times \frac{1 \text{ capsule}}{25 \text{ mg}} = 2 \text{ capsules}$$

Answer: Because 4 tsp of elixir contain 50 mg of diphenhydramine and the capsules contain 25 mg of diphenhydramine, the patient will need to take two capsules to provide the proper amount of medication.

Example 5.2.7

Name Exchange

Biaxin is a brand name for the generic drug clarithromycin.

How many milligrams of medication are in 1 tbsp of a clarithromycin oral suspension that contains 125 mg/5 mL?

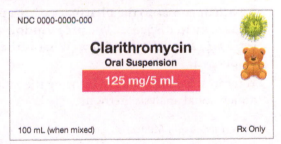

NDC 0000-0000-000

Clarithromycin
Oral Suspension

125 mg/5 mL

100 mL (when mixed)   Rx Only

You can solve this problem by using the ratio-proportion method or by using the dimensional analysis method.

Ratio-Proportion Method

To begin, convert the household units of measurement to metric units of measurement.

$$1 \text{ tbsp} = 15 \text{ mL}$$

Then set up a proportion of the unknown quantity (x mg) over the conversion (15 mL) on the left side of the equation, and the milligrams per milliliter of the available stock medication on the right side of the equation. Remember that the units of measurement in the numerators and in the denominators must match. Then solve for x.

$$\frac{x\text{ mg}}{15\text{ mL}} = \frac{125\text{ mg}}{5\text{ mL}}$$

$$x\text{ mg (5 mL)} = 125\text{ mg (15 mL)}$$

$$x = 375\text{ mg}$$

Dimensional Analysis Method

$$\frac{1\text{ tbsp}}{1} \times \frac{15\text{ mL}}{1\text{ tbsp}} \times \frac{125\text{ mg}}{5\text{ mL}} = 375\text{ mg}$$

Answer: There are 375 mg of medication in 1 tbsp of clarithromycin oral suspension.

Determining Quantity to Dispense for Liquid Oral Dosage Forms

Liquid medications are typically ordered and billed by volume (in most cases, milliliters). The volume dispensed is often indicated by the prescriber on a prescription or a medication order. However, some prescriptions and medication orders may not have explicit instructions on how much medication to dispense. For example, you may see a prescription that states the following: *Take 2 tsp every morning for 10 days*. This prescription does not specify the quantity to dispense. You may also see a prescription or a medication order that uses the abbreviation *QS*, which means to dispense a "quantity sufficient" to meet the needs of the patient given the dosing instructions. In these situations, the volume of medication to dispense can be calculated by determining the volume needed for a single day and multiplying this volume by the duration of therapy. Both the ratio-proportion and dimensional analysis methods can be used to determine the quantity to dispense.

Example 5.2.8

A patient comes to the pharmacy with a prescription that does not indicate a quantity to dispense. The prescription states the following: *amoxicillin 125 mg/5 mL, 1 tsp TID for 10 days.* **What is the total volume of medication to be dispensed?**

You can solve this problem by using the ratio-proportion method or by using the dimensional analysis method.

Ratio-Proportion Method

To begin, convert the household unit of measurement to a metric unit of measurement.

$$1\text{ tsp} = 5\text{ mL}$$

Therefore, 1 tsp/dose equals 5 mL/dose. You also know that the patient is to take that 5 mL dose three times a day (TID).

Next, use that information to calculate how many milliliters of medication are taken each day. Remember that the units of measurement in the numerators and in the denominators must match. Then solve for x.

$$\frac{x \text{ mL}}{3 \text{ doses}} = \frac{5 \text{ mL}}{1 \text{ dose}}$$

$$x \text{ mL (1 dose)} = 5 \text{ mL (3 doses)}$$

$$x = 15 \text{ mL}$$

Now, determine how many milliliters of medication are taken over the course of therapy—in this case, 10 days. To do so, set up a proportion of the unknown quantity (x mL) over the duration of therapy (10 days) on the left side of the equation and the number of milliliters taken each day (15 mL) on the right side of the equation. Remember that the units of measurement in the numerators and in the denominators must match. Then solve for x.

$$\frac{x \text{ mL}}{10 \text{ days}} = \frac{15 \text{ mL}}{1 \text{ day}}$$

$$x \text{ mL (1 day)} = 15 \text{ mL (10 days)}$$

$$x = 150 \text{ mL}$$

Dimensional Analysis Multi-Step Method

To begin, convert the household unit of measurement to a metric unit of measurement.

$$1 \text{ tsp} = 5 \text{ mL}$$

Using that conversion, you know that 1 tsp/dose equals 5 mL/dose.

Next, calculate how much medication is needed for one day if the patient is to take the medication three times a day (TID).

$$\frac{5 \text{ mL}}{\text{dose}} \times \frac{3 \text{ doses}}{\text{day}} = \frac{15 \text{ mL}}{\text{day}}$$

Finally, determine the volume of medication to dispense.

$$\frac{15 \text{ mL}}{\text{day}} \times 10 \text{ days} = 150 \text{ mL}$$

Dimensional Analysis One-Step Method

$$\frac{1 \text{ tsp}}{\text{dose}} \times \frac{3 \text{ doses}}{\text{day}} \times \frac{10 \text{ days}}{1} \times \frac{5 \text{ mL}}{1 \text{ tsp}} = 150 \text{ mL}$$

Answer: The total volume of medication to be dispensed is 150 mL.

Example 5.2.9

A patient is to take 2 tsp of fluoxetine hydrochloride each morning for 30 days. How many milliliters will be needed? How many bottles with the label shown will be required to fill this prescription?

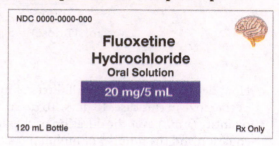

NDC 0000-0000-000

Fluoxetine Hydrochloride
Oral Solution

20 mg/5 mL

120 mL Bottle   Rx Only

You can solve this problem by using the ratio-proportion method or by using the dimensional analysis method.

Ratio-Proportion Method

To begin, convert the household unit of measurement to a metric unit of measurement.

$$1 \text{ tsp} = 5 \text{ mL}$$

Now, calculate the volume of medication the patient should take each day. You know that 1 tsp = 5 mL and that the patient is to take 2 tsp/day.

$$\frac{x \text{ mL}}{2 \text{ tsp}} \times \frac{5 \text{ mL}}{1 \text{ tsp}}$$

$$x \text{ mL } (1 \text{ tsp}) = 5 \text{ mL } (2 \text{ tsp})$$

$$x = 10 \text{ mL}$$

Next, calculate how much medication is needed for the duration of therapy, which is 30 days. Remember that the units of measurement in the numerators and in the denominators must match. Then solve for x.

$$\frac{x \text{ mL}}{30 \text{ days}} \times \frac{10 \text{ mL}}{1 \text{ day}}$$

$$x \text{ mL } (1 \text{ day}) = 10 \text{ mL } (30 \text{ days})$$

$$x = 300 \text{ mL}$$

Now, determine the number of bottles needed to dispense 300 mL. The volume of each bottle can be found on the medication label above. Set up a proportion to solve for x.

$$\frac{x \text{ bottles}}{300 \text{ mL}} = \frac{1 \text{ bottle}}{120 \text{ mL}}$$

$$x \text{ bottles } (120 \text{ mL}) = 1 \text{ bottle } (300 \text{ mL})$$

$$x = 2.5 \text{ bottles, rounded to 3 full bottles}$$

Dimensional Analysis Multi-Step Method

To begin, convert the household unit of measurement to a metric unit of measurement.

$$1 \text{ tsp} = 5 \text{ mL}$$

Now, calculate the volume of medication the patient should take each day. You know that 1 tsp = 5 mL and that the patient is to take 2 tsp/day.

$$\frac{2 \text{ tsp}}{\text{day}} \times \frac{5 \text{ mL}}{1 \text{ tsp}} = 10 \text{ mL/day}$$

Next, calculate how much medication is needed for the duration of therapy, which is 30 days.

$$\frac{10 \text{ mL}}{\text{day}} \times 30 \text{ days} = 300 \text{ mL}$$

Finally, calculate the number of bottles of medication needed. The label indicates that each bottle contains 120 mL.

$$\frac{300 \text{ mL}}{1} \times \frac{1 \text{ bottle}}{120 \text{ mL}} = 2.5 \text{ bottles, rounded to 3 full bottles}$$

Dimensional Analysis One-Step Method

This problem has two questions: *How many milliliters will be needed?* and *How many bottles will be required to fill this prescription?* Therefore, the one-step method must be performed twice.

To determine the number of milliliters needed, set up the following calculation.

$$\frac{2 \text{ tsp}}{\text{dose}} \times \frac{1 \text{ dose}}{\text{day}} \times \frac{30 \text{ day}}{1} \times \frac{5 \text{ mL}}{\text{tsp}} = 300 \text{ mL}$$

To determine the number of bottles required to fill the prescription, set up the following calculation.

$$\frac{300 \text{ mL}}{1} \times \frac{1 \text{ bottle}}{120 \text{ mL}} = 2.5 \text{ bottles, rounded to 3 bottles}$$

Answer: The patient will need 300 mL of fluoxetine hydrochloride for 30 days of therapy. Three of the 120 mL bottles are necessary to dispense 300 mL of this medication.

Determining Days' Supply for Liquid Oral Dosage Forms

A related calculation to the quantity to dispense is determining the number of days a dispensed volume will last, or days' supply. In Chapter 3, days' supply was calculated for solid dosage forms. The following examples calculate days' supply for liquid oral dosage forms. While both the ratio-proportion method and dimensional analysis methods can be used, only the dimensional analysis method is shown.

Example 5.2.10

A patient is taking 2 tsp of medication every 8 hours. The patient has a 6 fl oz bottle of medication. How many days will the medication last?

Dimensional Analysis Multi-Step Method

To begin, convert the household units of measurement to metric units of measurement.

$$1 \text{ tsp} = 5 \text{ mL; therefore, } \frac{2 \text{ tsp}}{\text{dose}} \times \frac{5 \text{ mL}}{\text{tsp}} = \frac{10 \text{ mL}}{\text{dose}}$$

$$1 \text{ fl oz} = 30 \text{ mL; therefore, } \frac{6 \text{ fl oz}}{\text{bottle}} \times \frac{30 \text{ mL}}{1 \text{ fl oz}} = \frac{180 \text{ mL}}{\text{bottle}}$$

Next, determine how much medication is needed for one day of treatment. If the patient takes a dose every 8 hours and there are 24 hours in a day, set up the following calculations.

$$\frac{24 \text{ hr}}{\text{day}} \times \frac{1 \text{ dose}}{8 \text{ hr}} = \frac{3 \text{ doses}}{\text{day}}$$

$$\frac{3 \text{ doses}}{\text{day}} \times \frac{10 \text{ mL}}{\text{dose}} = \frac{30 \text{ mL}}{\text{day}}$$

Finally, calculate the number of days the medication will last.

$$\frac{180 \text{ mL}}{\text{bottle}} \times \frac{1 \text{ day}}{30 \text{ mL}} = \frac{6 \text{ days}}{\text{bottle}}$$

Dimensional Analysis One-Step Method

$$\frac{6 \text{ fl oz}}{\text{bottle}} \times \frac{30 \text{ mL}}{1 \text{ fl oz}} \times \frac{1 \text{ tsp}}{5 \text{ mL}} \times \frac{8 \text{ hr}}{2 \text{ tsp}} \times \frac{1 \text{ day}}{24 \text{ hr}} = \frac{6 \text{ days}}{\text{bottle}}$$

Answer: The 6 fl oz bottle will last 6 days.

Example 5.2.11

A patient is to take 1 tsp of a medication twice daily. The patient has a 4 fl oz bottle of medication. How many milliliters of medication will the patient take in one day? How many days will the medication last?

To begin, convert the household units of measurement to metric units of measurement.

$$1 \text{ tsp} = 5 \text{ mL; therefore, } \frac{1 \text{ tsp}}{\text{dose}} \times \frac{5 \text{ mL}}{\text{tsp}} = \frac{5 \text{ mL}}{\text{dose}}$$

$$1 \text{ fl oz} = 30 \text{ mL; therefore, } \frac{4 \text{ fl oz}}{\text{bottle}} \times \frac{30 \text{ mL}}{1 \text{ fl oz}} = \frac{120 \text{ mL}}{\text{bottle}}$$

Next, determine how much medication is needed for one day. The dose is taken twice daily, so there are 2 doses/day.

$$\frac{2 \text{ doses}}{\text{day}} \times \frac{5 \text{ mL}}{\text{dose}} = \frac{10 \text{ mL}}{\text{day}}$$

Finally, calculate the number of days the medication will last.

$$\frac{120 \text{ mL}}{\text{bottle}} \times \frac{1 \text{ day}}{10 \text{ mL}} = \frac{12 \text{ days}}{\text{bottle}}$$

Answer: The patient will take 10 mL/day, and the medication will last 12 days.

Example 5.2.12

A patient has a prescription that states the following: *Take Magic Cough Syrup 1–2 tsp every 4–6 hours prn cough. Disp: 8 fl oz.* **If the patient uses the maximum prescribed amount, how many days will the cough syrup last?**

Dimensional Analysis Multi-Step Method

To begin, convert the household units of measurement to metric units of measurement. As prescribed, the patient will take up to 2 teaspoonfuls/dose. Using 2 teaspoonfuls/dose for the calculation will provide the maximum volume of cough syrup in a dose.

$$1 \text{ tsp} = 5 \text{ mL; therefore,} \frac{2 \text{ tsp}}{\text{dose}} \times \frac{5 \text{ mL}}{\text{tsp}} = \frac{10 \text{ mL}}{\text{dose}}$$

$$1 \text{ fl oz} = 30 \text{ mL; therefore, an} \frac{8 \text{ fl oz}}{\text{bottle}} \times \frac{30 \text{ mL}}{1 \text{ fl oz}} = \frac{240 \text{ mL}}{\text{bottle}}$$

Next, determine how much medication is needed for one day. As prescribed, the patient will take the medication up to 6 times a day (every 4 hours). Using 6 doses a day for the calculation will provide the minimum number of days the medication will last.

$$\frac{6 \text{ doses}}{\text{day}} \times \frac{10 \text{ mL}}{\text{dose}} = \frac{60 \text{ mL}}{\text{day}}$$

Finally, determine the number of days the medication will last.

$$\frac{240 \text{ mL}}{\text{bottle}} \times \frac{1 \text{ day}}{60 \text{ mL}} = \frac{4 \text{ days}}{\text{bottle}}$$

Dimensional Analysis One-Step Method

$$\frac{8 \text{ fl oz}}{1} \times \frac{30 \text{ mL}}{1 \text{ fl oz}} \times \frac{1 \text{ tsp}}{5 \text{mL}} \times \frac{4 \text{ hr}}{2 \text{ tsp}} \times \frac{1 \text{ day}}{24 \text{ hr}} = 4 \text{ days}$$

Answer: The minimum number of days one bottle of the medication will last is 4 days. Note that the medication may last longer if the patient uses the prescription less than 6 times a day or uses 1 teaspoonful a dose instead of 2 teaspoonfuls/dose.

Determining Pediatric Doses Using Dosing Tables

The methods in which doses are determined for pediatric patients are often different from the methods used for adult patients. Consider the over-the-counter (OTC) analgesic acetaminophen. A typical adult dose of acetaminophen is 325 mg. However, there is no single, typical pediatric dose. The pediatric dose of acetaminophen varies and depends on specific factors. One resource that provides assistance in determining acetaminophen doses in pediatric patients is a dosing table.

A **dosing table** is a guide that includes an age range and/or a weight range with corresponding doses. Dosing tables are used for both oral liquids and solid dosage forms, but oral liquids are easier for young patients to take and, therefore, are more commonly prescribed.

Dosing tables often appear on OTC packaging for products used for children older than age two. For medications used for children under age two, the labels instruct caregivers to consult the child's physician. The table for children under age two is available to healthcare providers in pharmacies and physicians' offices. Physicians often instruct parents to purchase OTC medications for small children, so appropriate dosing instructions must be provided for these patients. Dosing may need to be translated from metric units of measurement to household units of measurement. Use the dosing information in Tables 5.2 and 5.3 to complete the following examples.

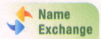

TABLE 5.2 Pediatric Acetaminophen Dosing

Age	Dose
0–3 mo	40 mg
4–11 mo	80 mg
1–2 yr	120 mg
2–3 yr	160 mg
4–5 yr	240 mg
6–8 yr	320 mg
9–10 yr	400 mg
11 yr to adult	480 mg
adult maximum	4,000 mg daily

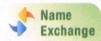

TABLE 5.3 Pediatric Ibuprofen Dosing

Age	Weight (lb)	Weight (kg)	Dose
6–11 mo	12–17 lb	5–7 kg	50 mg
12–23 mo	18–23 lb	8–10 kg	75 mg
2–3 yr	24–35 lb	11–16 kg	100 mg
4–5 yr	36–47 lb	17–21 kg	150 mg
6–8 yr	48–59 lb	22–27 kg	200 mg
9–10 yr	60–71 lb	28–32 kg	250 mg
11 yr	72–95 lb	33–43 kg	300 mg

Example 5.2.13

A 12-month-old child weighing 22 lb is to receive one dose of acetaminophen. According to the dosing information in Table 5.2, what is the appropriate dose?

Answer: Because the acetaminophen dosing is by age, not weight, you would use the dosing information for the age category 1–2 yr. The appropriate dose would be 120 mg.

Example 5.2.14

A parent wants to give her 15-month-old child, who weighs 21 lb, an appropriate dose of OTC ibuprofen. The package provides the dosing information shown in Table 5.3. What is the appropriate dose?

Answer: The dose can be determined by either age or weight, and, for this child, the dosing would be the same. The appropriate dose would be 75 mg.

Example 5.2.15

A parent is instructed to give his 4-year-old child acetaminophen alternating with ibuprofen. What is the appropriate dose for each drug?

Answer: The acetaminophen dose would be 240 mg, and the ibuprofen dose would be 150 mg.

5.2 Problem Set

1. A patient has brought in a prescription for a diabetes medication. The prescription states the following: *Take 1 tablet before breakfast, 1 tablet before lunch, and 1 tablet before dinner.* Determine the quantity to dispense for a 30 days' supply.

2. How many prednisone 5 mg tablets are needed to fill the following prescription?

 Prednisone 5 mg
Take 4 tablets × 2 days.
Take 3 tablets × 2 days.
Take 1 tablet × 1 day.

Applications

Solve these oral dose calculation problems. Round your answers to the nearest tenth as necessary.

3. A patient takes 1 tsp daily of a medication, and the drug has a concentration of 80 mg/15 mL. How many milligrams are in one dose?

4. A patient needs to have 60 mg of medication, and the drug has a concentration of 120 mg/5 mL. How many teaspoonfuls will the patient take?

5. If there are 24 mg in a teaspoonful of liquid medication, how many grams are in 8 fl oz of the medication?

6. How many milligrams are in 4 fl oz of a liquid medication with a concentration of 65 mg/tbsp?

7. How many milligrams are in a 2 tsp dose of liquid medication if there are 2.5 g in 2 fl oz?

8. How many milligrams are in a 1 tbsp dose of liquid medication if there are 260 mg in 600 mL?

9. A prescription states the following: *Take 2 tsp of medication BID.* The required strength of the medication is 25 mg/tsp. How many grams are needed to prepare 20 fl oz?

10. A prescription states the following: *Take 1 tbsp of medication qam.* The available strength of the drug is 30 mg/5 mL. How many milligrams are in a 1 tbsp dose?

11. A prescription states the following: *Take 1 tbsp of medication BID.* The available strength of the medication is 40 mg/mL. How many grams are needed to prepare 1 pt of medication?

12. A patient is taking $^3/_4$ tsp of an antibiotic suspension three times a day.

    a. How long will a 150 mL bottle of antibiotic suspension last this patient?

    b. How many milliliters will remain in the bottle after 10 days?

13. An antibiotic suspension is available in 80 mL, 150 mL, and 200 mL bottles.

    a. What size bottle of antibiotic suspension will a patient need in order to take 1 tsp twice daily for 14 days?

    b. How many milliliters will remain in the bottle after 14 days?

14. How many days will a 12 fl oz bottle last if a patient takes 1 tbsp TID?

15. A patient is on an alternate-day therapy consisting of 2 tsp of a medication one day and 1 tbsp the next day. How many days will a 300 mL bottle last?

16. If there are 25 mg in 1 tbsp of liquid medication, how many grams are in 20 fl oz?

17. A patient uses 1 fl oz of an antacid TID and hs. How many 12 fl oz bottles will this patient need to last 14 days?

18. How many prednisone 5 mg tablets are needed to fill the following prescription?

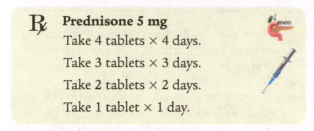

℞ **Prednisone 5 mg**
Take 4 tablets × 4 days.
Take 3 tablets × 3 days.
Take 2 tablets × 2 days.
Take 1 tablet × 1 day.

19. How many milliliters of nystatin must be dispensed for the following prescription?

℞ **Nystatin Oral Suspension**
Dosing instructions: Use 1 mL in each cheek pouch q3h
Quantity to dispense: qs 10 days

20. There are 25 mg in 1 tsp of liquid medication. You are dispensing 12 fl oz. How many milligrams will be in the bottle?

21. For the prescription below, how many fluid ounces of nystatin must be dispensed?

℞ **Nystatin Oral Suspension**
Take ii teaspoonfuls 3 times daily for 15 days.

22. A prescription states the following: *Take 2 tbsp of an oral elixir three times daily for 20 days.* How many milliliters should be dispensed?

Use the following label to answer questions 23 and 24.

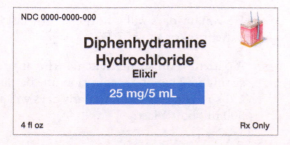

NDC 0000-0000-000

Diphenhydramine Hydrochloride
Elixir

25 mg/5 mL

4 fl oz   Rx Only

23. A mother has two children who have poison ivy. One child takes 1 tsp TID, and the other child takes 2 tsp TID. How many bottles of diphenhydramine hydrochloride elixir will be needed to supply both children for 4 days?

24. How many milligrams are contained in each child's dose?

Use the following label to answer questions 25–28.

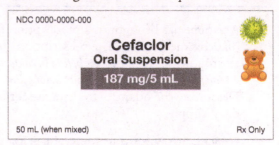

NDC 0000-0000-000

Cefaclor
Oral Suspension

187 mg/5 mL

50 mL (when mixed)   Rx Only

25. How many milligrams are in ³/₄ tsp?

26. How many milligrams are in 1 ¹/₂ tsp?

27. How many milliliters are needed to provide 125 mg?

28. How many milliliters are needed to provide 500 mg?

29. The following order for absolute (dehydrated) alcohol has been brought into the compounding pharmacy. How many syringes can be made from a 12 oz bottle of absolute alcohol?

℞ 1. Obtain a 12 fl oz bottle of absolute alcohol from the narcotics cabinet.
2. Filter through a 0.2 micron filter.
3. Fill 60 mL syringes with filtered absolute alcohol.

Complete the following calculations regarding aspirin dosing.

Aspirin is typically contraindicated in children. If a child is unable to take acetaminophen or ibuprofen, however, aspirin may be used. Additionally, aspirin is indicated for some conditions in children such as antiplatelet therapy and antirheumatic therapy. Items 30–33 identify the age of a child. For each child, determine the milligram dose of aspirin every 4 hours using the dosing table provided.

Aspirin Dosing Table

Age (years)	Weight (lb)	Weight (kg)	Dose (every 4 hr)
2–3	24–35	10.6–15.9	162 mg
4–5	36–47	16–21.4	243 mg
6–8	48–59	21.5–26.8	324 mg
9–10	60–71	26.9–32.3	405 mg
11	72–95	32.4–43.2	486 mg
12–14	≥ 96	≥ 43.3	648 mg

30. 4 years

31. 7 years

32. 10 years

33. 14 years

Complete the following calculations regarding levothyroxine dosing.

Levothyroxine is indicated for children who have hypothyroidism. Many states require infants to be tested for hypothyroidism shortly after birth so that therapy can begin immediately if needed. In adult patients, the dose is adjusted up or down based on blood titers and clinical signs and symptoms. Newborn patients are more difficult to assess, so a standard dosing table based on kilograms has been developed. For items 35–38, determine the daily dose of levothyroxine for each child using the dosing table provided.

Levothyroxine Dosing Table

Age	Daily Dose Per Kilogram
0 to 3 mo	10–15 mcg
3 to 6 mo	8–10 mcg
6 to 12 mo	6–8 mcg
1 to 5 yr	5–6 mcg
6 to 12 yr	4–5 mcg
> 12 yr	2–3 mcg

34. newborn (6 lb)

35. newborn (7 lb, 12 oz)

36. 11-month-old (23 lb)

37. 15-month-old (18 lb)

Self-check your work in Appendix A

5.3 Patient-Specific Dose Calculations

Medications are typically prescribed by indicating a specific amount on a prescription or a medication order. For example, a prescription for the cholesterol-lowering medication rosuvastatin may indicate that a patient is to take 10 mg by mouth daily. Other times, a prescription or a medication order may indicate that a drug is to be dosed based on a patient-specific factor (such as weight or body surface area). The anticoagulant enoxaparin, for example, may be dosed based on a patient's weight. A medication order for enoxaparin may simply state 1 mg/kg instead of offering a specific dosage. In these cases, it may be necessary for the pharmacist or pharmacy technician to calculate or verify a patient-specific dose.

Calculating Doses Based on Weight

A patient's weight may be especially important when calculating a customized dose of a medication. This practice is especially common for pediatric patients (newborn to age 18) whose weight differs from the weight of young adult and middle-age patients, an age range that is used by manufacturers to establish medication prescribing guidelines. In addition to wide-ranging weights, the physiology of pediatric patients may not metabolize or eliminate medications at the same rate as patients in other age groups. In these cases, manufacturers will often offer prescribing guidelines for medications based upon a therapeutic amount or range per unit of body weight. The most common unit used is milligram of a medication per kilogram of body weight (or mg/kg).

There are instances where medications for adult patients are dosed based on body weight. Medications that have a small difference between toxic and therapeutic doses (called *narrow therapeutic index drugs*) may be dosed this way. For example, the narrow therapeutic index drug phenytoin (an anticonvulsant) may be dosed based on a patient's weight.

The following examples demonstrate calculations used to customize a dose. When calculating a patient's weight and a dose associated with that weight, round to the nearest tenth, unless greater accuracy can be measured, as indicated in the example or question provided.

Example 5.3.1

A medication order indicates that a patient is to receive 15 mg/kg of a medication. The patient weighs 60 kg, and the medication is available in a 300 mg capsule. What dose should the patient receive? How many capsules will be dispensed for one dose?

You can solve this problem by using the ratio-proportion method or by using the dimensional analysis method.

Ratio-Proportion Method

To begin, ask yourself the following question: *What am I looking for to solve the problem?* In this scenario, you are looking for two components: the dose and the number of capsules to dispense for one dose.

To determine the dose, set up a proportion. Place the unknown amount (x mg) over the patient's weight (60 kg) on the left side of the proportion and the prescribed dose (15 mg/kg) on the right side of the proportion. Be sure that the units in the numerators and in the denominators match. Then solve for x.

$$\frac{x \text{ mg}}{60 \text{ kg}} = \frac{15 \text{ mg}}{1 \text{ kg}}$$

$$x \text{ mg (1 kg)} = 15 \text{ mg (60 kg)}$$

$$x = 900 \text{ mg}$$

Next, determine the number of capsules to be dispensed for one dose. Set up a proportion by placing the unknown amount (*x* capsules) over the dose (900 mg) on the left side of the proportion and the known amount (1 capsule contains 300 mg) on the right side of the proportion. Be sure that the units in the numerators and in the denominators match. Then solve for *x*.

$$\frac{x \text{ capsules}}{900 \text{ mg}} = \frac{1 \text{ capsule}}{300 \text{ mg}}$$

$$x \text{ capsules (300 mg)} = 1 \text{ capsule (900 mg)}$$

$$x = 3 \text{ capsules}$$

Dimensional Analysis Multi-Step Method

To begin, determine the dose.

$$\frac{60 \text{ kg}}{1} \times \frac{15 \text{ mg}}{\text{kg}} = 900 \text{ mg}$$

Then determine the number of capsules to be dispensed for one dose.

$$\frac{900 \text{ mg}}{1} \times \frac{1 \text{ capsule}}{300 \text{ mg}} = 3 \text{ capsules}$$

Answer: The patient will receive a dose of 900 mg, and 3 capsules should be dispensed for one dose.

Example 5.3.2

A medication order indicates that a patient is to receive a dose of 0.4 mg/kg of medication. The patient weighs 74 kg. What dose will the patient receive? If the medication is available in a 15 mg/10 mL solution, how many milliliters of medication will the patient receive in one dose? Round to the nearest tenth of a milliliter.

You can solve this problem by using the ratio-proportion method or by using the dimensional analysis method.

Ratio-Proportion Method

To begin, ask yourself the following question: *What am I looking for to solve the problem?* In this scenario, you are looking for two components: the dose and the number of milliliters to dispense for one dose.

To determine the dose, set up a proportion. Place the unknown amount (*x* mg) over the patient's weight (74 kg) on the left side of the proportion and the prescribed amount (0.4 mg/kg) on the right side of the proportion. Be sure that the units in the numerators and in the denominators match. Then solve for *x*.

$$\frac{x \text{ mg}}{74 \text{ kg}} = \frac{0.4 \text{ mg}}{1 \text{ kg}}$$

$$x \text{ mg (1 kg)} = 0.4 \text{ mg (74 kg)}$$

$$x = 29.6 \text{ mg}$$

Next, determine the number of milliliters to be dispensed for one dose. Set up a proportion by placing the unknown amount (x mL) over the dose (29.6 mg) on the left side of the proportion and the available concentration (15 mg/10 mL) on the right side of the proportion. Be sure that the units in the numerators and in the denominators match. Then solve for x.

$$\frac{x \text{ mL}}{29.6 \text{ mg}} = \frac{10 \text{ mL}}{15 \text{ mg}}$$

$$x \text{ mL } (15 \text{ mg}) = 10 \text{ mL } (29.6 \text{ mg})$$

$$x = 19.73 \text{ mL, rounded to } 19.7 \text{ mL}$$

Dimensional Analysis Multi-Step Method

To begin, determine the dose.

$$\frac{74 \text{ kg}}{1} \times \frac{0.4 \text{ mg}}{\text{kg}} = 29.6 \text{ mg}$$

Then determine the number of milliliters to be dispensed for one dose.

$$\frac{29.6 \text{ mg}}{1} \times \frac{10 \text{ mL}}{15 \text{ mg}} = 19.73 \text{ mL, rounded to } 19.7 \text{ mL}$$

Dimensional Analysis One-Step Method

$$\frac{74 \text{ kg}}{1} \times \frac{0.4 \text{ mg}}{\text{kg}} \times \frac{10 \text{ mL}}{15 \text{ mg}} = 19.73 \text{ mL, rounded to } 19.7 \text{ mL}$$

Answer: The patient will receive a dose of 29.6 mg, and 19.7 mL should be dispensed for one dose.

Calculating Doses Based on Body Surface Area

Body surface area (BSA) is a measurement based on weight and height variables and is expressed as meters squared (m^2). BSA takes a patient's overall size into account. Dosing based on BSA may help a patient receive the optimal amount of a drug, while minimizing toxicity. Chemotherapy, for example, may be dosed based on BSA.

BSA is calculated using a formula. A commonly used BSA formula is the Mosteller formula, shown below.

$$\text{BSA (in meters squared or } m^2) = \sqrt{\frac{\text{height (cm)} \times \text{weight (kg)}}{3,600}}$$

BSA is often provided in a patient's electronic health record. It is unusual for a pharmacy technician to need to calculate BSA. However, a pharmacy technician may need to use a patient's provided BSA to calculate specific doses. Medication doses based on BSA are often given in the following units: milligrams of medication per meters squared of BSA (or mg/m^2). The following examples use the ratio-proportion and dimensional analysis methods to determine a dose based on BSA.

Example 5.3.3

A patient is to receive a medication with the dose based on 50 mg/m². If the patient has a BSA of 0.90 m², what will the dose be? If the medication is available only in 15 mg tablets, how many tablets will be dispensed for one dose?

You can solve this problem by using the ratio-proportion method or by using the dimensional analysis method.

Ratio-Proportion Method

To determine the dose, set up a proportion. Place the unknown amount (x mg) over the patient's BSA (0.90 m²) on the left side of the proportion and the prescribed dose (50 mg/m²) on the right side of the proportion. Be sure that the units in the numerators and in the denominators match. Then solve for x.

$$\frac{x \text{ mg}}{0.90 \text{ m}^2} = \frac{50 \text{ mg}}{1 \text{ m}^2}$$

$$x \text{ mg} (1 \text{ m}^2) = 50 \text{ mg} (0.90 \text{ m}^2)$$

$$x = 45 \text{ mg}$$

Next, determine the number of tablets to be dispensed for one dose. Set up a proportion by placing the unknown amount (x tablets) over the dose (45 mg) on the left side of the proportion and the known amount (15 mg/1 tab) on the right side of the proportion. Be sure that the units in the numerators and in the denominators match. Then solve for x.

$$\frac{x \text{ tablets}}{45 \text{ mg}} = \frac{1 \text{ tablet}}{15 \text{ mg}}$$

$$x \text{ tablets} (15 \text{ mg}) = 45 \text{ mg} (1 \text{ tablet})$$

$$x = 3 \text{ tablets}$$

Dimensional Analysis Multi-Step Method

To begin, multiply the patient's BSA (in this case, 0.90 m²) by the medication dose based on BSA (in this case, 50 mg/m²).

$$\frac{0.90 \text{ m}^2}{1} \times \frac{50 \text{ mg}}{\text{m}^2} = 45 \text{ mg}$$

Then use this dose to determine the number of tablets to dispense.

$$\frac{45 \text{ mg}}{1} \times \frac{1 \text{ tablet}}{15 \text{ mg}} = 3 \text{ tablets}$$

Answer: The patient will receive a dose of 45 mg, and 3 tablets will be dispensed for one dose.

Example 5.3.4

A patient with a BSA of 1.30 m² is to receive a medication with the dose based on 0.80 mg/m². The prescription is to be divided into three equal doses. How much will each dose be? Round to the nearest hundredth of a milligram. If the medication is available only as 50 mcg tablets, how many tablets will be dispensed?

You can solve this problem by using the ratio-proportion method or by using the dimensional analysis method.

Ratio-Proportion Method

To determine the dose, set up a proportion. Place the unknown amount (x mg) over the patient's BSA (1.30 m²) on the left side of the proportion and the prescribed dose (0.80 mg/m²) on the right side of the proportion. Be sure that the units in the numerators and in the denominators match. Then solve for x.

$$\frac{x \text{ mg}}{1.30 \text{ m}^2} = \frac{0.80 \text{ mg}}{1 \text{ m}^2}$$

$$x \text{ mg} (1 \text{ m}^2) = 0.80 \text{ mg} (1.30 \text{ m}^2)$$

$$x = 1.04 \text{ mg}$$

Then divide the daily dose by 3 to determine the amount of each dose.

$$\frac{1.04 \text{ mg}}{3} = 0.346 \text{ mg, rounded to } 0.35 \text{ mg}$$

Now convert the dose in milligrams (0.35 mg) into the available tablet size in micrograms (mcg).

$$\frac{x \text{ mcg}}{0.35 \text{ mg}} = \frac{1,000 \text{ mcg}}{1 \text{ mg}}$$

$$x \text{ mcg} (1 \text{ mg}) = 1,000 \text{ mcg} (0.35 \text{ mg})$$

$$x = 350 \text{ mcg}$$

Next, determine the number of tablets to be dispensed for one dose. Set up a proportion by placing the unknown amount (x tablets) over the dose (350 mcg) on the left side of the proportion and the known amount (1 tablet/50 mcg) on the right side of the proportion. Be sure that the units in the numerators and in the denominators match. Then solve for x.

$$\frac{x \text{ tablets}}{350 \text{ mcg}} = \frac{1 \text{ tablet}}{50 \text{ mcg}}$$

$$x \text{ tablets} (50 \text{ mcg}) = 1 \text{ tablet} (350 \text{ mcg})$$

$$x = 7 \text{ tablets}$$

Dimensional Analysis Multi-Step Method

To begin, multiply the patient's BSA (in this case, 1.30 m²) by the medication dose based on BSA (in this case, 0.80 mg/m²).

$$\frac{1.30 \text{ m}^2}{1} \times \frac{0.80 \text{ mg}}{\text{m}^2} = 1.04 \text{ mg}$$

Next, divide the dose (1.04 mg) by 3 to determine three equal doses.

$$1.04 \text{ mg} \div 3 \text{ doses} = \frac{0.346 \text{ mcg}}{\text{dose}}, \text{ rounded to } \frac{0.35 \text{ mg}}{\text{dose}}$$

Then convert the dose from milligrams to micrograms (the units of the tablets) by using the equivalency 1 mg equals 1,000 mcg.

$$\frac{0.35 \text{ mg}}{1} \times \frac{1,000 \text{ mcg}}{1 \text{ mg}} = 350 \text{ mcg}$$

Now that you know that one dose is 350 mcg and each tablet is 50 mcg, you can determine how many tablets will be dispensed.

$$\frac{350 \text{ mcg}}{1} \times \frac{1 \text{ tablet}}{50 \text{ mcg}} = 7 \text{ tablets}$$

Answer: Each dose of medication contains 350 mcg, and 7 tablets will be dispensed.

5.3 Problem Set

Applications

1. Cortisone is dosed at 0.5 mg/kg per day. If the patient weighs 56 kg, what dose will the patient receive?

2. A postsurgical patient is to receive 125 mg/kg per day of cephalosporin divided into six doses daily. What will each dose be for a patient weighing 87 kg?

3. A premature infant is to receive 4 mL/kg of a medication. If the infant weighs 1.4 kg, how much medication will be administered?

4. A drug is to be given at a dose of 0.625 mg/kg.

   a. If a patient weighs 80 kg, what dose will be administered?

   b. If the dose you just calculated is to be divided and given three times over the course of 24 hours, what is the size of each dose? Round your answer to the nearest hundredth of a milligram.

5. A newborn weighs 6 kg and is to be given medication at 5 mg/kg per day in two divided doses. How much will each dose be?

6. A patient weighs 68.64 kg and is to receive 125 mg/kg of medication per day. How many milligrams are in this dose?

7. A child weighs 10 kg and is to receive a medication dose of 10 mg/kg per day. The medication should be administered in equal doses every 12 hours. How many milligrams are in each dose?

Calculate the following BSA-based doses.

8. A patient is to receive a medication dose based on the BSA of 25 mg/m² per day, divided into two equal doses. The patient has a BSA of 1.1 m². How much will each dose be?

9. A patient is to receive a medication dose based on the BSA of 0.75 mg/m². The patient has a BSA of 0.67 m². How much of the medication will you prepare? Round your answer to the nearest tenth.

10. The medication order for a patient states that a dose is to be based on the BSA of 100 mg/m². If this patient has a BSA of 0.85 m², what dose will be prepared?

11. A child is to receive acyclovir at 250 mg/m². The child's BSA is 0.71 m². What will the dose be?

12. Methotrexate is to be given at 3.3 mg/m². The patient has a BSA of 0.83 m². What will the dose be? Round your answer to the nearest tenth of a milligram.

Determine if the following doses are safe according to the manufacturer's recommended doses.

13. A pediatric patient has a BSA of 0.7 m². The manufacturer of vincristine has a recommended dose of 2 mg/m². The physician has ordered 1.9 mg of vincristine. Is the physician's order safe according to the recommended dose?

14. A pediatric patient has a BSA of 0.48 m². The manufacturer of methotrexate has a recommended dose of 3.3 mg/m². The physician has ordered 2.5 mg of methotrexate. Is the physician's order safe according to the recommended dose?

15. A pediatric patient has a BSA of 0.47 m². The manufacturer of acyclovir has a recommended dose of 250 mg/m² every 8 hours. The physician has ordered 200 mg of acyclovir TID. Is the physician's order safe according to the recommended dose?

16. A patient weighs 40.9 kg and is 58" in height. The manufacturer of erythromycin has a recommended dose of 50 mg/kg per day. The physician has ordered 300 mg of erythromycin TID. Is the physician's order safe according to the recommended dose?

Calculate dosage ranges for the following and determine whether the prescribed dose is in the recommended safe range.

17. A pediatric patient weighs 36.4 kg and is 48" in height. The manufacturer of cefazolin has a recommended dose of 50–100 mg/kg per day. The physician has prescribed 250 mg TID.

   a. Calculate the minimum daily dose for this pediatric patient.

   b. Calculate the maximum daily dose for this pediatric patient.

   c. Is the physician's dose within the recommended safe range?

   d. How many milliliters will be prepared for one prescribed dose if the product is available as a 500 mg/50 mL solution?

18. A pediatric patient weighs 5.45 kg and has a length of 21". The manufacturer of amoxicillin has a recommended dose of 20–40 mg/kg per day. The physician has ordered 125 mg TID.

   a. Calculate the minimum daily dose for this pediatric patient.

   b. Calculate the maximum daily dose for this pediatric patient.

   c. Is the physician's dose within the recommended safe range?

   d. How many milliliters will be prepared for one prescribed dose if the product is available as a 125 mg/5 mL suspension?

19. A pediatric patient weighs 11.8 kg and is 31″ in height. The physician has ordered acetaminophen with codeine, and safe dosing of acetaminophen with codeine is based on the amount of codeine. The manufacturer of codeine has a recommended dose of 0.5–1 mg/kg per dose. The physician has ordered 10 mL of 12 mg codeine/5 mL oral elixir.

    a. Calculate the minimum daily dose for this pediatric patient.

    b. Calculate the maximum daily dose for this pediatric patient.

    c. How many milligrams of codeine are in the 10 mL of oral elixir?

    d. Is the physician's dose within the recommended safe range?

20. A pediatric patient weighs 9.32 kg and is 28″ in length. The manufacturer of ibuprofen has a recommended dose of 5–10 mg/kg every 6 to 8 hours. The physician has ordered 125 mg q8h.

    a. Calculate the minimum daily dose for this pediatric patient.

    b. Calculate the maximum daily dose for this pediatric patient.

    c. Is the physician's dose within the recommended safe range?

    d. How many milliliters will be prepared for one prescribed dose if the product is available as a 100 mg/5 mL suspension?

21. A pediatric patient weighs 50 kg and is 65″ in height. The manufacturer of cephalexin has a recommended dose of 25–50 mg/kg per day in two or four equal doses. The physician has ordered 500 mg BID.

    a. Calculate the minimum daily dose for this pediatric patient.

    b. Calculate the maximum daily dose for this pediatric patient.

    c. Is the physician's dose within the recommended safe range?

    d. How many milliliters will be prepared for one prescribed dose if the product is available as a 250 mg/5 mL suspension?

22. A pediatric patient weighs 28.6 kg and is 50″ in height. The manufacturer of acetaminophen has a recommended dose of 10–15 mg/kg per dose. The physician has ordered 325 mg/dose.

    a. Calculate the minimum dose for this pediatric patient.

    b. Calculate the maximum dose for this pediatric patient.

    c. Is the physician's dose within the recommended safe range?

    d. How many milliliters will be prepared for one dose if the product is available as a 160 mg/5 mL suspension?

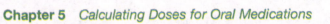

Review and Assessment

 CHAPTER SUMMARY

- When solving a story problem, remember to identify the question being asked.

- When using the ratio-proportion method to solve pharmacy problems, designate the unknown value with a variable (for example, the letter *x*) when writing your calculations.

- When setting up a proportion, verify that the units in the numerators and in the denominators match.

- The ratio-proportion method and the dimensional analysis method are commonly used to calculate medication doses.

- When solving for the unknown variable *x*, cancel similar terms (like terms) to verify that you are left with the correct unit.

- Quantity to dispense may need to be calculated for solid and liquid dosage forms.

- Dosing tables may be used to indicate doses for pediatric patients.

- Pediatric patients often need customized doses based on their weights.

- Body surface area is used to calculate doses for certain patients.

 FORMULAS FOR SUCCESS

Ratio-Proportion Setup to Compare Desired Dose to Available Medication Strength (Section 5.1)

$$\frac{\text{active ingredient (desired)}}{\text{vehicle (desired)}} = \frac{\text{active ingredient (on hand)}}{\text{vehicle (on hand)}}$$

Mosteller Formula (Section 5.3)

$$\text{BSA (in meters squared or m}^2) = \sqrt{\frac{\text{height (cm)} \times \text{weight (kg)}}{3{,}600}}$$

Take a moment to review what you have learned in this chapter and answer the following questions.

1. Common OTC medication doses for children are determined by
   a. referring to a manufacturer-provided dosing table or instructions on the packaging.
   b. contacting the primary care physician to identify an appropriate dose.
   c. calculating the dose based on the child's age.
   d. using a standard.

2. Most medications that are dosed based on a patient's weight use _____ as the unit of weight for the patient.
   a. pounds
   b. pounds and ounces
   c. kilograms
   d. grams

3. If a patient takes 1 tsp TID, how many milliliters will be needed for a 7-day course of therapy?
   a. 90 mL
   b. 100 mL
   c. 105 mL
   d. 125 mL

4. BSA is best described as a
   a. conversion method in which the given number and unit are multiplied by a ratio.
   b. formula used to determine an appropriate pediatric dose by using the child's age and the normal adult dose.
   c. measurement related to a patient's weight and height.
   d. measurement system based on subdivisions and multiples of ten.

5. A patient is to receive 6.25 mg of diphenhydramine. If the available dosage strength is 12.5 mg/5 mL, how many milliliters would be needed?
   a. 2 mL
   b. 2.5 mL
   c. 5 mL
   d. 7.5 mL

6. Which of the following is a way to convert pounds to kilograms?
   a. add 2.2
   b. divide by 2.2
   c. multiply by 2.2
   d. subtract 2.2

7. What does the abbreviation *QS* indicate on a prescription order?
   a. You should fill a quantity sufficient to meet the needs of the patient with the instructions given.
   b. You should refill the prescription as many times as needed to meet the needs of the patient.
   c. You should calculate the dose based on given patient-specific factors.
   d. You may not refill the prescription unless you receive the prescriber's permission.

8. You have dispensed a 250 mL bottle of oxcarbazepine. How many doses are in the bottle if the patient takes 1½ tsp at each dose?
   a. 25
   b. 30
   c. 33
   d. 40

9. A patient has been prescribed prednisone with the following instructions:

 Prednisone 5 mg

Take 5 tablets for 2 days.

Take 4 tablets for 1 day.

Take 3 tablets for 2 days.

Take 2 tablets for 1 day.

Take 1 tablet for 2 days.

How many tablets will the patient need to complete the course of therapy?
   a. 21 tablets
   b. 23 tablets
   c. 24 tablets
   d. 33 tablets

10. How many milligrams of medication are in 3 tsp of a clarithromycin oral suspension that contains 125 mg/tsp?

a. 125 mg
b. 250 mg
c. 375 mg
d. 500 mg

 # FIND SOLUTIONS

Take a moment to consider what you have learned in this chapter and respond thoughtfully to the prompts.

Note: *To indicate your answer for Scenario A, Question 4, ask your instructor for the handout depicting an oral syringe.*

Scenario A: Lucy Ramirez, a 14-month-old patient in the pediatric unit, weighs 22 lb. She has just been diagnosed with gastroesophageal reflux disease (GERD). Her physician has prescribed Pepcid Oral Suspension, which is dosed at 1 mg/kg per day, divided into two doses. Pepcid Oral Suspension is available in a 40 mg/5 mL strength.

1. How many kilograms does Lucy weigh?

2. How many milligrams should Lucy be taking each day?

3. How many milligrams will be given at each dose?

4. How many milliliters will be given at each dose? Round down to the nearest tenth of a milliliter. On the handout that you obtained from your instructor, indicate on the measuring device the amount of medication that should be administered to the child.

5. Is this dose more or less than a teaspoonful?

6. List one advantage of using an oral syringe versus a teaspoon to measure the needed dose.

Scenario B: Jordan Jay is a 38-year-old patient who brings a prescription to your community pharmacy for amoxicillin capsules (an antibiotic). The dose is 500 mg three times a day. The pharmacy has 500 mg capsules in stock.

7. What would be the quantity to dispense if the prescription indicated the patient should use the medication for 7 days?

8. What would be the quantity to dispense if the prescription indicated the patient should use the medication for 10 days?

9. What would be the days' supply if the prescription indicated that 15 capsules should be dispensed?

10. What would be the days' supply if the prescription indicated that 42 capsules should be dispensed?

 The online course includes additional review and assessment resources.

Calculating Doses for Injectable Medications

6

Learning Objectives

1. Perform dose calculations for subcutaneous, intramuscular, and intravenous injections. (Section 6.1)

2. Measure injection components and calculate the quantity of medication in a given volume. (Section 6.1)

3. Calculate ratio strength, or the parts of active drug in a liquid solution. (Section 6.1)

4. Perform powder reconstitution dose calculations using formulas for final volume, powder volume, and diluent volume. (Section 6.2)

5. Calculate the volume of a substance that has an electrolyte as its primary ingredient. (Section 6.3)

6. Determine the quantity of units in a given concentration and dose. (Section 6.3)

7. Calculate the volume of insulin to be administered. (Section 6.3)

For a key to the body system icons that appear in each chapter of this textbook, refer to the Preface.

ASHP/ACPE Accreditation Standards
To view the *ASHP/ACPE Accreditation Standards* addressed in this chapter, refer to Appendix D.

Now that Chapter 5 has provided you with a solid foundation for dose calculations for oral medications, Chapter 6 will build upon this instruction. This chapter has you apply your knowledge of the ratio-proportion and dimensional analysis methods to injectable medications. To that end, injectable liquid and powder reconstitution dose calculations are addressed. In addition, variant unit dose calculations for certain injectable medications—such as vitamins, electrolytes, heparin, and insulin products—are explained.

6.1 Injectable Dose Calculations

Injection is the act of administering a medication or other substance into the body. In injections, a needle or cannula (a small tube) attached to a syringe penetrates the skin or a membrane to deposit medication into the tissue, muscle, or vessel below. An **infusion** is a type of injection in which a large volume of fluid is administered into a blood vessel (typically through a vein). Unlike an injection, an infusion is used for both small and large volumes of fluid. Medications given as injections or infusions are considered **parenteral**, which literally means "occurring outside the intestines." In other words, the medications do not pass through the gastrointestinal system.

Injecting Medications

There are three main types of injections: subcutaneous injections, intramuscular injections, and intravenous infusions. All three types of injections are administered by healthcare professionals on a regular basis.

A **subcutaneous (subcut, SC, or SQ) injection** is administered into the vascular, fatty layer of tissue under the layers of skin. Most medications given by this route of administration are quickly absorbed. Patients can self-administer medications such as insulin by subcut injection.

An **intramuscular (IM) injection** is administered into the muscle tissue. Water-soluble medications are absorbed rapidly when given intramuscularly, whereas oil-based medications are absorbed slowly. With proper training, patients can self-administer medications by IM injection, but this route requires more skill and coordination than the subcut route of administration.

An **intravenous (IV) infusion** is administered into a vein. Large-volume IV infusions, such as 500–1,000 mL, may be administered over a period of hours. IV infusions of 50–100 mL are often given over a period of 30–60 minutes. A smaller volume, such as 5–30 mL, may be given via a syringe as an IV push medication over a few minutes. Most IV infusions are administered to inpatients, although these infusions can also be given in a clinic or at home with proper training of home healthcare personnel.

Measuring Injection Components

Because injectable medications are administered directly into the body, these medications must be specially compounded in a controlled environment that is as sterile, or germ-free, as possible. The preparation of injectable medications requires special training and the use of specific supply items. Most medications are combined with base solutions prior to injection. A **base solution** is a sterile solution compatible with human blood that serves as a vehicle for the delivery of medications. Commonly used base solutions include sterile water for injection (SWFI) as well as manufactured mixtures of dextrose in water (often dextrose 5% in water [D_5W]) or sodium chloride solutions (often sodium chloride [NaCl] 0.9% or 0.45% solutions).

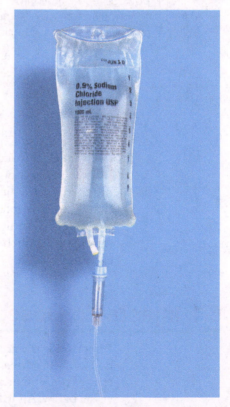

This image shows a manufactured mixture of 0.9% sodium chloride. This base solution may be administered with or without a medication added.

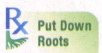

Put Down Roots

The word *subcutaneous* comes from two Latin roots: *sub*, meaning "under," and *cutis*, meaning "skin." Therefore, a subcutaneous injection is given "under the skin."

Put Down Roots

The word *intramuscular* comes from two Latin roots: *intra*, meaning "inward," and *musculus*, meaning "little mouse" because the shape and movement of the biceps resemble a mouse. Therefore, an intramuscular injection is given "within the muscle."

Name Exchange

Injectable 0.9% sodium chloride solution is often referred to as *normal saline* (abbreviated as *NS*) in healthcare settings.

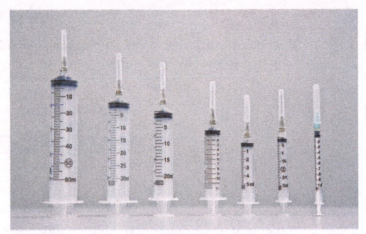

Syringes range in both volume and marked increments.

Volumes of medications and, at times, base solutions must be measured. Syringes are typically used for the volumetric measurement of injectable products. A **syringe** is a device that contains a hollow barrel (with calibration marks) and a piston plunger to withdraw or inject liquid. Syringes are available in a variety of sizes. Typical syringe sizes include 1 mL, 3 mL, 5 mL, 10 mL, 20 mL, or 50 mL. Smaller syringes are marked to indicate volume using fifths, tenths, or other fractions of a milliliter. Larger syringes are marked in 1 mL or 2 mL increments. For accuracy, it is best to select the smallest syringe that will hold the desired volume.

WORKPLACE WISDOM

Ideally, you should choose a syringe that provides the most accurate volume measurement. Typically, the smaller the syringe, the more accurate its measurement. The total volume to be prepared should generally fill at least half of the syringe barrel. For example, when measuring 2.8 mL of medication, the selection of a 3 mL or 5 mL syringe would be appropriate because the 2.8 mL would fill half or more of either syringe. If you chose the 10 mL syringe for dispensing 2.8 mL, the volume of fluid might not be measured as accurately as it would be in the smaller syringes.

Safety Alert

Because all syringes are not marked using the same increments, pharmacy technicians should become familiar with the demarcations (calibrations) of syringe sizes before using these measuring devices.

Calculating the Volume of an Injectable Solution

Medications given by injection are often ordered in milligrams, and the pharmacy or nursing staff must select and prepare an appropriate concentration of medication from the available stock medication. The volume of medication to be used (either directly administered to a patient or added to a base solution) must be calculated.

The following examples demonstrate how to calculate the volume of medication using the ratio-proportion and dimensional analysis methods. A small volume (less than 20 mL) is rounded to the nearest tenth or hundredth of a milliliter, depending on the size of the syringe barrel and its degree of accuracy. Larger volumes are rounded to the nearest tenth or whole milliliter.

Example 6.1.1

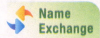

Name Exchange

The generic medication midazolam is commonly known as the brand name Versed.

How many milliliters of the medication shown in the label below must be prepared to provide 12.5 mg to a patient?

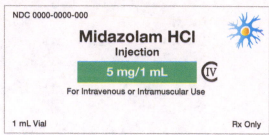

NDC 0000-0000-000

Midazolam HCl

Injection

5 mg/1 mL C-IV

For Intravenous or Intramuscular Use

1 mL Vial   Rx Only

You can solve this problem by using the ratio-proportion method or by using the dimensional analysis method.

Ratio-Proportion Method

To begin, set up a proportion with the desired medication amount on one side and the available drug concentration on the other side. Remember that the units of measurement in the numerators and in the denominators must match. Then, cross multiply, cancel similar units (like terms), and divide to solve for the unknown variable *x*.

$$\frac{12.5 \text{ mg}}{x \text{ mL}} = \frac{5 \text{ mg}}{1 \text{ mL}}$$

$$x \text{ mL} (5 \text{ mg}) = 1 \text{ mL} (12.5 \text{ mg})$$

$$x = 2.5 \text{ mL}$$

Dimensional Analysis Method

$$\frac{12.5 \text{ mg}}{1} \times \frac{1 \text{ mL}}{5 \text{ mg}} = 2.5 \text{ mL}$$

Answer: To provide 12.5 mg of midazolam to the patient, you must prepare 2.5 mL in a 3 mL syringe (see Figure 6.1).

FIGURE 6.1

2.5 mL of medication in a 3 mL syringe

Example 6.1.2

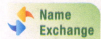

Name Exchange

The generic medication ondansetron is commonly known by the brand name Zofran.

How many milliliters of the medication shown in the label below must be prepared to provide 8 mg of ondansetron to a patient?

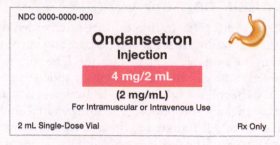

NDC 0000-0000-000

Ondansetron

Injection

4 mg/2 mL

(2 mg/mL)

For Intramuscular or Intravenous Use

2 mL Single-Dose Vial   Rx Only

You can solve this problem by using the ratio-proportion method or by using the dimensional analysis method.

Ratio-Proportion Method

To begin, set up a proportion with the desired medication amount on one side and the available drug concentration on the other side. Remember that the units of measurement in the numerators and in the denominators must match. Then, cross multiply, cancel similar units (like terms), and divide to solve for the unknown variable x.

$$\frac{8\text{ mg}}{x\text{ mL}} = \frac{4\text{ mg}}{2\text{ mL}}$$

$$x\text{ mL }(4\text{ mg}) = 2\text{ mL }(8\text{ mg})$$

$$x = 4\text{ mL}$$

Dimensional Analysis Method

$$\frac{8\text{ mg}}{1} \times \frac{2\text{ mL}}{4\text{ mg}} = 4\text{ mL}$$

Answer: To provide 8 mg of ondansetron to the patient, you must prepare 4 mL in a 5 mL syringe (see Figure 6.2).

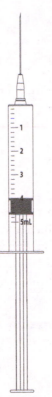

FIGURE 6.2

4 mL of medication in a 5 mL syringe

Example 6.1.3

How many milliliters of medication shown in the label below must be prepared to provide 10 mg of adenosine?

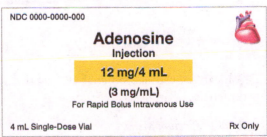

NDC 0000-0000-000

Adenosine
Injection

12 mg/4 mL

(3 mg/mL)

For Rapid Bolus Intravenous Use

4 mL Single-Dose Vial   Rx Only

You can solve this problem by using the ratio-proportion method or by using the dimensional analysis method.

Ratio-Proportion Method

To begin, set up a proportion with the desired medication amount on one side and the available drug concentration on the other side. Remember that the units of measurement in the numerators and in the denominators must match. Then, cross multiply, cancel similar units (like terms), and divide to solve for the unknown variable x.

$$\frac{10\text{ mg}}{x\text{ mL}} = \frac{12\text{ mg}}{4\text{ mL}}$$

$$x\text{ mL }(12\text{ mg}) = 4\text{ mL }(10\text{ mg})$$

$$x = 3.3\text{ mL}$$

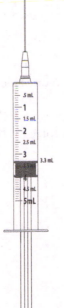

FIGURE 6.3

3.3 mL of medication in a 5 mL syringe

Dimensional Analysis Method

$$\frac{10 \text{ mg}}{1} \times \frac{4 \text{ mL}}{12 \text{ mg}} = 3.3 \text{ mL}$$

Answer: To provide 10 mg of adenosine to the patient, you must prepare 3.3 mL in a 5 mL syringe (see Figure 6.3).

Calculating the Quantity of Medication in an Injectable Solution

The previous examples demonstrated how to calculate the volume of an injectable solution needed to obtain a desired quantity of medication. As a pharmacy technician, you will also have situations in which you need to perform the opposite calculation. You will need to determine the quantity of medication in a given volume of an injectable solution.

Example 6.1.4

How many milligrams of progesterone are in 2 mL of the solution shown in the label below?

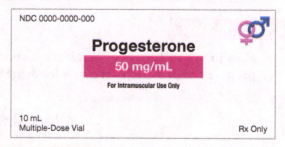

NDC 0000-0000-000

Progesterone

50 mg/mL

For Intramuscular Use Only

10 mL
Multiple-Dose Vial

Rx Only

You can solve this problem by using the ratio-proportion method or by using the dimensional analysis method.

Ratio-Proportion Method

To begin, set up a proportion with the desired medication volume on one side and the available drug concentration on the other side. Remember that the units of measurement in the numerators and in the denominators must match. Then, cross multiply, cancel similar units (like terms), and divide to solve for the unknown variable x.

$$\frac{x \text{ mg}}{2 \text{ mL}} = \frac{50 \text{ mg}}{1 \text{ mL}}$$

$$x \text{ mg } (1 \text{ mL}) = 50 \text{ mg } (2 \text{ mL})$$

$$x = 100 \text{ mg}$$

Dimensional Analysis Method

$$\frac{2 \text{ mL}}{1} \times \frac{50 \text{ mg}}{1 \text{ mL}} = 100 \text{ mg}$$

Answer: There are 100 mg of progesterone in 2 mL of the solution.

Example 6.1.5

How many milligrams of carboplatin are in 30 mL of the solution shown in the label below?

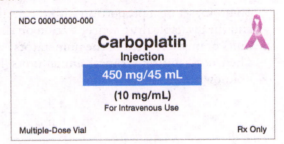

NDC 0000-0000-000

Carboplatin
Injection

450 mg/45 mL

(10 mg/mL)
For Intravenous Use

Multiple-Dose Vial   Rx Only

You can solve this problem by using the ratio-proportion method or by using the dimensional analysis method.

Ratio-Proportion Method

To begin, set up a proportion with the desired medication volume on one side and the available drug concentration on the other side. Remember that the units of measurement in the numerators and in the denominators must match. Then, cross multiply, cancel similar units (like terms), and divide to solve for the unknown variable *x*.

$$\frac{x \text{ mg}}{30 \text{ mL}} = \frac{450 \text{ mg}}{45 \text{ mL}}$$

$$x \text{ mg } (45 \text{ mL}) = 450 \text{ mg } (30 \text{ mL})$$

$$x = 300 \text{ mg}$$

Dimensional Analysis Method

$$\frac{30 \text{ mL}}{1} \times \frac{450 \text{ mg}}{45 \text{ mL}} = 300 \text{ mg}$$

Answer: There are 300 mg of carboplatin in 30 mL of the solution.

Example 6.1.6

How many milligrams of furosemide are in 6 mL of the solution shown in the label below?

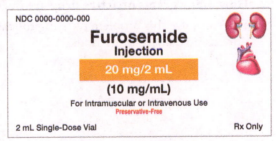

NDC 0000-0000-000

Furosemide
Injection

20 mg/2 mL

(10 mg/mL)
For Intramuscular or Intravenous Use
Preservative-Free

2 mL Single-Dose Vial   Rx Only

You can solve this problem by using the ratio-proportion method or by using the dimensional analysis method.

Ratio-Proportion Method

To begin, set up a proportion with the desired medication volume on one side and the available drug concentration on the other side. Remember that the units of measurement in the numerators and in the denominators must match. Then, cross multiply, cancel similar units (like terms), and divide to solve for the unknown variable *x*.

$$\frac{x \text{ mg}}{6 \text{ mL}} = \frac{20 \text{ mg}}{2 \text{ mL}}$$

$$x \text{ mg } (2 \text{ mL}) = 20 \text{ mg } (6 \text{ mL})$$

$$x = 60 \text{ mg}$$

Dimensional Analysis Method

$$\frac{6 \text{ mL}}{1} \times \frac{20 \text{ mg}}{2 \text{ mL}} = 60 \text{ mg}$$

Answer: There are 60 mg of furosemide in 6 mL of the solution.

Calculating Ratio Strength

As you learned in Chapter 2, a ratio can be used to express the strength or concentration of a drug. For example, a 1% solution could be written as 1:100. The ratio 1:100 is referred to as a *ratio strength* and is an alternate way to indicate medication strength for liquids.

Ratio strength is expressed by the ratio *a:b* (read as "a to b"). In this ratio, *a* represents parts of active drug, and *b* represents parts of a liquid solution. Therefore, **ratio strength** is defined as the parts of active drug in a liquid solution. The units indicated in a ratio strength are always *a* grams:*b* milliliters. Consequently, the ratio 1:100 represents 1 g of active drug in 100 mL of solution.

The following examples utilize methods to determine the quantity of active drug or volume for medications expressed in ratio strength.

Example 6.1.7

How many grams of active drug are in 500 mL of a 1:200 solution?

You can solve this problem by using the ratio-proportion method or by using the dimensional analysis method.

Ratio-Proportion Method

To begin, set up a proportion with the medication volume on one side and the available drug's ratio strength on the other side. Remember that the units of measurement in the numerators and in the denominators must match. Then, cross multiply, cancel similar units (like terms), and divide to solve for the unknown variable x.

$$\frac{x \text{ g}}{500 \text{ mL}} = \frac{1 \text{ g}}{200 \text{ mL}}$$

$$x \text{ g } (200 \text{ mL}) = 1 \text{ g } (500 \text{ mL})$$

$$x = 2.5 \text{ g}$$

Dimensional Analysis Method

$$\frac{500 \text{ mL}}{1} \times \frac{1 \text{ g}}{200 \text{ mL}} = 2.5 \text{ g}$$

Answer: There are 2.5 g of active drug in 500 mL of a 1:200 solution.

Example 6.1.8

How many grams of active drug are in 500 mL of a 1:3,000 solution?

You can solve this problem by using the ratio-proportion method or by using the dimensional analysis method.

Ratio-Proportion Method

To begin, set up a proportion with the medication volume on one side and the available drug's ratio strength on the other side. Remember that the units of measurement in the numerators and in the denominators must match. Then, cross multiply, cancel similar units (like terms), and divide to solve for the unknown variable x.

$$\frac{x \text{ g}}{500 \text{ mL}} = \frac{1 \text{ g}}{3,000 \text{ mL}}$$

$$x \text{ g } (3,000 \text{ mL}) = 1 \text{ g } (500 \text{ mL})$$

$$x = 0.17 \text{ g}$$

Dimensional Analysis Method

$$\frac{500 \text{ mL}}{1} \times \frac{1 \text{ g}}{3000 \text{ mL}} = 0.17 \text{ g}$$

Answer: There is 0.17 g of active drug in 500 mL of a 1:3,000 solution.

Example 6.1.9

 How many milligrams of active drug are in 1.5 mL of a 1:1,000 solution of epinephrine?

You can solve this problem by using the ratio-proportion method or by using the dimensional analysis method.

Ratio-Proportion Method

First, convert the ratio strength from units of grams per milliliter to milligrams per milliliter.

$$\frac{x \text{ mg}}{1 \text{ g}} = \frac{1{,}000 \text{ mg}}{1 \text{ g}}$$

$$x \text{ mg} (1 \text{ g}) = 1{,}000 \text{ mg} (1 \text{ g})$$

$$x = 1{,}000 \text{ mg}$$

We now can rewrite the drug's ratio strength as 1,000 mg/1,000 ml.

Now, set up a proportion with the medication volume on one side and the available drug's ratio strength on the other side. Remember that the units of measurement in the numerators and in the denominators must match. Then, cross multiply, cancel similar units (like terms), and divide to solve for the unknown variable x.

$$\frac{x \text{ mg}}{1.5 \text{ mL}} = \frac{1{,}000 \text{ mg}}{1{,}000 \text{ mL}}$$

$$x \text{ mg} (1{,}000 \text{ mL}) = 1{,}000 \text{ mg} (1.5 \text{ mL})$$

$$x = 1.5 \text{ mg}$$

Dimensional Analysis Method

$$\frac{1.5 \cancel{\text{ mL}}}{1} \times \frac{1 \cancel{\text{ g}}}{1{,}000 \cancel{\text{ mL}}} \times \frac{1{,}000 \text{ mg}}{1 \cancel{\text{ g}}} = 1.5 \text{ mg}$$

Answer: There are 1.5 mg of active drug in 1.5 mL of a 1:1,000 solution of epinephrine.

Example 6.1.10

How many milligrams of active drug are in 3 mL of a 1:2,500 solution?

You can solve this problem by using the ratio-proportion method or by using the dimensional analysis method.

Ratio-Proportion Method

To begin, set up your calculation using grams. Create a proportion with the medication volume on one side and the available drug's ratio strength on the other side. Remember that the units of measurement in the numerators and in the denominators must match. Then, cross multiply, cancel similar units (like terms), and divide to solve for the unknown variable x.

$$\frac{x\,g}{3\text{ mL}} = \frac{1\text{ g}}{2{,}500\text{ mL}}$$

$$x\,g\,(2{,}500\text{ mL}) = 1\text{ g }(3\text{ mL})$$

$$x = 0.0012\text{ g}$$

Next, use your answer in the first calculation (0.0012 g) and set up a conversion from grams to milligrams.

$$\frac{x\,\text{mg}}{0.0012\text{ g}} = \frac{1{,}000\text{ mg}}{1\text{ g}}$$

$$x\,\text{mg }(1\text{ g}) = 1{,}000\text{ mg }(0.0012\text{ g})$$

$$x = 1.2\text{ mg}$$

Alternatively, you can use your answer in the first calculation (0.0012 g) and simply move the decimal point three places to the right.

$$0.0012\text{ g} = 1.2\text{ mg}$$

Dimensional Analysis Method

$$\frac{3\text{ mL}}{1} \times \frac{1\text{ g}}{2{,}500\text{ mL}} \times \frac{1{,}000\text{ mg}}{1\text{ g}} = 1.2\text{ mg}$$

Answer: There are 1.2 mg of active drug in 3 mL of a 1:2,500 solution.

Example 6.1.11

How many milliliters are needed to provide 0.75 g of a medication if the solution available is 1:2,000?

You can solve this problem by using the ratio-proportion method or by using the dimensional analysis method.

Ratio-Proportion Method

To begin, set up a proportion with the medication amount on one side and the available drug's ratio strength on the other side. Remember that the units of measurement in the numerators and in the denominators must match. Then, cross multiply, cancel similar units (like terms) and divide to solve for the unknown variable x.

$$\frac{0.75\text{ g}}{x\text{ mL}} = \frac{1\text{ g}}{2{,}000\text{ mL}}$$

$$x\text{ mL }(1\text{ g}) = 2{,}000\text{ mL }(0.75\text{ g})$$

$$x = 1{,}500\text{ mL}$$

Dimensional Analysis Method

$$\frac{0.75\ g}{1} \times \frac{2{,}000\ \text{mL}}{1\ g} = 1{,}500\ \text{mL}$$

Answer: For a 1:2,000 solution, a volume of 1,500 mL is needed to provide 0.75 g of a medication.

Example 6.1.12

How many milliliters are needed to provide 20 mg of a medication if the solution available is 1:500?

You can solve this problem by using the ratio-proportion method or by using the dimensional analysis method.

Ratio-Proportion Method

To begin, convert the desired dose units from milligrams to grams.

$$\frac{x\ g}{20\ \text{mg}} = \frac{1\ g}{1{,}000\ \text{mg}}$$

$$x\ g\ (1{,}000\ \text{mg}) = 1\ g\ (20\ \text{mg})$$

$$x = 0.02\ g$$

Next, set up a proportion with the medication amount on one side and the available drug's ratio strength on the other side. Remember that the units of measurement in the numerators and in the denominators must match. Then, cross multiply, cancel similar units (like terms), and divide to solve for the unknown variable x.

$$\frac{0.02\ g}{x\ \text{mL}} = \frac{1\ g}{500\ \text{mL}}$$

$$x\ \text{mL}\ (1\ g) = 500\ \text{mL}\ (0.02\ g)$$

$$x = 10\ \text{mL}$$

Dimensional Analysis Method

$$\frac{20\ \text{mg}}{1} \times \frac{1\ g}{1{,}000\ \text{mg}} \times \frac{500\ \text{mL}}{1\ g} = 10\ \text{mL}$$

Answer: For a 1:500 solution, a volume of 10 mL is needed to provide 20 mg of a medication.

6.1 Problem Set

Determine the volume to be prepared for each ordered injectable solution using the labels provided. Round your answer to the nearest hundredth.

> **Note:** Questions 1–10 have accompanying handouts that you must obtain from your instructor.

1. How many milliliters of solution are needed to provide 50 mg of Xylocaine? On the handout that you obtained from your instructor, indicate the correct volume on the measuring device.

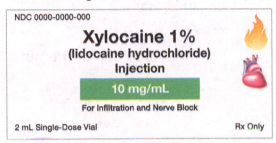

2. How many milliliters of solution are needed to provide 60 mg of furosemide? On the handout that you obtained from your instructor, indicate the correct volume on the measuring device.

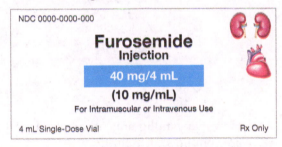

3. How many milliliters of solution are needed to provide 80 mg of furosemide? On the handout that you obtained from your instructor, indicate the correct volume on the measuring device.

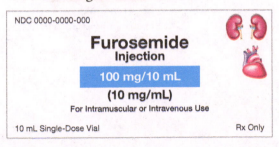

4. How many milliliters of solution are needed to provide 0.75 mg of indomethacin in this 1 mg/1 mL vial? On the handout that you obtained from your instructor, indicate the correct volume on the measuring device.

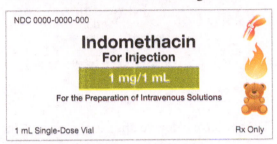

5. How many milliliters of solution are needed to provide 100 mg of diphenhydramine hydrochloride? On the handout that you obtained from your instructor, indicate the correct volume on the measuring device.

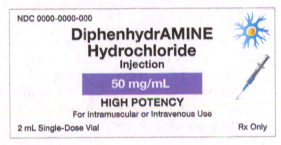

6. How many milliliters of solution are needed to provide 30 mg of famotidine? On the handout that you obtained from your instructor, indicate the correct volume on the measuring device.

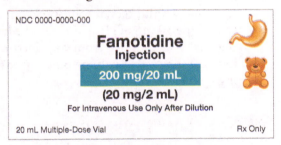

7. How many milliliters of solution are needed to provide 40 mg of famotidine? On the handout that you obtained from your instructor, indicate the correct volume on the measuring device.

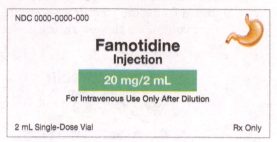

NDC 0000-0000-000

Famotidine
Injection

20 mg/2 mL

For Intravenous Use Only After Dilution

2 mL Single-Dose Vial   Rx Only

Use the label below to answer questions 8 and 9.

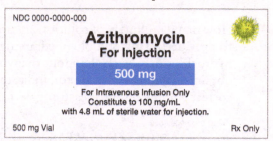

NDC 0000-0000-000

Azithromycin
For Injection

500 mg

For Intravenous Infusion Only
Constitute to 100 mg/mL
with 4.8 mL of sterile water for injection.

500 mg Vial   Rx Only

8. How many milliliters of solution are needed to provide 250 mg of azithromycin? On the handout that you obtained from your instructor, indicate the correct volume on the measuring device.

9. How many milliliters of solution are needed to provide 400 mg of azithromycin? On the handout that you obtained from your instructor, indicate the correct volume on the measuring device.

10. How many milliliters of solution are needed to provide 50 mg of cisplatin? On the handout that you obtained from your instructor, indicate the correct volume on the measuring device.

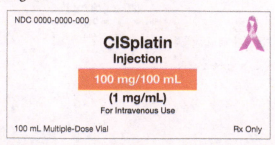

NDC 0000-0000-000

CISplatin
Injection

100 mg/100 mL
(1 mg/mL)
For Intravenous Use

100 mL Multiple-Dose Vial   Rx Only

Calculate the quantity of medication in the injectable solution using the provided vial labels.

11. How many milligrams of ketorolac are contained in 0.5 mL?

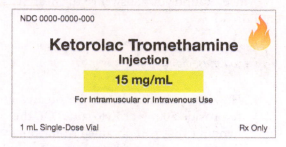

NDC 0000-0000-000

Ketorolac Tromethamine
Injection

15 mg/mL

For Intramuscular or Intravenous Use

1 mL Single-Dose Vial   Rx Only

12. How many milligrams of ketorolac are contained in 1.75 mL?

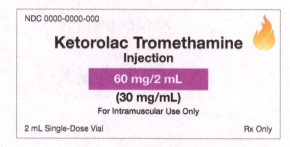

NDC 0000-0000-000

Ketorolac Tromethamine
Injection

60 mg/2 mL
(30 mg/mL)
For Intramuscular Use Only

2 mL Single-Dose Vial   Rx Only

13. How many milligrams of lidocaine HCl are contained in 3.75 mL?

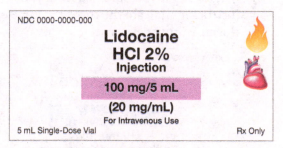

NDC 0000-0000-000

Lidocaine HCl 2%
Injection

100 mg/5 mL
(20 mg/mL)
For Intravenous Use

5 mL Single-Dose Vial   Rx Only

14. How many milligrams of midazolam HCl are contained in 1.3 mL?

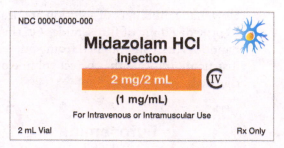

NDC 0000-0000-000

Midazolam HCl
Injection

2 mg/2 mL   (IV)
(1 mg/mL)
For Intravenous or Intramuscular Use

2 mL Vial   Rx Only

15. How many milligrams of midazolam HCl are contained in 5 mL?

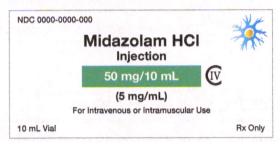

16. How many milligrams of midazolam HCl are contained in 5 mL?

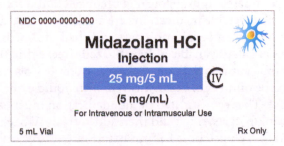

17. How many milligrams of midazolam HCl are contained in 5 mL?

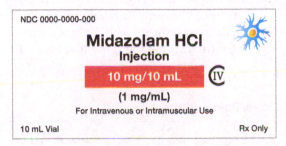

18. How many milligrams of dexamethasone are contained in 8 mL?

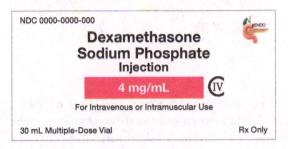

19. How many milligrams of ondansetron are contained in 1.5 mL?

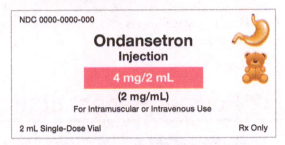

20. How many milligrams of progesterone are contained in 2.5 mL?

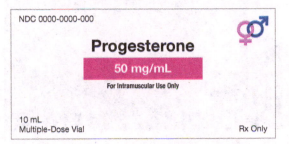

Calculate the amount of active drug in a ratio-strength solution.

21. How many milligrams are in 2 mL of a 1:1,000 solution?

22. How many micrograms are in 1 mL of a 1:5,000 solution?

23. How many micrograms are in 1.5 mL of a 1:10,000 solution?

24. How many micrograms are in 1.4 mL of a 1:2,000 solution?

25. How many micrograms are in 2.5 mL of a 1:10,000 solution?

Calculate the volume of solution needed for each requested dose to be infused intravenously.

26. How many milliliters of 1:1,000 solution are needed to provide a 500 mg dose?

27. How many milliliters of 1:10,000 solution are needed to provide a 50 mg dose?

28. How many milliliters of 1:300 solution are needed to provide a 600 mg dose?

29. How many milliliters of 1:500 solution are needed to provide a 250 mg dose?

30. How many milliliters of 1:750 solution are needed to provide a 0.01 g dose?

Self-check your work in Appendix A.

6.2 Powder Reconstitution Dose Calculations

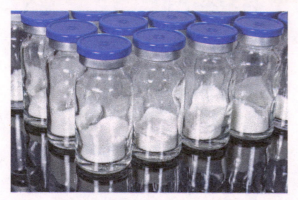

Some medications are supplied as lyophilized powders that must be reconstituted prior to use.

In the preparation of solutions, the active ingredient is discussed in terms of weight, but it also occupies a certain amount of space. Although some injectables are commercially available in a premixed liquid form, not all injectable medications are available as liquids. Often to extend expiration date and shelf life, medications are also available as **lyophilized** (freeze-dried) pharmaceuticals that are packaged in sterile vials that must be diluted, or reconstituted, with liquid prior to use. The reconstituted liquid medication must be drawn up in a syringe and then added to an IV bag or used for IV push or IM administration.

To reconstitute a lyophilized powder, a specified volume of **diluent** (a substance used to dilute) must be added to the vial. The amount of space the lyophilized drug takes up is the **powder volume (pv)**. Powder volume equals the difference between the **final volume (fv)** and the volume of the diluting ingredient, or the **diluent volume (dv)**. This equation can be rearranged algebraically so you can solve for final volume or diluent volume. To learn these formulas, see Table 6.1.

TABLE 6.1 Formulas for Powder Reconstitution Dose Calculations

Variable Desired	Formula	Abbreviated Formula
powder volume	powder volume = final volume − diluent volume	pv = fv − dv
diluent volume	diluent volume = final volume − powder volume	dv = fv − pv
final volume	final volume = powder volume + diluent volume	fv = pv + dv

Example 6.2.1

A powdered antibiotic must be reconstituted for use. The label states that the dry powder occupies 0.5 mL. Determine the diluent volume (the amount of solvent added) for each pairing of final volume and powder volume listed below.

Final Volume	Powder Volume
2 mL	0.5 mL
5 mL	0.5 mL
10 mL	0.5 mL

To begin, recognize the information provided in the problem: the final volume and the powder volume. Then ask yourself the following question: *What am I looking for to solve the problem?* In this problem, you are looking for the *diluent volume*. With that in mind, choose the formula from Table 6.1 that is appropriate for solving the problem.

$$\text{diluent volume (dv)} = \text{final volume (fv)} - \text{powder volume (pv)}$$

$$dv = fv - pv$$

Then set up your calculations to determine diluent volume by subtracting the powder volume from the final volume for the volumes listed above.

$$dv = 2 \text{ mL} - 0.5 \text{ mL} = 1.5 \text{ mL}$$

$$dv = 5 \text{ mL} - 0.5 \text{ mL} = 4.5 \text{ mL}$$

$$dv = 10 \text{ mL} - 0.5 \text{ mL} = 9.5 \text{ mL}$$

Answer: The diluent volumes are 1.5 mL, 4.5 mL, and 9.5 mL.

Example 6.2.2

You are to reconstitute 1 g of dry powder. The label states that you are to add 9.3 mL of diluent to make a desired concentration of 100 mg/1 mL. What is the powder volume?

You can solve this problem by using the ratio-proportion method or by using the dimensional analysis method.

Ratio-Proportion Method

To begin, convert 1 g to milligrams so that you can work with similar units when performing calculations.

$$1 \text{ g} = 1{,}000 \text{ mg}$$

Then ask yourself the following question: *What am I looking for to solve the problem?* In this problem, you are looking for the *powder volume*. You know that you have the diluent volume (9.3 mL), but you do not have the final volume in milliliters. To find the final volume, place your conversion (1,000 mg) over the unknown variable (x mL) on the left side of the proportion and the desired concentration of the solution (100 mg/1 mL) on the right side of the proportion. Be sure that the units in the numerators and in the denominators match. Then, cross multiply, cancel similar units (like terms), and divide to solve for the unknown variable x.

$$\frac{1{,}000 \text{ mg}}{x \text{ mL}} = \frac{100 \text{ mg}}{1 \text{ mL}}$$

$$x \text{ mL } (100 \text{ mg}) = 1 \text{ mL } (1{,}000 \text{ mg})$$

$$x = 10 \text{ mL}$$

Now that you have the final volume (10 mL) and the diluent volume provided in the problem (9.3 mL), choose the formula from Table 6.1 that is appropriate for finding the powder volume.

$$\text{powder volume (pv)} = \text{final volume (fv)} - \text{diluent volume (dv)}$$

$$pv = fv - dv$$

Finally, subtract the diluent volume from the final volume to determine the powder volume.

$$pv = 10 \text{ mL} - 9.3 \text{ mL}$$

$$pv = 0.7 \text{ mL}$$

Dimensional Analysis Method

$$\frac{1 \cancel{g}}{1} \times \frac{1000 \cancel{mg}}{1 \cancel{g}} \times \frac{1 \text{ mL}}{100 \cancel{mg}} = 10 \text{ mL}$$

Now that you have the final volume (10 mL) and the diluent volume provided in the problem (9.3 mL), choose the formula from Table 6.1 that is appropriate for finding the powder volume.

powder volume (pv) = final volume (fv) − diluent volume (dv)

$$pv = fv - dv$$

Finally, find the difference of your final volume and your diluent volume.

$$pv = 10 \text{ mL} - 9.3 \text{ mL}$$

$$pv = 0.7 \text{ mL}$$

Answer: The powder volume is 0.7 mL.

Example 6.2.3

A label states that a 5 g quantity of an antibiotic in a bottle should be reconstituted with 8.7 mL of saline for injection. The resulting concentration will be 500 mg/1 mL. What is the powder volume contained in the vial?

You can solve this problem by using the ratio-proportion method or by using the dimensional analysis method.

Ratio-Proportion Method

To begin, convert 5 g to milligrams so that you can work with similar units when performing calculations.

$$5 \text{ g} = 5{,}000 \text{ mg}$$

Then ask yourself the following question: *What am I looking for to solve the problem?* In this problem, you are looking for the *powder volume*. You know that you have the diluent volume (8.7 mL), but you do not have the final volume in milliliters. To find the final volume, place your conversion (5,000 mg) over the unknown variable (x mL) on the left side of the proportion and the desired concentration of the solution (500 mg/1 mL) on the right side of the proportion. Be sure that the units in the numerators and in the denominators match. Then, cross multiply, cancel similar units (like terms), and divide to solve for the unknown variable x.

$$\frac{5{,}000 \text{ mg}}{x \text{ mL}} = \frac{500 \text{ mg}}{1 \text{ mL}}$$

$$x \text{ mL } (500 \text{ mg}) = 1 \text{ mL } (5{,}000 \text{ mg})$$

$$x = 10 \text{ mL}$$

Now that you have the final volume (10 mL) and the diluent volume provided in the problem (8.7 mL), choose the formula from Table 6.1 that is appropriate for finding the powder volume.

$$\text{powder volume (pv)} = \text{final volume (fv)} - \text{diluent volume (dv)}$$

$$pv = fv - dv$$

Finally, subtract the diluent volume from the final volume to determine the powder volume.

$$pv = 10 \text{ mL} - 8.7 \text{ mL}$$

$$pv = 1.3 \text{ mL}$$

Dimensional Analysis Method

$$\frac{5\ \cancel{g}}{1} \times \frac{1{,}000\ \cancel{mg}}{1\ \cancel{g}} \times \frac{1 \text{ mL}}{500\ \cancel{mg}} = 10 \text{ mL}$$

Now that you have the final volume (10 mL) and the diluent volume provided in the problem (8.7 mL), choose the formula from Table 6.1 that is appropriate for finding the powder volume.

$$\text{powder volume (pv)} = \text{final volume (fv)} - \text{diluent volume (dv)}$$

$$pv = fv - dv$$

Finally, find the difference of your final volume and your diluent volume.

$$pv = 10 \text{ mL} - 8.7 \text{ mL}$$

$$pv = 1.3 \text{ mL}$$

Answer: The powder volume is 1.3 mL.

Example 6.2.4

A 6 g vial must have 10 mL of diluent added to it. It has a powder volume of 2 mL. How many milligrams will be in each milliliter of the final solution?

To begin, ask yourself the following question: *What am I looking for to solve the problem?* You know that you are looking for the desired concentration (mg/mL) of the solution. You also know that you have the diluent volume (10 mL) and the powder volume (2 mL), but you do not have the final volume. Therefore, you can easily determine the *final volume* by using the appropriate formula from Table 6.1.

$$\text{final volume (fv)} = \text{powder volume (pv)} + \text{diluent volume (dv)}$$

$$fv = pv + dv$$

Next, plug in the powder volume and the diluent volume that were stated in the problem.

$$fv = 2 \text{ mL} + 10 \text{ mL}$$

$$fv = 12 \text{ mL}$$

Now that you have the final volume, you can determine the desired concentration of the solution.

You can solve this problem by using the ratio-proportion method or by using the dimensional analysis method.

Ratio-Proportion Method

To determine the desired concentration of the solution, set up a proportion to determine the number of grams in each milliliter. Place the unknown quantity (x g) over 1 mL on the left side of the proportion and the number of grams (6 g) over the final volume you just calculated (12 mL) on the right side of the proportion. Be sure that the units are the same in the numerators and in the denominators. Then, cross multiply, cancel similar units (like terms), and divide to solve for the unknown variable x.

$$\frac{x\,g}{1\,mL} = \frac{6\,g}{12\,mL}$$

$$x\,g\,(12\,mL) = 6\,g\,(1\,mL)$$

$$x = 0.5\,g \text{ in each milliliter}$$

Finally, you need to convert grams in each milliliter (in this case, 0.5 g) to milligrams in each milliliter. To do so, set up another proportion by placing the unknown quantity (x mg) over the number of grams on the left side and the conversion factor on the right side (1 g equals 1,000 mg) on the right side of the equation. Be sure that the units are the same in the numerators and in the denominators. Then, cross multiply, cancel similar units (like terms), and divide to solve for the unknown variable x.

$$\frac{x\,mg}{0.5\,g} = \frac{1{,}000\,mg}{1\,g}$$

$$x\,mg\,(1\,g) = 1{,}000\,mg\,(0.5\,g)$$

$$x = 500\,mg \text{ in each milliliter}$$

Alternatively, you can use your answer in the first calculation (0.5 g) and simply move the decimal point three places to the right.

$$0.500\,g = 500\,mg \text{ in each milliliter}$$

Dimensional Analysis Method

$$\frac{6\,\cancel{g}}{12\,mL} \times \frac{1{,}000\,mg}{1\,\cancel{g}} = \frac{500\,mg}{mL}$$

Answer: There are 500 mg in each milliliter of the final solution.

Example 6.2.5

The label of a 10 g vancomycin vial states the following: *Add 95 mL of sterile water to the vial's contents to achieve a concentration of 1 g/10 mL.* **What will be the concentration if you add 45 mL of sterile water to the vial's contents?**

You can solve this problem by using the ratio-proportion method or by using the dimensional analysis method.

Ratio-Proportion Method

To begin, ask yourself the following question: *What am I looking for to solve the problem?* You know that you are first looking for the final volume of the known solution. Then set up your proportion by placing the known amount (10 g) over the unknown amount (*x* mL) on the left side and the known concentration of the solution (1 g/10 mL) on the right side. Be sure that the units in the numerators and in the denominators match. Then, cross multiply, cancel similar units (like terms), and divide to solve for the unknown variable *x*.

$$\frac{10 \text{ g}}{x \text{ mL}} = \frac{1 \text{ g}}{10 \text{ mL}}$$

$$x \text{ mL } (1 \text{ g}) = 10 \text{ mL } (10 \text{ g})$$

$$x = 100 \text{ mL}$$

Now that you have the final volume (100 mL) of the known solution and the diluent volume (95 mL) provided in the problem, you can determine the powder volume of the solution. With that in mind, choose the appropriate formula from Table 6.1.

powder volume (pv) = final volume (fv) − diluent volume (dv)

$$pv = fv - dv$$

Next, plug in the final volume and the diluent volume to this formula.

$$pv = 100 \text{ mL} - 95 \text{ mL}$$

$$pv = 5 \text{ mL}$$

Then determine the final volume using 45 mL of diluent instead of 95 mL of diluent. Use the appropriate formula from the box above.

final volume (fv) = powder volume (pv) + diluent volume (dv)

$$fv = pv + dv$$

$$fv = 5 \text{ mL} + 45 \text{ mL}$$

$$fv = 50 \text{ mL}$$

Now convert the known amount of vancomycin (10 g) to mg. Place the unknown amount (*x* mg) over the known known amount (10 g) on the left side and the known conversion (1,000 mg/1 g) on the right side. Be sure that the units in the numerators and in the denominators match. Then, cross multiply, cancel similar units (like terms), and divide to solve for the unknown variable *x*.

$$\frac{x \text{ mg}}{10 \text{ g}} = \frac{1{,}000 \text{ mg}}{1 \text{ g}}$$

$$x \text{ mg } (1 \text{ g}) = 1{,}000 \text{ mg } (10 \text{ g})$$

$$x = 10{,}000 \text{ mg}$$

Finally, determine the new concentration of the solution by dividing your answer by the final volume.

$$\frac{10{,}000 \text{ mg}}{50 \text{ mL}} = \frac{200 \text{ mg}}{\text{mL}}$$

Dimensional Analysis Method

To begin, determine the final volume of the known solution.

$$\frac{10 \text{ g}}{1} \times \frac{10 \text{ mL}}{1 \text{ g}} = 100 \text{ mL}$$

Now that you have the final volume of the known solution, you can determine the powder volume of the solution. With that in mind, choose the appropriate formula from Table 6.1.

powder volume (pv) = final volume (fv) − diluent volume (dv)

$$pv = fv - dv$$

Next, plug in the final volume and the diluent volume to this formula.

$$pv = 100 \text{ mL} - 95 \text{ mL}$$

$$pv = 5 \text{ mL}$$

Then determine the final volume using 45 mL of diluent instead of 95 mL of diluent. Use the appropriate formula from the box above.

final volume (fv) = powder volume (pv) + diluent volume (dv)

$$fv = pv + dv$$

Next, plug in the powder volume and the diluent volume that were stated in the problem.

$$fv = 5 \text{ mL} + 45 \text{ mL}$$

$$fv = 50 \text{ mL}$$

Finally, determine the new concentration of the solution.

$$\frac{10 \text{ g}}{50 \text{ mL}} \times \frac{1{,}000 \text{ mg}}{1 \text{ g}} = \frac{200 \text{ mg}}{\text{mL}}$$

Answer: With the addition of 45 mL of sterile water, the concentration of the solution becomes 200 mg/mL.

6.2 Problem Set

1. You need to make an injectable solution with a final concentration of 375 mg/mL. After checking your available stock medication, you see that you have a vial that contains 1.5 g with the instructions to add 3.3 mL. What is the powder volume?

2. You must add water to an oral suspension before it can be dispensed to a patient. The dose is to be 250 mg/tsp, and the dry powder is 5 g with a powder volume of 8.6 mL. How much water must you add?

3. An injectable preparation comes packaged as a 1 g vial, and you want a final concentration of 125 mg/2 mL. The vial states that you are to add 14.4 mL of diluent. What is the powder volume?

4. The label of a 2 g vial states that you are to add 6.8 mL to get a concentration of 250 mg/mL. What is the powder volume?

5. Using the medication vial from question 4, how much diluent do you need to add to make a medication with a final concentration of 125 mg/mL?

6. The label of a 4 g vial states that you are to add 11.7 mL to get a concentration of 250 mg/mL. What is the powder volume?

7. The label of a 6 g vial states that adding 12.5 mL of diluent to the vial's contents will achieve a concentration of 1 g/2.5 mL. What concentration (mg/mL) will you achieve if you add 2.5 mL?

8. You have added 3.3 mL of diluent to a 1 g vial and now have a final volume of 4 mL. What is the powder volume?

9. Using the medication concentration from question 8, what is the volume of medication needed for a 100 mg dose?

10. If you add 8.8 mL of diluent to a 2 g vial and get a final concentration of 200 mg/mL, what is the powder volume?

11. A 10 g vial must have 45 mL of diluent added to it. It has a powder volume of 5 mL. How many milligrams will be in each milliliter of the reconstituted solution?

12. For an oral suspension, you add 170 mL of fluid and get a final volume of 200 mL. There is a total of 8 g of medication in the reconstituted solution. How many milligrams will be in 1 tsp?

13. A 20 g bulk vial label states that if you add 106 mL of diluent, the concentration will be 1 g/6 mL. How much diluent would you add to get a desired concentration of 1 g/3 mL?

14. You need a concentration of 375 mg/mL. Your vial contains 2 g with instructions to add 3.5 mL of diluent. What is the powder volume?

15. An oral medication requires reconstitution. The concentration of the reconstituted medication is 300 mg/tsp. The dry powder is 2.5 g with a volume of 9.6 mL. How much water do you add?

16. A 5 g vial requires that 8.6 mL of diluent be added to achieve a desired concentration of 250 mg/mL. What is the powder volume?

17. A 10 g vial label states to add 20 mL of diluent to achieve a desired concentration of 1 g/2.5 mL. What concentration (mg/mL) would you achieve if you added 35 mL?

18. You add 4.3 mL of diluent to a 1 g vial and have a final volume of 5 mL. What is the powder volume?

19. A 5 g vial requires 25 mL to be added. It has a powder volume of 5 mL. How many milligrams are in each milliliter of the reconstituted solution?

20. A 20 g vial must have 90 mL of diluent added. It has a powder volume of 10 mL. How many milligrams are in each milliliter of the reconstituted solution?

21. A 3 g vial requires 20 mL of diluent to be added. It has a powder volume of 5 mL. How many milligrams are in each milliliter of the reconstituted solution?

22. A pediatric antibiotic requires 67 mL to be added to the bottle for reconstitution. The final volume will be 100 mL. What is the powder volume?

23. If the pediatric antibiotic in question 22 is reconstituted and there are 35 g of active ingredient in the medication bottle, what will the resulting strength be in milligrams per milliliters?

Self-check your work in Appendix A.

6.3 Variant Unit Dose Calculations

Most medications are dosed using the metric system units of measurement, such as milligrams or grams. However, certain substances are dosed using other units of measurement, including units based on the number of particles in a substance, units based on the electrical charge of a substance, and units based on the activity of a medication. Electrolytes, such as potassium phosphate and potassium chloride, may use units based on the number of particles or electrical charge. Medications that use units based on activity include vitamins, such as ergocalciferol; complicated proteins, such as epoetin alfa; and hormones, such as insulin. Although these medications do have weights, they are dosed based on variant units, and their weights are often disregarded.

Calculating Milliequivalents and Millimoles

Many fluids in the pharmacy contain dissolved mineral salts known as *electrolytes*. An **electrolyte** separates into smaller molecules and is capable of transporting an electrical charge. Electrolytes are required for normal body functions and are typically obtained through nutrition. When administered as medications, electrolytes are used to restore a natural electrolyte balance and may affect many body systems.

Electrolytes are not measured using standard metric system units of measurement. Rather, these substances are measured using milliequivalents and millimoles. These units of measurement are particularly important when preparing IV solutions. Therefore, knowledge of a few basic chemistry concepts is helpful in understanding milliequivalents and millimoles.

Name Exchange

Potassium chloride may be referred to by one of its brand names, *Klor-Con*, or by its molecular abbreviation, *KCl*.

An **element** is a substance that cannot be chemically broken down into a simpler substance. Elements have **valence**, which is the ability to bond with other charged molecules. Valence is indicated by a positive or a negative symbol after a chemical abbreviation. Consider the element potassium, which has a positive valence of 1 (indicated by the abbreviation K^+). The valence of substances used in pharmacy preparations is most commonly plus or minus 1, 2, or 3. **The atomic weight** of an element is the weight of a single atom of that element compared with the weight of a single atom of hydrogen. The atomic weight of potassium (K^+) is 39.10 atomic mass units (amu). The **molecular weight** is the sum of the atomic weights of all atoms in one molecule of a compound. When potassium is combined with chlorine to make potassium chloride (KCl), the molecular weight is 74.55 amu. This value is obtained by adding the molecular weight of potassium, 39.10, to the molecular weight of chlorine, 35.45.

A **mole (mol)** is a unit of measurement based on the number of particles in a given substance. The mass of one mole of a substance is its molecular weight in grams. The number of grams in one mole differs among substances. For example, a mole of potassium (K^+) is 39.10 g, and a mole of chlorine (Cl^-) is 35.45 g. A **millimole (mmol)** is one-thousandth of a mole, or the molecular weight expressed in milligrams.

An **equivalent** is a unit that takes into account both moles and valence. Equivalents give you information about how one substance interacts with another. An equivalent represents both the amount of active substance and the likelihood that the substance, once in the body, will cause a change in the way two compounds are bonded. An equivalent can be calculated by multiplying the number of moles of charged particles in a substance by the valence of those particles. A **milliequivalent (mEq)** is one-thousandth of an equivalent. Potassium is a common medication that is measured in milliequivalents.

Fortunately, medications commonly used today are standardized. The calculations needed in the pharmacy will involve determining the volume of a substance that has an electrolyte as its primary ingredient rather than calculating the number of millimoles or milliequivalents in a substance.

Example 6.3.1

 You are asked to add 44 mEq of sodium chloride (NaCl) to an IV bag. Sodium chloride is available as a 4 mEq/mL solution. How many milliliters will you add to the bag?

You can solve this problem by using the ratio-proportion method or by using the dimensional analysis method.

Ratio-Proportion Method

To determine the number of milliliters to add to the bag, set up a proportion. Place the milliequivalents of sodium chloride over the unknown quantity (x mL) on the left side of the proportion and the available solution on the right side of the proportion. Be sure that the units are the same in the numerators and in the denominators. Then, cross multiply, cancel similar units (like terms), and divide to solve for the unknown variable x.

$$\frac{44 \text{ mEq}}{x \text{ mL}} = \frac{4 \text{ mEq}}{1 \text{ mL}}$$

$$x \text{ mL} (4 \text{ mEq}) = 1 \text{ mL} (44 \text{ mEq})$$

$$x = 11 \text{ mL}$$

Dimensional Analysis Method

$$\frac{44 \text{ mEq}}{1} \times \frac{1 \text{ mL}}{4 \text{ mEq}} = 11 \text{ mL}$$

Answer: You will add 11 mL of sodium chloride to the IV bag.

Example 6.3.2

 Math Morsel

Medications used to replace potassium can be administered intravenously as a solution or administered orally as tablets or a solution. No matter the route of administration, pharmacy technicians perform the calculations using the same process.

A patient needs to take a solution of potassium chloride to replace potassium lost due to diuresis. The available solution is shown in the label below. The physician has indicated that the patient needs 15 mEq of potassium chloride solution. How many milliliters should you prepare for the patient?

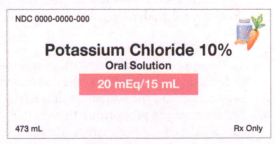

NDC 0000-0000-000

Potassium Chloride 10%
Oral Solution

20 mEq/15 mL

473 mL   Rx Only

You can solve this problem by using the ratio-proportion method or by using the dimensional analysis method.

Ratio-Proportion Method

To determine the number of milliliters to prepare, set up a proportion. Place the ordered dose (15 mEq) over the unknown quantity (x mL) on the left side of the proportion and the available solution (indicated on the medication label) on the right side of the proportion. Be sure that the units are the same in the numerators and in the denominators. Then, cross multiply, cancel similar units (like terms), and divide to solve for the unknown variable x.

$$\frac{15 \text{ mEq}}{x \text{ mL}} = \frac{20 \text{ mEq}}{15 \text{ mL}}$$

$$x \text{ mL } (20 \text{ mEq}) = 15 \text{ mL } (15 \text{ mEq})$$

$$x = 11.25 \text{ mL, rounded to } 11.3 \text{ mL}$$

Dimensional Analysis Method

$$\frac{15 \text{ mEq}}{1} \times \frac{15 \text{ mL}}{20 \text{ mEq}} = 11.25 \text{ mL, rounded to } 11.3 \text{ mL}$$

Answer: You will prepare 11.3 mL of potassium chloride solution for the patient.

Example 6.3.3

You are instructed to add 20 mEq of potassium chloride to a patient's IV solution bag. Using the multiple-dose vial label provided, how many milliliters should be prepared?

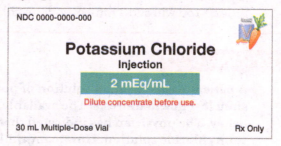

You can solve this problem by using the ratio-proportion method or by using the dimensional analysis method.

Ratio-Proportion Method

To determine the number of milliliters to prepare, set up a proportion. Place the ordered dose (20 mEq) over the unknown quantity (x mL) on the left side of the proportion and the available solution (indicated on the medication label) on the right side of the proportion. Be sure that the units are the same in the numerators and in the denominators. Then, cross multiply, cancel similar units (like terms), and divide to solve for the unknown variable x.

$$\frac{20 \text{ mEq}}{x \text{ mL}} = \frac{2 \text{ mEq}}{1 \text{ mL}}$$

$$x \text{ mL } (2 \text{ mEq}) = 1 \text{ mL } (20 \text{ mEq})$$

$$x = 10 \text{ mL}$$

Dimensional Analysis Method

$$\frac{20 \;\cancel{\text{mEq}}}{1} \times \frac{1 \text{ mL}}{2 \;\cancel{\text{mEq}}} = 10 \text{ mL}$$

Answer: You will prepare 10 mL of potassium chloride.

Example 6.3.4

You are instructed to add 16 mEq of potassium chloride to a patient's IV bag. Using the single-dose vial labels below, select the correct vial and then calculate how many milliliters you will prepare.

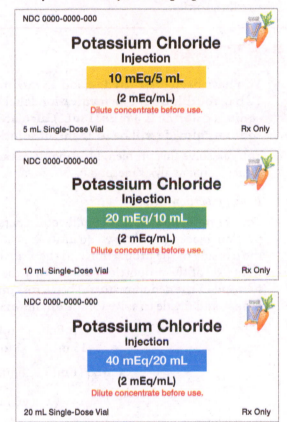

To begin, analyze the total milliequivalents in each vial to choose the correct vial. Because the order calls for 16 mEq, you will select the potassium chloride vial labeled 20 mEq/10 mL. The total volume of the selected vial is 10 mL.

Then determine the number of milliliters needed to fill this order.

You can solve this problem by using the ratio-proportion method or by using the dimensional analysis method.

Ratio-Proportion Method

To determine the number of milliliters needed for this order, set up a proportion. Place the ordered dose (16 mEq) over the unknown quantity (x mL) on the left side of the proportion and the available solution (indicated on the medication label) on the right side of the proportion. Be sure that the units are the same in the numerators and in the denominators. Then, cross multiply, cancel similar units (like terms), and divide to solve for the unknown variable x.

$$\frac{16\ \text{mEq}}{x\ \text{mL}} = \frac{20\ \text{mEq}}{10\ \text{mL}}$$

$$x\ \text{mL}\ (20\ \text{mEq}) = 10\ \text{mL}\ (16\ \text{mEq})$$

$$x = 8\ \text{mL}$$

Dimensional Analysis Method

$$\frac{16\ \cancel{\text{mEq}}}{1} \times \frac{10\ \text{mL}}{20\ \cancel{\text{mEq}}} = 8\ \text{mL}$$

Answer: You will select the vial containing 20 mEq/10 mL and will prepare 8 mL to fill the order.

Example 6.3.5

 You have been instructed to add 15 mL of sodium chloride to a patient's IV bag for dilution. The medication label states that the concentration of sodium chloride is 4 mEq/1 mL. Calculate how many milliequivalents of sodium chloride will be in 15 mL of solution.

You can solve this problem by using the ratio-proportion method or by using the dimensional analysis method.ç

Ratio-Proportion Method

To determine the number of milliequivalents of sodium chloride, set up a proportion. Place the unknown quantity (x mEq) over the ordered dose (15 mL) on the left side of the proportion and the available solution (4 mEq/1 mL) on the right side of the proportion. Be sure that the units are the same in the numerators and in the denominators. Then, cross multiply, cancel similar units (like terms), and divide to solve for the unknown variable x.

$$\frac{x\ \text{mEq}}{15\ \text{mL}} = \frac{4\ \text{mEq}}{1\ \text{mL}}$$

$$x\ \text{mEq}\ (1\ \text{mL}) = 4\ \text{mEq}\ (15\ \text{mL})$$

$$x = 60\ \text{mEq}$$

Dimensional Analysis Method

$$\frac{15\ \cancel{\text{mL}}}{1} \times \frac{4\ \text{mEq}}{1\ \cancel{\text{mL}}} = 60\ \text{mEq}$$

Answer: There are 60 mEq of sodium chloride in 15 mL of solution.

Example 6.3.6

 You must add 9 mmol of an inorganic phosphate to an IV solution. You have 15 mmol/5 mL available. How many milliliters should you add?

You can solve this problem by using the ratio-proportion method or by using the dimensional analysis method.

Ratio-Proportion Method

To determine the number of milliliters to add to this solution, set up a proportion. Place the ordered dose (9 mmol) over the unknown quantity (x mL) on the left side of the proportion and the available solution (15 mmol/5 mL) on the right side of the proportion. Be sure that the units are the same in the numerators and in the denominators. Then, cross multiply, cancel similar units (like terms), and divide to solve for the unknown variable x.

$$\frac{9 \text{ mmol}}{x \text{ mL}} = \frac{15 \text{ mmol}}{5 \text{ mL}}$$

$$x \text{ mL } (15 \text{ mmol}) = 5 \text{ mL } (9 \text{ mmol})$$

$$x = 3 \text{ mL}$$

Dimensional Analysis Method

$$\frac{9 \text{ mmol}}{1} \times \frac{5 \text{ mL}}{15 \text{ mmol}} = 3 \text{ mL}$$

Answer: You will need to add 3 mL of the inorganic phosphate to the solution.

Calculating Units

A number of medications are measured in units. A **unit** is a standardized measurement that describes medication activity irrespective of weight. Medications that are derived mainly from biological products, such as insulin, heparin, corticotropin (ACTH), Factor VIII, penicillin, and some vitamins, are expressed in international units or United States Pharmacopeia (USP) units. Both expressions include the term *units*.

Each medication's unique properties define its unit of activity. For example, heparin units are based on the amount of heparin required to keep blood from clotting. When performing calculations for medications measured in units, you typically consider units and volume, not weight.

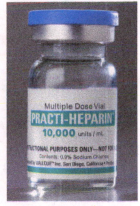

Heparin is a medication that is dosed in units.

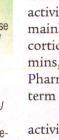
Example 6.3.7

A patient is to receive a bolus (concentrated) dose of heparin. If the dose is 7,500 units and you have a vial with the label shown below, how many milliliters will you prepare?

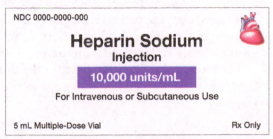

NDC 0000-0000-000

Heparin Sodium
Injection

10,000 units/mL

For Intravenous or Subcutaneous Use

5 mL Multiple-Dose Vial   Rx Only

You can solve this problem by using the ratio-proportion method or by using the dimensional analysis method.

Ratio-Proportion Method

To determine the number of milliliters to prepare, set up a proportion. Place the ordered dose (7,500 units) over the unknown quantity (x mL) on the left side of the proportion and the available concentration (10,000 units/1 mL) on the right side of the proportion. Be sure that the units are the same in the numerators and in the denominators. Then, cross multiply, cancel similar units (like terms), and divide to solve for the unknown variable x.

$$\frac{7{,}500 \text{ units}}{x \text{ mL}} = \frac{10{,}000 \text{ units}}{1 \text{ mL}}$$

$$x \text{ mL } (10{,}000 \text{ units}) = 1 \text{ mL } (7{,}500 \text{ units})$$

$$x = 0.75 \text{ mL}$$

Dimensional Analysis Method

$$\frac{7{,}500 \text{ units}}{1} \times \frac{1 \text{ mL}}{10{,}000 \text{ units}} = 0.75 \text{ mL}$$

Answer: You will prepare 0.75 mL of heparin.

Example 6.3.8

Safety Alert

Pharmacy technicians need to pay close attention to the heparin concentration stated on a vial's label. The misinterpretation of 1,000 units/mL for 10,000 units/mL has led to serious medication errors and patient harm.

An infant is to receive an injection of 75 units/kg of heparin. The infant weighs 6.4 kg. If you have a vial with the label shown below, how many milliliters will you prepare?

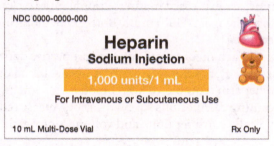

NDC 0000-0000-000

Heparin
Sodium Injection

1,000 units/1 mL

For Intravenous or Subcutaneous Use

10 mL Multi-Dose Vial   Rx Only

You can solve this problem by using the ratio-proportion method or by using the dimensional analysis method.

Ratio-Proportion Method

To begin, determine the number of units in the dose based on the patient's weight of 6.4 kg. To do so, set up a proportion by placing the unknown quantity (x units) over the patient's weight on the left side of the proportion and the dose on the right side of the proportion. Be sure that the units are the same in the numerators and in the denominators. Then, cross multiply, cancel similar units (like terms), and divide to solve for the unknown variable x.

$$\frac{x \text{ units}}{6.4 \text{ kg}} = \frac{75 \text{ units}}{1 \text{ kg}}$$

$$x \text{ units } (1 \text{ kg}) = 75 \text{ units } (6.4 \text{ kg})$$

$$x = 480 \text{ units}$$

Then calculate the number of milliliters needed to prepare the dose. To do so, set up a proportion by placing the ordered dose (480 units) over the unknown quantity (x mL) on the left side of the proportion and the available concentration (1,000 units/1 mL) on the right side of the proportion. Be sure that the units are the same in the numerators and in the denominators. Then, cross multiply, cancel similar units (like terms), and divide to solve for the unknown variable x.

$$\frac{480 \text{ units}}{x \text{ mL}} = \frac{1,000 \text{ units}}{1 \text{ mL}}$$

$$x \text{ mL } (1,000 \text{ units}) = 1 \text{ mL } (480 \text{ units})$$

$$x = 0.48 \text{ mL}$$

Dimensional Analysis Method

$$\frac{6.4 \text{ kg}}{1} \times \frac{75 \text{ units}}{\text{kg}} \times \frac{1 \text{ mL}}{1,000 \text{ units}} = 0.48 \text{ mL}$$

Answer: You will prepare 0.48 mL of heparin.

Example 6.3.9

A patient is to receive 1,000 units/kg of bacitracin IM indicated on the label below. The patient weighs 15 kg. How many milliliters of bacitracin are needed?

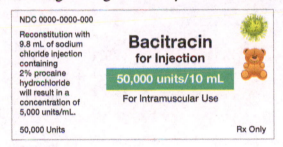

You can solve this problem by using the ratio-proportion method or by using the dimensional analysis method.

Ratio-Proportion Method

To begin, determine the number of units in the dose based on the patient's weight of 15 kg. To do so, set up a proportion by placing the unknown quantity (x units) over the patient's weight on the left side of the proportion and the dose given on the right side of the proportion. Be sure that the units are the same in the numerators and in the denominators. Then, cross multiply, cancel similar units (like terms), and divide to solve for the unknown variable x.

$$\frac{x \text{ units}}{15 \text{ kg}} = \frac{1,000 \text{ units}}{1 \text{ kg}}$$

$$x \text{ units } (1 \text{ kg}) = 1,000 \text{ units } (15 \text{ kg})$$

$$x = 15,000 \text{ units}$$

Then calculate the number of milliliters needed to prepare the dose. To do so, set up a proportion by placing the ordered dose (15,000 units) over the unknown quantity (*x* mL) on the left side of the proportion and the available concentration (50,000 units/10 mL) on the right side of the proportion. Be sure that the units are the same in the numerators and in the denominators. Then, cross multiply, cancel similar units (like terms), and divide to solve for the unknown variable *x*.

$$\frac{15,000 \text{ units}}{x \text{ mL}} = \frac{50,000 \text{ units}}{10 \text{ mL}}$$

$$x \text{ mL } (50,000 \text{ units}) = 10 \text{ mL } (15,000 \text{ units})$$

$$x = 3 \text{ mL}$$

Dimensional Analysis Method

$$\frac{15 \text{ kg}}{1} \times \frac{1,000 \text{ units}}{\text{kg}} \times \frac{10 \text{ mL}}{50,000 \text{ units}} = 3 \text{ mL}$$

Answer: The patient will receive 3 mL of bacitracin.

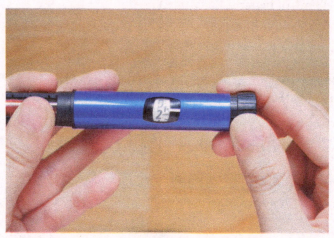

Insulin can be administered via an insulin pen. The numbers on the insulin pen pictured indicate the number of units that will be administered.

Safety Alert

Insulin syringes should only be used to administer the standard concentration of insulin (100 units/mL).

Insulin is dosed in units based on the amount of glucose that a specific amount of insulin can make available to the cells of the body. Different types and brands of insulin have different weights, but all insulins are measured using a common unit of activity. Thus, the metric weight can be disregarded, and the unit becomes a universal dose for insulin.

Many types of insulin products are available. Some insulin products require the patient to withdraw medication from a vial into a syringe. Other insulin products come in a prefilled syringe or "pen" with a disposable needle on the tip. Insulin syringes should be used to administer or dispense the standard concentration of insulin (100 units/mL). Insulin syringes are available in standard unit sizes, as illustrated in Figure 6.4.

Reading insulin labels can be challenging because there may be only slight variations from one product to another. *However, it is critical to select the correct insulin product because insulin products are not interchangeable.* Insulin products differ by onset and duration of action and have the potential to harm a patient who uses the wrong brand or type. Consequently, when preparing an insulin dose or prescription, you must triple-check the medication's label against the printed label and the ordered medication. Confirm that the NDC numbers match. If the pharmacy is equipped with a bar code scanner, use the device to confirm that the correct medication has been selected.

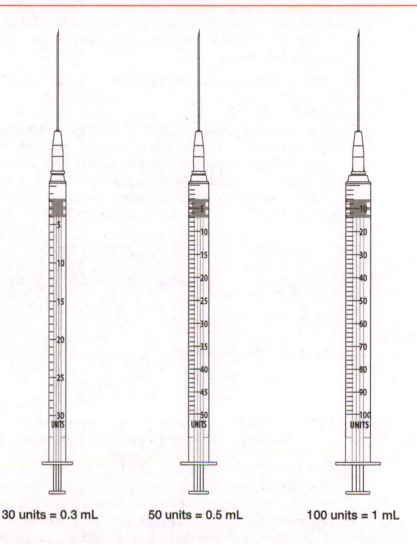

30 units = 0.3 mL   50 units = 0.5 mL   100 units = 1 mL

The following examples demonstrate how to calculate a volume of insulin in milliliters (vs standard units). Calculating the volume of insulin in milliliters is helpful when determining how long an insulin vial or pen will last a patient. Volume is also useful when insulin is added to a parenteral solution, such as parenteral nutrition.

Example 6.3.10

A patient is to receive 32 units of regular insulin each morning before breakfast. Insulin comes in a concentration of 100 units/mL. How many milliliters will the patient receive with each dose? How many days will the insulin vial last if the patient takes one dose per day?

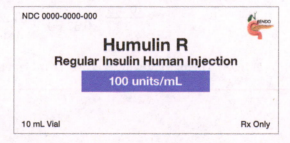

NDC 0000-0000-000

Humulin R
Regular Insulin Human Injection
100 units/mL

10 mL Vial   Rx Only

You can solve this problem by using the ratio-proportion method or by using the dimensional analysis method. You will need to perform two different sets of calculations. First, you need to determine the number of milliliters the patient will receive with each dose; second, you need to determine how many days the insulin vial will last.

Step 1. Determine the volume per dose.

Ratio-Proportion Method

To determine how many milliliters the patient will receive with each dose, set up a proportion. Place the ordered dose (32 units) over the unknown quantity (x mL) on the left side of the proportion and the available concentration (100 units/mL) on the right side of the proportion. Be sure that the units are the same in the numerators and in the denominators. Then, cross multiply, cancel similar units (like terms), and divide to solve for the unknown variable x.

$$\frac{32 \text{ units}}{x \text{ mL}} = \frac{100 \text{ units}}{1 \text{ mL}}$$

$$x \text{ mL} (100 \text{ units}) = 1 \text{ mL} (32 \text{ units})$$

$$x = 0.32 \text{ mL}$$

Dimensional Analysis Method

$$\frac{32 \text{ units}}{1} \times \frac{1 \text{ mL}}{100 \text{ units}} = 0.32 \text{ mL}$$

Step 2. Using the volume per dose you just calculated, determine the number of days a single vial will last if the patient takes one dose per day.

Ratio-Proportion Method

To determine the number of days a single vial will last, set up a proportion. Place the unknown quantity (x days) over the vial size (10 mL) on the left side of the proportion and the dose the patient will receive (0.32 mL) on the right side of the proportion. Be sure that the units are the same in the numerators and in the denominators. Then, cross multiply, cancel similar units (like terms), and divide to solve for the unknown variable x.

$$\frac{x \text{ days}}{10 \text{ mL}} = \frac{1 \text{ day}}{0.32 \text{ mL}}$$

$$x \text{ days} (0.32 \text{ mL}) = 1 \text{ day} (10 \text{ mL})$$

$$x = 31.25 \text{ days, rounded down to the nearest whole day or 31 days}$$

Dimensional Analysis Method

$$\frac{10 \text{ mL}}{1} \times \frac{1 \text{ day}}{0.32 \text{ mL}} = 31.25 \text{ days, rounded down to the nearest whole day or 31 days}$$

Answer: The patient will receive 0.32 mL at each dose. The vial will last 31 days.

Example 6.3.11

A patient is to receive 49 units of Humulin 70/30 insulin twice daily. The insulin comes in a concentration of 100 units/mL. How many milliliters will the patient receive in each dose? How many vials will the patient need to last 30 days (1 month)?

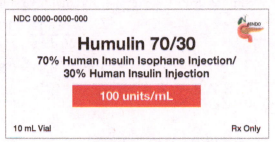

You can solve this problem by using the ratio-proportion method or by using the dimensional analysis method. You will need to perform two different sets of calculations. First, you need to determine the number of milliliters the patient will receive with each dose; second, you need to determine how many vials the patient will need to last 30 days.

Step 1. Determine the volume per dose.

Ratio-Proportion Method

To determine how many milliliters the patient will receive with each dose, set up a proportion. Place the patient's prescribed dose (49 units) over the unknown quantity (x mL) on the left side of the proportion and the concentration of the product (100 units/mL) on the right side of the proportion. Be sure that the units are the same in the numerators and in the denominators. Then, cross multiply, cancel similar units (like terms), and divide to solve for the unknown variable x.

$$\frac{49 \text{ units}}{x \text{ mL}} = \frac{100 \text{ units}}{1 \text{ mL}}$$

$$x \text{ mL } (100 \text{ units}) = 1 \text{ mL } (49 \text{ units})$$

$$x = 0.49 \text{ mL}$$

Dimensional Analysis Method

$$\frac{49 \text{ units}}{1} \times \frac{1 \text{ mL}}{100 \text{ units}} = 0.49 \text{ mL}$$

Step 2. Using the volume per dose you just calculated, determine the number of milliliters the patient will need for twice daily dosing.

$$\frac{0.49 \text{ mL}}{\text{dose}} \times \frac{2 \text{ doses}}{\text{day}} = \frac{0.98 \text{ mL}}{\text{day}}$$

Now that you know how many milliliters the patient will need each day, you can use the ratio-proportion method to determine the number of milliliters the patient will need for 30 days.

Ratio-Proportion Method

Set up a proportion by placing the unknown quantity (x mL) over the number of days (30) on the left side of the proportion and the dose the patient will receive (0.98 mL/day) on the right side of the proportion. Be sure that the units are the same in the numerators and in the denominators. Then, cross multiply, cancel similar units (like terms), and divide to solve for the unknown variable x.

$$\frac{x \text{ mL}}{30 \text{ days}} = \frac{0.98 \text{ mL}}{1 \text{ day}}$$

$$x \text{ mL} (1 \text{ day}) = 0.98 \text{ mL} (30 \text{ days})$$

$$x = 29.4 \text{ mL}$$

Dimensional Analysis Method

$$\frac{30 \text{ days}}{1} \times \frac{0.98 \text{ mL}}{1 \text{ day}} = 29.4 \text{ mL}$$

Answer: The patient will receive 0.49 mL in each dose. Because one vial contains 10 mL, the patient will need three vials to last 30 days.

Example 6.3.12

How many units are in the Humalog Mix 75/25 KwikPen with the following label? If a patient uses 23 units daily, how many days will this KwikPen last?

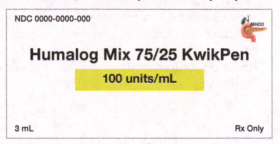

You can solve this problem by using the ratio-proportion method or by using the dimensional analysis method. You will need to perform two different sets of calculations. First, you need to determine the number of units in a single pen; second, you need to determine the number of days a single pen will last.

Step 1. Determine the number of units in a single pen.

Ratio-Proportion Method

To begin, calculate the total number of units in a single pen. Set up a proportion by placing the unknown amount (x units) over the number of milliliters in one pen (3 mL) on the left side of the proportion and the concentration of the product (100 units/mL) on the right side of the proportion. Be sure that the units are the same in the numerators and in the denominators. Then, cross multiply, cancel similar units (like terms), and divide to solve for the unknown variable x.

$$\frac{x \text{ units}}{3 \text{ mL}} = \frac{100 \text{ units}}{1 \text{ mL}}$$

$$x \text{ units } (1 \text{ mL}) = 100 \text{ units } (3 \text{ mL})$$

$$x = 300 \text{ units}$$

Dimensional Analysis Method

$$\frac{3 \text{ mL}}{1} \times \frac{100 \text{ units}}{1 \text{ mL}} = 300 \text{ units}$$

Part 2. Now that you know how many units are in a single pen, you can calculate the number of days that a single pen will last.

Ratio-Proportion Method

Set up a proportion by placing the unknown quantity (*x* days) over the number of units in a single pen (300 units) on the left side of the proportion and the prescribed units (23 units/day) on the right side of the proportion. Be sure that the units are the same in the numerators and in the denominators. Then, cross multiply, cancel similar units (like terms), and divide to solve for the unknown variable *x*.

$$\frac{x \text{ days}}{300 \text{ units}} = \frac{1 \text{ day}}{23 \text{ units}}$$

$$x \text{ days } (23 \text{ units}) = 1 \text{ day } (300 \text{ units})$$

$$x = 13.04 \text{ days, rounded down to the nearest whole day or 13 days}$$

Dimensional Analysis Method

$$\frac{300 \text{ units}}{1} \times \frac{1 \text{ day}}{23 \text{ units}} = 13.04 \text{ days, rounded down to the nearest whole day or 13 days}$$

Answer: There are 300 units of insulin in the pen. The pen will last 13 days.

Example 6.3.13

A patient is to receive 100 units of regular insulin twice daily. The insulin comes in a concentration of 500 units/mL. How many milliliters will the patient receive with each dose?

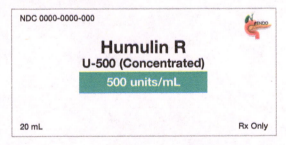

NDC 0000-0000-000

Humulin R
U-500 (Concentrated)
500 units/mL

20 mL   Rx Only

You can solve this problem by using the ratio-proportion method or by using the dimensional analysis method.

Ratio-Proportion Method

To begin, set up a proportion by placing the unknown amount (*x* mL) over the patient's prescribed dose (100 units) on the left side of the proportion and the concentration of the product (500 units/mL) on the right side of the proportion. Be sure that the units are the same in the numerators and in the denominators. Then, cross multiply, cancel similar units (like terms), and divide to solve for the unknown variable *x*.

$$\frac{x \text{ mL}}{100 \text{ units}} = \frac{1 \text{ mL}}{500 \text{ units}}$$

$$x \text{ mL } (500 \text{ units}) = 1 \text{ mL } (100 \text{ units})$$

$$x = 0.2 \text{ mL}$$

Dimensional Analysis Method

$$\frac{100 \text{ units}}{1} \times \frac{1 \text{ mL}}{500 \text{ units}} = 0.2 \text{ mL}$$

Answer: The patient will receive 0.2 mL with each dose.

A 1 mL tuberculin syringe can be used to administer a concentrated insulin, such as U-500 insulin. Simply draw up the insulin to the calculated 0.2 mL mark to measure the appropriate dose (see Figure 6.5).

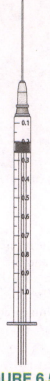

FIGURE 6.5

0.2 mL of medication in a 1 mL tuberculin syringe

WORKPLACE WISDOM

The most common insulin concentration is 100 units/mL (U-100). However, some types of insulin come in 200 units/mL (U-200), 300 units/mL (U-300), and 500 units/mL (U-500) formulations. When drawing up insulin into a syringe, pharmacy technicians should ensure that they have selected the correct concentration. Patients can be harmed by receiving too much or too little insulin because the vial selected contained a concentration different from the concentration that was prescribed.

6.3 Problem Set

Perform the necessary calculations to answer each of the following. Round your answer to the nearest tenth.

Note: Questions 1, 2, 4, 6, 7, 8, 13, 14, and 16 have accompanying handouts depicting measuring devices. Be sure to obtain these handouts from your instructor.

1. An order requires 30 mEq of potassium phosphate. You have a 4.4 mEq/mL solution available. How many milliliters of potassium phosphate should be used to fill the order? On the handout that you obtained from your instructor, indicate the correct volume on the measuring device.

2. An order requires 44 mEq of potassium phosphate. You have a 4.4 mEq/mL solution available. How many milliliters should you put in the IV solution? On the handout that you obtained from your instructor, indicate the correct volume on the measuring device(s).

3. A prescription states that a patient must take 32 mEq of potassium. The potassium replacement selected has 8 mEq per tablet. How many tablets would the patient need to take?

4. A patient is to use a sugar-free, alcohol-free solution of potassium that contains 40 mEq/15 mL. The patient is to take 30 mEq daily in two equally divided doses. How many milliliters will each dose be? On the handout that you obtained from your instructor, indicate the correct volume on the measuring device(s).

5. A prescription has been filled for 15 mL Rum-K with breakfast. Rum-K contains 20 mEq/10 mL. How many milliequivalents is the patient taking with each dose?

6. A patient needs to take 36 mEq of potassium orally. The solution on hand has 20 mEq/15 mL. How much solution should be prepared for the patient? On the handout that you obtained from your instructor, indicate the correct volume on the measuring device.

For questions 7–10, select the vial that is needed to fill each order with the required number of milliequivalents of potassium chloride, and then calculate the volume to be withdrawn from the selected vial for the order.

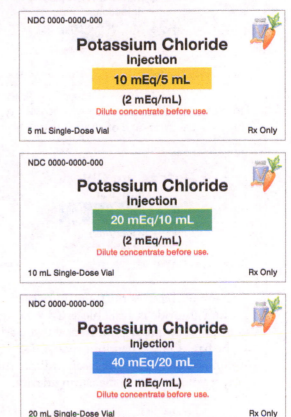

7. Add 14 mEq of potassium chloride to the patient's IV solution. On the handout that you obtained from your instructor, indicate the correct volume on the measuring device.

8. Add 20 mEq of potassium chloride to the patient's IV solution. On the handout that you obtained from your instructor, indicate the correct volume on the measuring device.

9. Add 27 mEq of potassium chloride to the patient's IV solution.

10. Add 50 mEq of potassium chloride to the patient's IV solution.

For questions 11 and 12, use the label provided to calculate the volume or amount requested.

11. How many milliequivalents of potassium chloride are in 8 mL of the solution?

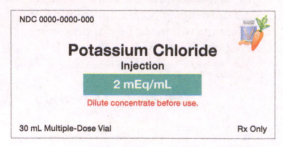

NDC 0000-0000-000

Potassium Chloride
Injection

2 mEq/mL

Dilute concentrate before use.

30 mL Multiple-Dose Vial   Rx Only

12. How many milliequivalents of potassium chloride are in 15 mL of the solution?

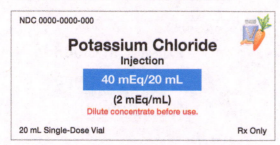

NDC 0000-0000-000

Potassium Chloride
Injection

40 mEq/20 mL

(2 mEq/mL)

Dilute concentrate before use.

20 mL Single-Dose Vial   Rx Only

13. A pharmacy receives the following order. Sodium chloride is available as a 4 mEq/mL solution. How many milliliters will you add to the bag? On the handout that you obtained from your instructor, indicate the correct volume on the measuring device.

> ℞   Give 132 mEq of sodium chloride in 100 mL.
>
> Infuse at 62 mL/hour.

14. A pharmacy receives an order indicating that you should add 120 mEq of sodium chloride to an IV bag of D_5W. Using a vial that is labeled 4 mEq/mL, how many milliliters should you add to the bag? On the handout that you obtained from your instructor, indicate the correct volume on the measuring device.

Use the following label to answer questions 15 and 16.

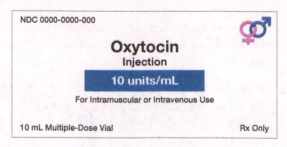

NDC 0000-0000-000

Oxytocin
Injection

10 units/mL

For Intramuscular or Intravenous Use

10 mL Multiple-Dose Vial   Rx Only

15. A patient is to receive 4 units of oxytocin. Using the vial with the label shown above, how many milliliters will be needed?

16. A patient has received 2.8 mL of the oxytocin solution shown in the label above. How many units did the patient receive? On the handout that you obtained from your instructor, indicate the correct volume on the measuring device.

17. A patient is to receive 3,500 units of heparin, and the following label shows the medication you are to dispense. How many milliliters will the patient receive?

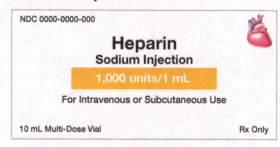

NDC 0000-0000-000

Heparin
Sodium Injection

1,000 units/1 mL

For Intravenous or Subcutaneous Use

10 mL Multi-Dose Vial   Rx Only

18. A patient needs an injection of heparin. An order for 0.43 mL has been prepared. How many units of heparin are in the dose if it contains 20,000 units/0.8 mL?

19. Prepare 7,000 units of heparin from the vial with the label shown below. How many milliliters will you prepare?

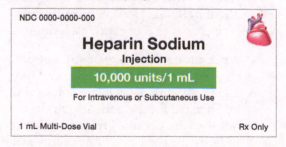

NDC 0000-0000-000

Heparin Sodium
Injection

10,000 units/1 mL

For Intravenous or Subcutaneous Use

1 mL Multi-Dose Vial   Rx Only

20. Prepare 24,000 units of heparin from the vial with the label shown below. How many milliliters will you prepare?

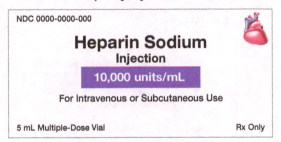

NDC 0000-0000-000

Heparin Sodium
Injection

10,000 units/mL

For Intravenous or Subcutaneous Use

5 mL Multiple-Dose Vial   Rx Only

21. Prepare two syringes for a patient on the orthopedic floor. Each syringe should contain 30 mg of Lovenox. How many milliliters does each syringe contain?

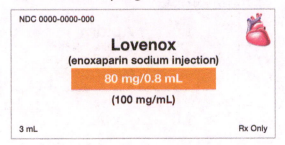

NDC 0000-0000-000

Lovenox
(enoxaparin sodium injection)

80 mg/0.8 mL

(100 mg/mL)

3 mL   Rx Only

Calculate the following volumes or number of units.

22. Penicillin G can be reconstituted to many different concentrations. You are filling an order for 175,000 units and have a stock medication with a concentration of 500,000 units/mL. How many milliliters is the dose?

23. Bicillin CR is a preparation administered as an IM injection. You have a stock medication with a concentration of 600,000 units/mL, and you are to prepare a dose of 1.2 million units. What volume will be administered?

24. A physician has ordered 385,000 units of penicillin G for a patient. You have a stock medication with a concentration of 50,000 units/mL. How many milliliters is the dose?

25. A patient is to receive Humulin 70/30 insulin at a dose of 45 units at 8:00 every morning. Using the vial with the following label, how many milliliters should be drawn into the syringe?

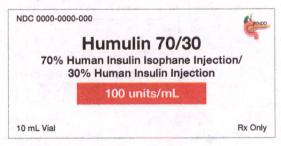

NDC 0000-0000-000

Humulin 70/30
70% Human Insulin Isophane Injection/
30% Human Insulin Injection

100 units/mL

10 mL Vial   Rx Only

26. A patient uses 18 units of insulin every morning and 10 units of insulin at 7:00 p.m. Using the label below, how long will the volume last?

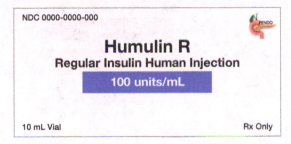

NDC 0000-0000-000

Humulin R
Regular Insulin Human Injection

100 units/mL

10 mL Vial   Rx Only

27. A patient uses 20 units of insulin every morning and 18 units of insulin every evening. Using the label below, answer the following questions.

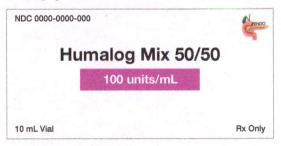

NDC 0000-0000-000

Humalog Mix 50/50

100 units/mL

10 mL Vial   Rx Only

a. How many total units does the patient use daily?

b. How many vials does the patient need for 30 days?

28. A patient uses 10 units of Humulin R each morning and 15 units of Humulin 70/30 at lunch and dinner. Using the labels below, determine the number of vials of each type of Humulin the patient will need for 30 days.

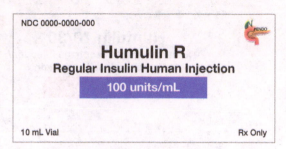

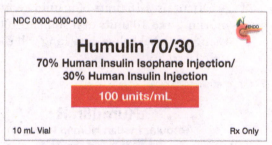

29. A patient uses 0.5 mL daily of Lantus shown in the following label. How many units does the patient receive?

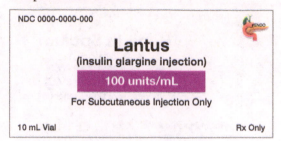

30. Using the label shown below, determine how long two vials of Apidra will last a patient who uses 20 units twice daily.

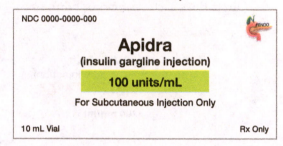

Self-check your work in Appendix A.

Review and Assessment

CHAPTER SUMMARY

- The three common types of injections are subcutaneous (subcut, SC, or SQ), intramuscular (IM), and intravenous (IV).

- Subcut and IM injections are small-volume injections given over a short period.

- IV infusions typically range from 50–1,000 mL and are administered in a vein over a period of minutes to hours, depending on the volume.

- Syringe barrel size is selected by choosing the smallest volume barrel that will accurately measure the desired amount.

- Ratio strength (e.g., 1:1,000) is used to represent the concentration when the amount of medication in the vehicle is very small.

- When a solid medication has been dissolved in a liquid, the units of measurement for a 1:100 ratio solution are 1 g:100 mL.

- Powder volume is the amount of space taken up by a lyophilized drug in a sterile vial. This type of medication is used for reconstitution.

- Electrolytes are measured in milliequivalents or millimoles.

- Milliequivalents represent the amount of active, charged electrolytes, not the amount of medication by weight.

- When a medication is measured in units, weight is not used to measure the medication.

- Insulin and heparin are the two most common medications dosed in units.

- Insulin is most often concentrated as standard U-100, which means that there are 100 units/1 mL.

- Even though there are many brands and types of insulin that use the standard U-100 concentration, they are not interchangeable.

FORMULAS FOR SUCCESS

Ratio Strength (Section 6.1)

a grams: *b* milliliters
a = parts of active drug
b = parts of liquid solution

Formulas for Powder Reconstitution (Section 6.2)

powder volume (pv) = final volume (fv) − diluent volume (dv)

or

pv = fv − dv

diluent volume (dv) = final volume (fv) − powder volume (pv)

or

dv = fv − pv

final volume (fv) = powder volume (pv) + diluent volume (dv)

or

fv = pv + dv

CHECK YOUR UNDERSTANDING

Take a moment to review what you have learned in this chapter and answer the following questions.

1. Injectable solutions are typically measured in the pharmacy using
   a. IV bags.
   b. syringes.
   c. graduated cylinders.
   d. ampules.

2. The final volume of a solution made with a lyophilized powder equals the diluent volume plus the
   a. vial volume.
   b. air volume.
   c. liquid volume.
   d. powder volume.

3. You need to prepare a 50 mg dose of enoxaparin. The medication is in a vial containing 80 mg/0.8 mL. How many milliliters will you need to prepare the medication?
   a. 0.5 mL
   b. 0.8 mL
   c. 1.5 mL
   d. 5 mL

4. You have an order for 10,000 units of heparin to be administered to a patient. The vial you have on hand contains 5,000 units/mL and contains 10 mL. How many milliliters will you need to fill the order?
   a. 1 mL
   b. 1.5 mL
   c. 2 mL
   d. 2.5 mL

5. A patient who is self-administering Humulin R uses 20 units in the morning and 15 units in the afternoon. How many days will a 10 mL vial of U-100 insulin last?
   a. 10 days
   b. 15 days
   c. 21 days
   d. 28 days

6. A patient is to receive 14,000 units of heparin *stat*. The vial on hand is a 10 mL bottle of 5,000 units/mL. How many milliliters will you need to fill this order?
   a. 2.8 mL
   b. 3.5 mL
   c. 5 mL
   d. 5.6 mL

7. A medication order for 40 mg of furosemide injection is received by the pharmacy. The pharmacy has furosemide 10 mg/mL in stock. How many milliliters will you need to fill this order?
   a. 1 mL
   b. 2 mL
   c. 3 mL
   d. 4 mL

8. How many grams of active drug are in 750 mL of a 1:200 solution?
   a. 2.5 g
   b. 3.75 g
   c. 5 g
   d. 6.25 g

9. A powdered antibiotic must be reconstituted for use. The label states the dry powder occupies 0.4 mL. What is the diluent volume if the final volume is 5 mL?
   a. 0.8 mL
   b. 1.6 mL
   c. 4.6 mL
   d. 5.4 mL

10. A 500 mg vial of lyophilized azithromycin injection states it should be reconstituted with 4.8 mL of water to make a 100 mg/mL concentration. What is the powder volume contained in the vial?
    a. 0.2 mL
    b. 0.4 mL
    c. 0.5 mL
    d. 0.6 mL

 FIND SOLUTIONS

Take a moment to consider what you have learned in this chapter and respond thoughtfully to the prompts.

Scenario A: Lauren Nickelson is a 38-year-old patient weighing 83 kg who is being admitted to the hospital from the emergency department. The admission orders include heparin 5,000 units subcut three times daily and penicillin G 2,000,000 units IV every 6 hours.

1. How many milliliters of heparin will the patient receive with each injection if the vial concentration is 10,000 units/mL?

2. How many milliliters of heparin will the patient receive with each injection if the vial concentration is 20,000 units/mL? Round your answer to the nearest hundredth of a milliliter.

3. How many milliliters of penicillin G will the patient receive with each dose if the stock product concentration is 60,000 units/mL? Round your answer to the nearest tenth of a milliliter.

4. How many milliliters of penicillin G will the patient receive each day if the stock product concentration is 60,000 units/mL? Round your answer to the nearest tenth of a milliliter.

5. How many milliliters of penicillin G will the patient receive with each dose if the stock product concentration is 20,000 units/mL?

6. How many milliliters of penicillin G will the patient receive each day if the stock product concentration is 20,000 units/mL?

Scenario B: Rahim Patel is a 56-year-old hospitalized patient with a lab value indicating a low potassium level. The physician orders 40 mEq of IV potassium chloride and 40 mEq of oral potassium chloride.

7. How many milliliters will be needed for the patient's IV dose if you have a 10 mL vial of potassium chloride 20 mEq?

8. How many milliliters will be needed for the patient's IV dose if you have a stock product of potassium chloride with a concentration of 20 mEq/50 mL?

9. How many milliliters will be needed for the patient's oral dose if you have a 20 mEq/15 mL potassium chloride oral solution?

10. After receiving a total of 80 mEq of potassium chloride, the patient's potassium level is still low. An additional IV infusion is started with potassium chloride 10 mEq/5 mL added. How many milliequivalents of potassium chloride will the patient receive if the amount added was 15 mL?

The online course includes additional review and assessment resources.

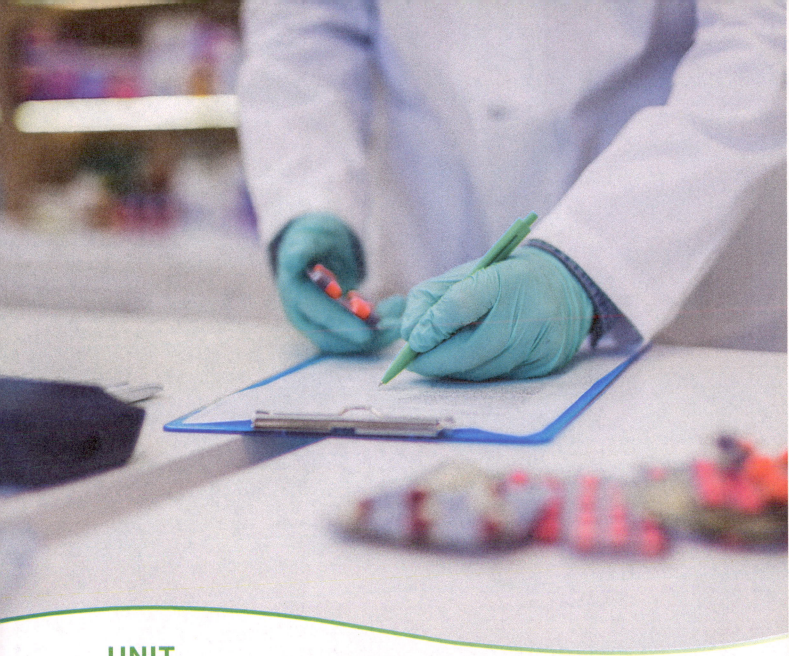

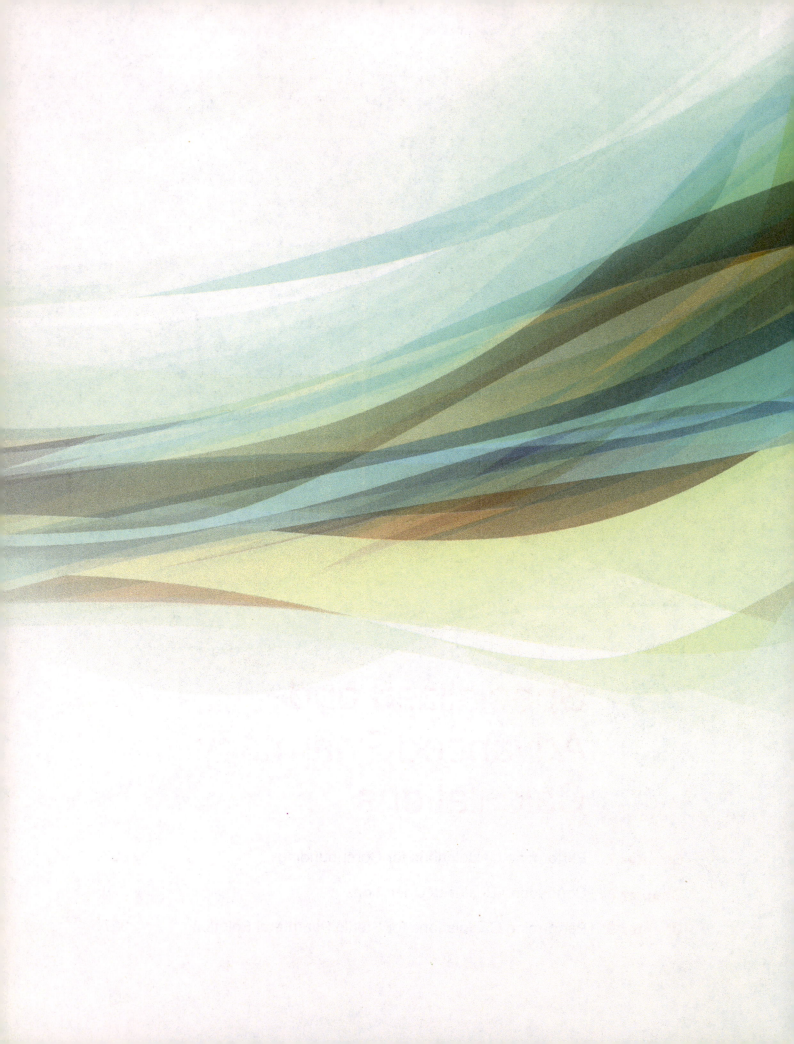

7

Performing Calculations for Compounding

Learning Objectives

1 Define the term *compounding* and the types of ingredients used in this process. (Section 7.1)

2 Distinguish between a compounded stock preparation and a compounded sterile preparation. (Section 7.1)

3 Calculate the amount of each ingredient needed to enlarge or reduce a formula stored in a pharmacy recipe book. (Section 7.1)

4 Describe the importance of setting up an alligation grid to help make the desired strength of a medication that is not commercially available or on hand in a pharmacy. (Section 7.2)

5 Compute the amount of two strengths of an active ingredient needed to prepare a product whose concentration lies between the two strengths. (Section 7.2)

6 Describe the weight-in-weight formula used when compounding two solid ingredients. (Section 7.3)

7 Calculate percentage strength for a weight-in-weight preparation. (Section 7.3)

8 Determine the amount of ingredients using the weight-in-weight formula. (Section 7.3)

For a key to the body system icons that appear in each chapter of this textbook, refer to the Preface.

ASHP/ACPE Accreditation Standards
To view the *ASHP/ACPE Accreditation Standards* addressed in this chapter, refer to Appendix D.

This chapter provides a foundation for the preparation of customized medications for patients. This process, referred to as *compounding*, is performed in both community and institutional pharmacy settings and includes the enlargement or reduction of a medication recipe, the utilization of available pharmacy products to produce a customized product, and the preparation of a medication using two solid ingredients. These different compounding scenarios require the use of specific calculation methods such as formulas for current and desired ratios, alligations, and weight-in-weight calculations.

7.1 Enlargement or Reduction of Formulas

Compounding is the process of using raw ingredients and/or prepared ingredients to create a medication for a patient. Compounding usually involves both **active ingredients** (components that provide pharmacologic activity) and

inactive ingredients (components that do not provide pharmacologic activity). The process of compounding is similar to making a cake from scratch by using ingredients such as butter, sugar, eggs, flour, and baking powder. Compounding is commonly performed by pharmacy personnel at specialized compounding pharmacies (pharmacies that primarily compound medications) and at institutional pharmacies. In addition, nonsterile compounding is performed by personnel in certain community pharmacies.

Compounding Formulas

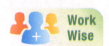

Work Wise

Pharmacy technicians who are interested in a career in a compounding pharmacy may want to complete specialized training in this practice area. Several professional organizations offer certifications in different types of compounding that pharmacy technicians can pursue.

A compounded medication is prepared using a formula or a recipe. The formula is a document prepared by a pharmacist that lists the ingredients and instructions needed to compound a specific medication. Formulas may be organized and maintained in a computerized file system or, simply, in a card file or binder. A pharmacy's set of formulas is often called the *pharmacy's recipe book*. Some pharmacies also have different formulas for different prescribers, as each prescriber may prefer a slightly different version of a specific compound.

Compounding formulas or recipes may be used in both sterile and nonsterile compounding. **Sterile compounding** is the practice of combining, admixing, diluting, pooling, reconstituting, repackaging, or otherwise altering a drug or bulk drug substance to create a sterile medication using aseptic technique. **Aseptic technique** is a method designed to minimize the risk of contamination. A medication made by sterile compounding is called a *compounded sterile preparation (CSP)*. Common CSPs include intravenous (IV) antibiotics and ophthalmic solutions. **Nonsterile compounding**, also known as *extemporaneous compounding*, is the compounding of commercially unavailable, noninjectable products. Prescription topical products (such as lotions and creams) are common examples of nonsterile compounded medications.

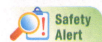

Safety Alert

Pharmacies that produce mass quantities of compounded medications have come under scrutiny due to contaminated products that resulted in serious illness and death. The FDA has since become more aggressive in its inspections of pharmacies and enforcement methods.

Some formulas are intended to prepare a single prescription, whereas others are intended to prepare a **compounded stock preparation**, or a larger amount to be divided and dispensed for individual prescription orders later. Compounded stock preparations may be made in pharmacies that routinely receive orders for the same formula. A pharmacy that prepares these compounds will often have a recipe for making a large amount to have on hand. It is not uncommon to prepare a compound that can be divided and dispensed to as many as 20 patients. Preparing larger batches is sometimes referred to as *batch compounding*.

The preparation of compounds in advance can be cost-effective for pharmacies by reducing the labor needed to make the product and can be time-saving for patients by providing the compound expediently. Although the US Food and Drug Administration (FDA) prohibits pharmacies from mass manufacturing compounded medications, anticipatory compounding is permitted in small quantities when a particular pharmacy is located near a physician's office that routinely orders certain compounded prescriptions.

Enlarging and Reducing Formulas

Enlarging or reducing formulas involves taking the recipe for a particular compounded medication and adjusting the amount of the ingredients to meet the needs of a prescriber's order. This practice is similar to doubling the ingredients in a recipe for cookies to make twice as many cookies or reducing the ingredients in half to make half as many cookies. Just as retaining the correct proportion of each ingredient in the cookie recipe is important to the final product, so too is the adjustment of a formula to prepare the final, compounded medication.

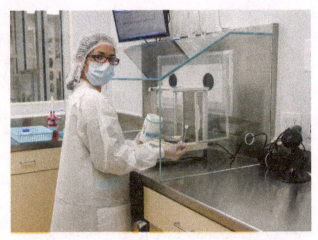

USP 800 compounding pharmacy during business hours.

To that end, it is essential for you to maintain accurate records and documentation of the mathematical calculations used in enlarging or reducing a formula. All amounts should be calculated and recorded before weighing, measuring, or mixing. The final prepared product must match the concentration (also referred to as the *strength* or *percent*) and amount ordered by the prescriber.

To accurately compound an order, you must locate the **current formula**, which is the formula that is kept on hand in the pharmacy's recipe book. In addition, you will need to know the **desired formula**, which is a specialized pharmaceutical recipe ordered by a prescriber that alters various components of a current formula. The desired formula is typically an enlarged or a reduced form of the current formula.

Compound formulas often include the abbreviation *QSAD*. This abbreviation is derived from the Latin term *quantum sufficit ad*, meaning "a quantity sufficient" or "a quantity sufficient to make." The abbreviation *QSAD* almost always refers to an inactive ingredient in a formula. It instructs the preparer to use an ingredient up to the specified quantity. For example, suppose that you are preparing 100 mL of a compounded medication that contains two ingredients (one active ingredient and one inactive ingredient). The formula calls for 5 g of the powdered form of the active ingredient. The formula also instructs QSAD 100 mL of the inactive ingredient (which is a liquid). To prepare the formula, you would first measure 5 g of the active ingredient. You would then add a sufficient amount of the inactive ingredient until the total volume of the compounded medication is 100 mL. The volume of the added inactive ingredient is actually less than 100 mL because the active ingredient takes up volume.

When you enlarge or reduce a compounding formula, you must manipulate the quantity of each ingredient in the formula. To accomplish this task, you must determine a ratio to compare the desired formula with the current formula. Consider the following compounding formula.

Put Down Roots

The abbreviation *QSAD* is derived from the Latin term *quantum sufficit ad*, meaning "a quantity sufficient" or "a quantity sufficient to make."

Math Morsel

When enlarging or reducing a formula for compounding, pharmacy technicians must always retain the correct proportion of ingredients from the current formula.

Pharmacy's Recipe Book Formula for Progesterone 50 mg/g in Cream Base (yields 100 g)		
Progesterone	5 g	
Pentylene glycol	10 g	
Topical cream base	QSAD 100 g	

Suppose that the desired quantity was 200 g. To determine how much of each ingredient is required for the desired quantity, the amount of each ingredient must be multiplied by the appropriate ratio. To determine the ratio, you compare the desired formula quantity to the current formula quantity.

$$\text{ratio to enlarge or reduce a formula} = \frac{\text{desired formula quantity}}{\text{current formula quantity}}$$

In this example, the desired formula quantity is 200 g, and the current formula quantity is 100 g.

$$\frac{200 \text{ g}}{100 \text{ g}} = 2$$

The determined ratio is 2 to 1 (2:1 or $\frac{2}{10}$). As a result, each ingredient in the current formula must be multiplied by 2 to achieve the desired formula.

progesterone	$5 \text{ g} \times 2 = 10 \text{ g}$
pentylene glycol	$10 \text{ g} \times 2 = 20 \text{ g}$
topical cream base	QSAD $100 \text{ g} \times 2 = $ QSAD to 200 g

To create the desired formula, you will need 10 g of progesterone, 20 g of pentylene glycol, and up to 200 g of topical cream base.

The following examples demonstrate the calculations for reducing or enlarging formulas.

Example 7.1.1

A prescriber has ordered 100 mL of a commonly used topical iodine solution. The pharmacy's recipe book lists a formula to prepare 1,000 mL of the solution. Determine how much of each ingredient will be needed to prepare 100 mL of the solution.

Pharmacy's Recipe Book Formula for a Topical Iodine Solution (yields 1,000 mL)

Iodine	30 g
Sodium iodide	25 g
Purified water	QSAD to 1,000 mL

Step 1. Determine the ratio to compare the desired formula quantity with the current formula quantity.

The desired formula requires you to provide 100 mL of the solution.

The current formula provides 1,000 mL of the solution.

Use this information to set up your ratio:

$$\text{ratio to enlarge or reduce a formula} = \frac{\text{desired formula quantity}}{\text{current formula quantity}}.$$

$$\frac{100 \text{ mL}}{1,000 \text{ mL}} = \frac{1}{10}$$

Therefore, you will need $\frac{1}{10}$ (i.e., 100 mL desired formula/1,000 mL current formula) of the amount of each ingredient listed in the current recipe. To find the amount of each ingredient, you will multiply each ingredient amount by $\frac{1}{10}$. This calculation is the same as dividing each ingredient amount by 10, as shown in Step 2.

Step 2. Calculate the amount of each ingredient by dividing each ingredient amount by 10.

Desired Formula (for 100 mL)

iodine	$\dfrac{30 \text{ g}}{10} = 3 \text{ g}$
sodium iodide	$\dfrac{25 \text{ g}}{10} = 2.5 \text{ g}$
purified water	QSAD to $\dfrac{1,000 \text{ mL}}{10} = 100 \text{ mL}$

Answer: You will need 3 g of iodine and 2.5 g of sodium iodide. Because the desired formula indicates QSAD to 100 mL, you will need to add enough purified water to achieve a final volume of 100 mL.

Example 7.1.2

You need to prepare 16 oz of coal tar ointment, a compounded medication, for a patient. The pharmacy's recipe book lists a formula to prepare 4 oz of the ointment. Determine how much of each ingredient you will need to prepare 16 oz of the ointment.

Pharmacy's Recipe Book Formula for Coal Tar Ointment (yields 4 oz)	
Coal tar	4 g
Salicylic acid	1 g
Triamcinolone 0.1%	15 g
Hydrophilic petrolatum base ointment	100 g

Step 1. Determine the ratio to compare the desired formula quantity with the current formula quantity.

The desired formula requires you to provide 16 oz of the ointment.

The current formula provides 4 oz of the ointment.

Use this information to set up your ratio:

$$\text{ratio to enlarge or reduce a formula} = \frac{\text{desired formula quantity}}{\text{current formula quantity}}$$

$$\frac{16\ oz}{4\ oz} = \frac{4}{1}$$

Therefore, you will need four times (i.e., 16 desired/4 formula = 4) the amount of each ingredient listed in the current formula. To find the amount of each ingredient, you will multiply each amount by 4, as shown in Step 2.

Step 2. Calculate the amount of each ingredient by multiplying each ingredient amount by 4.

Desired Formula (for 16 oz)

coal tar	$4\ g \times 4 = 16\ g$
salicylic acid	$1\ g \times 4 = 4\ g$
triamcinolone 0.1%	$15\ g \times 4 = 60\ g$
hydrophilic petrolatum base ointment	$100\ g \times 4 = 400\ g$

Answer: You will need 16 g of coal tar, 4 g of salicylic acid, 60 g of triamcinolone 0.1%, and 400 g of hydrophilic petrolatum base ointment to prepare 16 oz of the ointment.

WORKPLACE WISDOM

Compounded medications provide many benefits for patients who have specific needs. For example, compounding can reformulate medications for individuals who have allergies to inactive ingredients such as lactose, gluten, or artificial colors. Compounding can also eliminate medication preservatives such as benzyl alcohol for individuals who are unable to tolerate these agents. In addition, compounding can tailor medications to a specific dose or strength. For example, compounded medications can be diluted to accommodate the special needs of pediatric patients. Finally, compounding can add flavorings to medications, making the drugs more palatable to children.

7.1 Problem Set

1. A pharmacy's recipe book provides a formula that yields 120 g of coal tar ointment. You are asked to prepare a 30 g jar of coal tar ointment. By what number do you need to divide each ingredient to make the desired formula? State how much of each ingredient you will need. Round your answer to the nearest hundredth of a gram.

Recipe Book Formula for Coal Tar Ointment (yields 120 g)	
Coal tar	4 g
Salicylic acid	1 g
Triamcinolone 0.1%	15 g
Hydrophilic petrolatum base ointment	100 g

2. A pharmacy's recipe book provides a formula that yields 30 vaginal suppositories. You are to prepare 150 vaginal suppositories. By what number do you need to multiply each ingredient to make the desired formula? State how much of each ingredient you will need. Round your answer to the nearest whole gram.

Pharmacy's Recipe Book Formula for Vaginal Suppositories (yields 30 vaginal suppositories)	
Progesterone	2.4 g
Polyethylene glycol 3350	30 g
Polyethylene glycol 1000	90 g

3. A pharmacy's recipe book provides a formula that yields 20 mL of solution for wart removal. You are to prepare 120 mL of the solution. State how much of each ingredient you will need. Round your answer to the nearest whole milliliter.

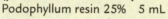

Pharmacy's Recipe Book Formula for Wart Removal Solution (yields 20 mL of solution)	
Podophyllum resin 25%	5 mL
Benzoin tincture	QSAD to 20 mL

4. A pharmacy's recipe book provides a formula that yields 8 oz of solution. You are to prepare 120 mL of the solution. State how much of each ingredient you will need. Round your answer to the nearest tenth of a milliliter.

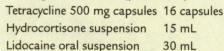

Pharmacy's Recipe Book Formula A for Magic Mouthwash (yields 8 oz)	
Tetracycline 500 mg capsules	16 capsules
Hydrocortisone suspension	15 mL
Lidocaine oral suspension	30 mL
Mylanta suspension	QSAD to 240 mL

5. A pharmacy's recipe book provides a formula to prepare one 30 mL dropper bottle of Oticaine. You are to prepare four 15 mL dropper bottles of Oticaine. State how much of each ingredient you will need to prepare the entire batch. Round your answer to the nearest tenth of a gram.

Pharmacy's Recipe Book Formula for Oticaine (yields 30 mL of solution)	
Antipyrine	1.8 g
Benzocaine	0.5 g
Glycerin	QSAD to 30 mL

Self-check your work in Appendix A.

7.2 Alligations

Safety Alert

Pharmacy technicians should always document calculations before compounding to reduce the potential for medication errors.

Occasionally, a prescriber will write a prescription for a medication strength that is not commercially available, or a medication strength that is not kept on hand in a pharmacy. In these instances, the pharmacy may be required to mix two different strengths of the same active ingredient of a drug or solution to make the desired strength. A higher-percent strength (i.e., the more concentrated ingredient) of a drug or solution is mixed with a lower-percent strength (i.e., the less concentrated ingredient) of a drug or solution to make the desired strength, which falls somewhere between the two extremes. This scenario requires you to employ a calculation called the **alligation method**, or simply *alligation*. Alligations are rarely performed by pharmacy technicians, but you may need to carry out this kind of calculation from time to time.

FIGURE 7.1 Alligation Grid

		D (parts of higher %; the difference of B − C)
A (higher %)		
	B (desired %)	
C (lower %)		E (parts of lower %; the difference of A − B)

KEY
A = higher concentration or strength (stated as a percent [%])
B = desired concentration or strength (stated as a percent [%])
C = lower concentration or strength (stated as a percent [%])
D = parts of higher concentration or strength (difference of B − C)
E = parts of lower concentration or strength (difference of A − B)

Math Morsel

To determine whether the alligation grid is set up properly, pharmacy technicians should check that the desired percent is a value in between the two concentrations being combined.

To understand how to solve an alligation problem, you will set up an alligation grid (see Figure 7.1). To begin, you must identify the desired concentration that was ordered (B% in the center square of the alligation grid) and the total volume (TV) needed. Next, you determine the currently available concentrations, which include a higher-percent strength (A% in the top left-hand square) and a lower-percent strength (C% in the bottom left-hand square). Then determine the number of parts needed of each component to make the desired concentration (B%). The number of parts of the higher-percent strength (D in the top right-hand square) is the difference between B and C. The number of parts of the lower-percent strength (E in the bottom right-hand square) is the difference between A and B. Then add the number of parts of each component (D and E) to determine the number of total parts (TP). Use the following formula to determine the volume of the higher-percent strength product needed to compound the desired concentration.

$$\frac{x}{TV} = \frac{D}{TP}$$

To determine the volume of the lower-percent strength product needed, use the following formula.

$$\frac{x}{TV} = \frac{E}{TP}$$

You can check your answer by adding the volume needed of the higher-percent strength and the lower-percent strength products. The sum should equal the total volume (TV) needed. The following examples outline this process.

Example 7.2.1

The CSP label shown below indicates that a prescriber has ordered 250 mL of dextrose 7% in water (D_7W). In your pharmacy, you have both dextrose 5% in water (D_5W) and dextrose 70% in water ($D_{70}W$). Because 7 falls between 5 and 70, you can use these two strengths to make the D_7W you need. How much D_5W and $D_{70}W$ do you combine to make an IV solution of D_7W and a total volume of 250 mL for infusion?

Note: The abbreviation *LVP* means "large-volume parenteral," and the abbreviation *BUD* means "beyond-use date."

IV Solution – LVP

Mercy Hospital

Pt. Name: Werekela, Francis   **Room:** PICU-4
ID#: 543678   **Rx#:** 420883

Dextrose 7% in Water (D_7W) 250 mL
Rate: 10 mL/hr

Keep refrigerated. Warm to room temperature
before administration.

BUD _____   Tech _____   RPh _____

Step 1. Identify the variables by determining the component concentrations. The desired concentration (B%) is what the prescriber has written on the medication order and, therefore, is indicated on the CSP label. The higher concentration (A%) and the lower concentration (C%) are determined by the stock IV base solution strengths on hand in your pharmacy. In this case, the desired concentration is 7%, the higher concentration is 70%, and the lower concentration is 5%.

Step 2. Using the alligation grid template from Figure 7.1, set up your own alligation grid by filling in the concentration strengths (given as percentages) in the Key section below the grid. Place the same strengths in their designated squares on the grid.

A (higher %) 70		D (parts of higher %; the difference of B − C)
	B (desired %) 7	
C (lower %) 5		E (parts of lower %; the difference of A − B)

KEY

A% = 70   D (parts of 70% solution) =

B% = 7   E (parts of 5% solution) =

C% = 5

Step 3. Determine the number of parts of each component (higher % and lower %).

To find the value of D in the top right-hand square, set up the equation B − C = D. Then fill in the values for B and C (found in Step 2) in the equation.

$$7 - 5 = D$$

$$D = 2 \text{ (number of parts of dextrose 70\%)}$$

Record the number 2 in the key and in the upper right-hand square as shown in the alligation grid below.

To find the value of E in the bottom right-hand square, set up the equation A − B = E. Then fill in the values for A and B (found in Step 2) in the equation.

$$70 - 7 = E$$

$$E = 63 \text{ (number of parts of dextrose 5\%)}$$

Record the number 63 in the key and in the bottom right-hand square as shown in the alligation grid below.

Check that your completed alligation grid now matches the grid shown below.

A (higher %) 70		D (parts of higher %) 2
	B (desired %) 7	
C (lower %) 5		E (parts of lower %) 63

KEY

A% = 70   D (parts of 70% solution) = 2

B% = 7   E (parts of 5% solution) = 63

C% = 5

Step 4. Set up a ratio using the values of D and E as shown in the right-hand column of your completed grid.

$$\frac{D}{E} = \frac{2}{63}$$

This ratio indicates that to prepare the desired concentration (in this case, a D_7W solution), $D_{70}W$ and D_5W must be mixed in a 2:63 ratio: 2 parts of $D_{70}W$ and 63 parts of D_5W.

Step 5. Using the ratio from Step 4, add D and E to obtain the total number of parts (TP).

$$D + E = TP$$

$$2 + 63 = TP$$

$$65 = TP$$

Math Morsel

Pharmacy technicians must add the parts of both strengths (determined in Step 5) to find the total number of parts. This number is then used as the divisor in Step 6.

Step 6. Now you need to determine the exact volume of each component needed to prepare 250 mL of D_7W. Because you already know the ratio in which the parts must be combined and the total number of parts, you can set up a ratio-proportion problem.

To find the volume of $D_{70}W$ needed for the CSP, use the following formula.

$$\frac{x}{TV} = \frac{D}{TP}$$

D = parts of the higher % solution
TP = total number of parts
TV = total volume of desired concentration

$$\frac{x}{250 \text{ mL}} = \frac{2}{65}$$

$$x = 7.69 \text{ mL (rounded to 7.7 mL)}$$
$$\text{of } D_{70}W$$

To find the volume of D_5W needed for the CSP, use the following formula.

$$\frac{x}{TV} = \frac{E}{TP}$$

E = parts of the lower % solution
TP = total number of parts
TV = total volume of desired concentration

$$\frac{x}{250 \text{ mL}} = \frac{63}{65}$$

$$x = 242.31 \text{ mL (rounded to 242.3 mL)}$$
$$\text{of } D_5W$$

Step 7. To verify the volume of each component (determined in Step 6), add the volumes of the two components. Your answer should equal the total volume of the desired concentration. Therefore, to make 250 mL of D_7W, mix 7.7 mL of $D_{70}W$ with 242.3 mL of D_5W.

$$7.7 \text{ mL } (D_{70}W) + 242.3 \text{ mL } (D_5W) = 250 \text{ mL (total volume of}$$
$$\text{desired concentration)}$$

Answer: To make 250 mL of D_7W, you will need to combine 7.7 mL of $D_{70}W$ and 242.3 mL of D_5W.

Example 7.2.2

A prescriber has ordered an IV infusion of 250 mL of dextrose 20% in water ($D_{20}W$). You have stock concentrations of dextrose 5% in water (D_5W) and dextrose 70% in water ($D_{70}W$) on hand in the pharmacy. How much D_5W and $D_{70}W$ must be combined to make an IV solution of $D_{20}W$ and a total volume of 250 mL for infusion?

IV Solution – LVP

Mercy Hospital

Pt. Name: Alvarez, Sara   **Room:** NICU-2
ID#: 543682   **Rx#:** 420923

Dextrose 20% in Water ($D_{20}W$) 250 mL
Rate: 10 mL/hr

Keep refrigerated. Warm to room temperature
before administration.

BUD _____   Tech _____   RPh _____

Step 1. Identify the variables. Determine the component concentrations by identifying the desired concentration (in this case, 20%); the higher concentration (in this case, 70%); and the lower concentration (in this case, 5%).

A (higher %) = 70
B (desired %) = 20
C (lower %) = 5

Reminder: The desired concentration (B%) is what the prescriber has written on the medication order, and it is also listed on the CSP label. The higher concentration (A%) and the lower concentration (C%) are determined by the stock IV base solution strengths that you have on hand in your pharmacy.

Step 2. Set up an alligation grid and key.

A (higher %) 70		D (parts of higher %; the difference of B − C)
	B (desired %) 20	
C (lower %) 5		E (parts of lower %; the difference of A − B)

KEY

A% = 70   D (parts of 70% solution) =
B% = 20   E (parts of 5% solution) =
C% = 5

Step 3. Determine the number of parts of each component (higher % and lower %).

Subtract the center number in the alligation grid from the number in the top left-hand square of the grid (A − B). Place this number in the bottom right-hand square of the grid (E).

$$A - B = E$$

$$70 - 20 = 50$$

Subtract the number in the bottom left-hand square of the alligation grid from the number in the center of the grid (B − C). Place this number in the top right-hand square of the grid (D).

$$B - C = D$$

$$20 - 5 = 15$$

D = 15 (parts of dextrose 70%)

E = 50 (parts of dextrose 5%)

Check that your completed alligation grid now matches the grid shown below.

A (higher %) 70		D (parts of higher %) 15
	B (desired %) 20	
C (lower %) 5		E (parts of lower %) 50

KEY

A% = 70   D (parts of 70% solution) = 15

B% = 20   E (parts of 5% solution) = 50

C% = 5

Step 4. Set up a ratio using the information you determined in Step 3.

$$\frac{D}{E} = \frac{15}{50}$$

This ratio indicates that to prepare the desired concentration (in this case, a $D_{20}W$ solution), $D_{70}W$ and D_5W must be mixed in a 15:50 ratio—in other words, 15 parts of $D_{70}W$ and 50 parts of D_5W.

Step 5. Determine the total number of parts (TP) in the ratio.

$$D + E = TP$$

$$15 + 50 = 65$$

$$65 = TP$$

Step 6. Determine the volume of each component.

To determine the volume of $D_{70}W$ needed for the CSP, use the following formula.

$$\frac{x}{TV} = \frac{D}{TP}$$

D = parts of the higher % solution

TP = total number of parts

TV = total volume of desired concentration

$$\frac{x}{250 \text{ mL}} = \frac{15}{65}$$

$$x = 57.7 \text{ mL of } D_{70}W$$

To determine the volume of D_5W needed for the CSP, use the following formula.

$$\frac{x}{TV} = \frac{E}{TP}$$

E = parts of the lower % solution

TP = total number of parts

TV = total volume of desired concentration

$$\frac{x}{250 \text{ mL}} = \frac{50}{65}$$

$$x = 192.3 \text{ mL of } D_5W$$

Therefore, to make 250 mL of $D_{20}W$, mix 57.7 mL of $D_{70}W$ with 192.3 mL of D_5W.

Step 7. To verify the volume of each component (determined in Step 6), add the volumes of the two components. Your answer should equal the total volume of the desired concentration.

$$57.7 \text{ mL } (D_{70}W) + 192.3 \text{ mL } (D_5W) = 250 \text{ mL}$$

Answer: To make 250 mL of $D_{20}W$, you will need to combine 57.7 mL of $D_{70}W$ and 192.3 mL of D_5W.

The alligation method may also be used in compounding situations that require you to mix two strengths of an active ingredient to compound a product whose desired strength lies between the two extremes.

Example 7.2.3

 A prescriber has ordered a topical preparation of 120 g of hydrocortisone 1.25% cream. The pharmacy carries hydrocortisone cream in the following concentrations: 2.5% and 1%. Determine how much of the 2.5% cream and how much of the 1% cream will be needed to prepare 120 g of the desired 1.25% concentration.

Step 1. Identify the variables. Determine the component concentrations by identifying the desired concentration (in this case, 1.25%); the higher concentration (in this case, 2.5%); and the lower concentration (in this case, 1%).

A (higher %) = 2.5%
B (desired %) = 1.25%
C (lower %) = 1%

Step 2. Set up the alligation grid.

A (higher %) 2.5		D (parts of higher %; the difference of B − C)
	B (desired %) 1.25	
C (lower %) 1		E (parts of lower %; the difference of A − B)

KEY

A% = 2.5   D (parts of hydrocortisone 2.5% cream) =

B% = 1.25   E (parts of 1% hydrocortisone cream) =

C% = 1

Step 3. Determine the number of parts of each component.

Subtract the number in the center square from the number in the upper left-hand square of the alligation grid (A − B); place this number in the lower right-hand square of the grid (E).

$$A - B = E$$

$$2.5 - 1.25 = 1.25$$

Subtract the number in the lower left-hand square of the alligation grid from the number in the center of the grid (B − C). Place this number in the upper right-hand square of the grid (D).

$$B - C = D$$

$$1.25 - 1 = 0.25$$

D = 0.25 (parts of hydrocortisone 2.5% cream)

E = 1.25 (parts of hydrocortisone 1% cream)

Fill in the values for D and E on the alligation grid.

A (higher %) 2.5		D (parts of higher %; the difference of B − C) 0.25
	B (desired %) 1.25	
C (lower %) 1		E (parts of lower %; the difference of A − B) 1.25

KEY

A% = 2.5

B% = 1.25

C% = 1

D (parts of hydrocortisone 2.5% cream) = 0.25

E (parts of 1% hydrocortisone cream) = 1.25

Step 4. Set up a ratio using the parts you determined in Step 3.

$$\frac{D}{E} = \frac{0.25}{1.25}$$

This ratio indicates that to prepare the desired concentration (in this case, hydrocortisone 1.25% cream), hydrocortisone 2.5% and hydrocortisone 1% must be mixed in a 0.25:1.25 ratio.

Step 5. Determine the total number of parts.

$$D + E = TP$$

$$0.25 + 1.25 = 1.5$$

$$1.5 = TP$$

Step 6. Determine the amount of each component.

To determine the amount of hydrocortisone 2.5% needed for the product, use the following formula.

$$\frac{x}{TA} = \frac{D}{TP}$$

D = parts of the higher % ingredient

TP = total number of parts

TA = total amount of desired concentration

$$\frac{x}{120 \text{ g}} = \frac{0.25}{1.5}$$

$$x = 20 \text{ g of 2.5\% hydrocortisone cream}$$

To determine the amount of hydrocortisone 1% cream needed for the product, use the following formula.

$$\frac{x}{TA} = \frac{E}{TP}$$

E = parts of the lower % ingredient

TP = total number of parts

TA = total amount of desired concentration

$$\frac{x}{120 \text{ g}} = \frac{1.25}{1.5}$$

$$x = 100 \text{ g of hydrocortisone 1\% cream}$$

Step 7. To verify the amount of each component (determined in Step 6), add the amounts of the two components. Your answer should equal the total amount of the desired concentration.

20 g (hydrocortisone 2.5%) + 100 g (hydrocortisone 1%) = 120 g

Answer: To make 120 g of hydrocortisone 1.25% cream, you will combine 20 g of hydrocortisone 2.5% with 100 g of hydrocortisone 1%.

7.2 Problem Set

Use the alligation method to solve the following problems. Round your answer to the nearest whole gram or whole milliliter.

1. You need to prepare 200 mL of $D_{7.5}W$ solution using D_5W and $D_{10}W$. How many milliliters of each solution will you need?

2. You need to prepare 400 mL of D_8W using D_5W and $D_{20}W$. How many milliliters of each solution will you need?

3. You need to prepare 500 mL of $D_{12.5}W$. You have on hand $D_{70}W$ and D_5W. How many milliliters of each solution will you need?

4. You need to prepare 250 mL of D_6W. You have on hand $D_{10}W$ and D_5W. How many milliliters of each solution will you need?

5. You need to prepare 500 mL of $D_{7.5}W$. You have on hand D_5W and $D_{50}W$. How many milliliters of each solution will you need?

6. You need to prepare 250 mL of D_8W from D_5W and $D_{20}W$. How many milliliters of each solution will you need?

7. You need to prepare 300 mL of $D_{7.5}W$ using D_5W and $D_{20}W$. How many milliliters of each solution will you need?

8. You need to prepare 500 mL of $D_{12.5}W$ using $D_{10}W$ and $D_{20}W$. How many milliliters of each solution will you need?

9. You need to prepare 150 mL of $D_{7.5}W$ from D_5W and $D_{10}W$. How many milliliters of each solution will you need?

10. A physician has ordered 250 mL of $D_{12.5}W$. You have $D_{10}W$ and $D_{20}W$ available. How many milliliters of each solution will you need?

11. You need to prepare 60 g of a 3% cream from a 1% cream and a 10% cream. How many grams of each cream will you need?

12. You need to prepare 30 g of a 7.5% cream from a 5% cream and a 15% cream. How many grams of each cream will you need?

13. The pharmacy has received an order that requires the batch preparation of four 30 g jars of hydrocortisone 3% cream. The pharmacy has a hydrocortisone 1% cream and a hydrocortisone 5% cream on hand. How many grams of each cream will you need to prepare the entire batch?

14. Prepare 45 g of zinc oxide 10% ointment using a zinc oxide 5% ointment and a zinc oxide 20% ointment. How many grams of each ointment will you need?

15. Prepare 100 g of an 8% cream from a 5% cream and a 10% cream. How many grams of each cream will you need?

Self-check your work in Appendix A.

7.3 Weight-in-Weight Calculations

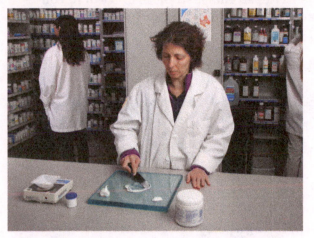

A pharmacy technician is compounding a medication made from two solid ingredients.

When compounding two solid ingredients—an active ingredient and an inactive ingredient—the weight-in-weight (w/w) formula is sometimes used to determine the amount of each ingredient needed for the preparation. The **weight-in-weight (w/w) formula** identifies the number of grams of medication per 100 g of the product. This concentration can be expressed as a ratio or as a fraction, as shown in the following formula.

$$\text{weight-in-weight (w/w)} = \frac{x \text{ g of medication}}{100 \text{ g of product}}$$

Percentage strength is related to the w/w formula. **Percentage strength** is a way of expressing strength as parts of 100 or percent of the whole. In pharmacy practice, percentage strength of a w/w preparation signifies the number of grams of active ingredient per 100 g of the product. The following formula may be used to determine the percentage strength of w/w preparations.

$$\text{percentage strength of w/w preparation} = \frac{x \text{ g of active ingredient}}{100 \text{ g of product}} \times 100$$

The following example illustrates how to calculate percentage strength of a w/w preparation.

Example 7.3.1

 You have a compound with a concentration of 5 g of hydrocortisone powder in 100 g of petrolatum. Determine the percentage strength of this compound.

To begin, use the formula for percentage strength of a w/w preparation.

$$\frac{x \text{ g of active ingredient}}{100 \text{ g of product}} \times 100$$

Then plug in the concentration of the available product into the formula.

$$\frac{5 \text{ g of hydrocortisone powder}}{100 \text{ g of product}} \times 100 = 5\%$$

Answer: The percentage strength of a compound with 5 g of hydrocortisone powder in 100 g of petrolatum is 5%.

When the percentage strength of the product is known, the w/w formula may also be used to determine how many grams of an active ingredient are in a defined amount of product. Apply either the ratio-proportion method or the dimensional analysis method to determine the number of grams of active ingredient needed to compound the preparation.

Example 7.3.2

If a compounded preparation has a percentage strength of 3% of miconazole, how many grams of medication are in 50 g of the preparation?

To begin, use the w/w formula to rewrite 3% as a w/w ratio.

$$3\% = \frac{3 \text{ g of miconazole}}{100 \text{ g of product}}$$

Next, determine the amount of active ingredient in 50 g of the preparation. You can solve this problem by using the ratio-proportion method or by using the dimensional analysis method.

Ratio-Proportion Method

$$\frac{x \text{ g}}{50 \text{ g}} = \frac{3 \text{ g}}{100 \text{ g}}$$

$$x \text{ g} (100 \text{ g}) = 3 \text{ g} (50 \text{ g})$$

$$x = 1.5 \text{ g}$$

Dimensional Analysis Method

$$\frac{50 \text{ g of product}}{1} \times \frac{3 \text{ g of miconazole}}{100 \text{ g of product}} = 1.5 \text{ g of miconazole}$$

Answer: There are 1.5 g of miconazole in 50 g of the preparation.

Example 7.3.3

A compounded preparation has a percentage strength of 0.4% of testosterone. The final product contains 15 g of medication. How many total grams of testosterone are in the final product?

To begin, use the w/w formula to rewrite 0.4% as a w/w ratio.

$$0.4\% = \frac{0.4 \text{ g of testosterone}}{100 \text{ g of product}}$$

Next, determine the amount of active ingredient in 15 g of the preparation. You can solve this problem by using the ratio-proportion method or by using the dimensional analysis method.

Ratio-Proportion Method

$$\frac{x \text{ g}}{15 \text{ g}} = \frac{0.4 \text{ g}}{100 \text{ g}}$$

$$x \text{ g} (100 \text{ g}) = 0.4 \text{ g} (15 \text{ g})$$

$$x = 0.06 \text{ g}$$

Dimensional Analysis Method

$$\frac{15 \text{ g of product}}{1} \times \frac{0.4 \text{ g of testosterone}}{100 \text{ g of product}} = 0.06 \text{ g}$$

Answer: There are 0.06 g of testosterone in 15 g of the final product.

7.3 Problem Set

Use the w/w method to solve the following problems.

1. You need to prepare a compound of hydro-cortisone cream in petrolatum with a concentration of 2%. How many grams of hydrocortisone are contained in 75 g of the cream? Round your answer to the nearest tenth of a gram.

2. You need to prepare a compound of zinc oxide using 8 g of zinc oxide powder in 454 g of hydrophilic petrolatum base ointment. What is the percentage strength of this compounded preparation? Round your answer to the nearest tenth of a percent.

3. You need to prepare a compound of 100 g of acyclovir cream 2.5%. How many grams of acyclovir will you need for this preparation? Round your answer to the nearest tenth of a gram.

4. You need to prepare a compound that mixes 10 g of acyclovir with 50 g of petrolatum. What is the percentage strength of this compounded preparation? Round your answer to the nearest tenth of a percent.

5. The pharmacy has received a prescription for 30 g of a triamcinolone 2% ointment. How many grams of triamcinolone will you need to prepare this prescription? Round your answer to the nearest tenth of a gram.

6. The pharmacy has received the following prescription. *Note:* The abbreviation *aaa* means "apply to the affected area"; the abbreviation *tid* means "three times daily"; and the abbreviation *prn* means "as needed."

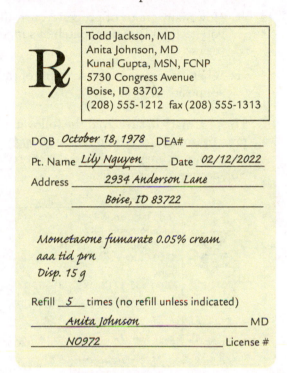

> **R̸**
>
> Todd Jackson, MD
> Anita Johnson, MD
> Kunal Gupta, MSN, FCNP
> 5730 Congress Avenue
> Boise, ID 83702
> (208) 555-1212 fax (208) 555-1313
>
> DOB *October 18, 1978*   DEA# _____
>
> Pt. Name *Lily Nguyen*   Date *02/12/2022*
>
> Address _____ *2934 Anderson Lane* _____
>
> _____ *Boise, ID 83722* _____
>
> *Mometasone fumarate 0.05% cream*
> *aaa tid prn*
> *Disp. 15 g*
>
> Refill __*5*__ times (no refill unless indicated)
>
> _____ *Anita Johnson* _____ MD
>
> _____ *N0972* _____ License #

How many grams of mometasone fumarate are contained in this prescription? Round your answer to the nearest ten-thousandth of a gram.

7. The pharmacy has received an order to compound a batch preparation of progesterone suppositories. You will need to prepare 100 suppositories, each containing 200 mg of progesterone. The total weight of each suppository is 1 g. Round your answers to the nearest whole gram and whole percent.

   a. How many grams of progesterone will you need for the entire batch of suppositories?

   b. What is the percentage strength of each suppository?

8. The pharmacy has received the following prescription. *Note:* The abbreviation *qid* means "four times daily," and the abbreviation *prn* means "as needed."

> R̸
>
> Todd Jackson, MD
> Anita Johnson, MD
> Kunal Gupta, MSN, FCNP
> 5730 Congress Avenue
> Boise, ID 83702
> (208) 555-1212 fax (208) 555-1313
>
> DOB _March 28, 1989_ DEA# _____
> Pt. Name _Eeva Novak_ Date _07/14/2022_
> Address _____ 4521 Birch Avenue _____
> _____ Boise, ID 83722 _____
>
> Metronidazole 0.75% cream
> Compound without benzyl alcohol
>
> Apply to affected facial areas qid prn rosacea flare
> Dispense 30 g
>
> Refill __2__ times (no refill unless indicated)
> ___Todd Jackson_____ MD
> ___HO786_____ License #

You look at the patient's profile in the computer and realize that the patient has an allergy to benzyl alcohol. Metronidazole 0.75% cream is commercially available; however, all formulations have benzyl alcohol as an ingredient and you need to compound the medication. How many grams of metronidazole will you need to prepare this prescription? Round your answer to the nearest hundredth of a gram.

9. The pharmacy has received the following medication order. *Note:* The abbreviation *bid* means "two times daily," and the abbreviation *utd* means "as directed."

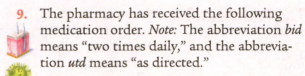

ID#: HYII897			Memorial Hospital
Name: Bishop, Walter			
DOB: 01/25/71			
Room: 717a			Physician's
Dr: Michal Nikolai, MD			Medication Order

ALLERGY OR SENSITIVITY		DIAGNOSIS	
ceftazidime		cellulitis	

DATE	TIME	ORDERS	PHYSICIAN'S SIG.
03/15/2022	1714	Clindamycin 0.05% topical gel	
		Apply 1 g to acne bid utd	
		Dispense 30 g tube	
			Michal Nikolai, MD

How many grams of clindamycin will be contained in this prescription? Round your answer to the nearest hundredth of a gram.

10. The pharmacy has received the following medication order. *Note:* The abbreviation *tid* means "three times daily," and the abbreviation *utd* means "as directed."

ID#: 7882993ZZ			Memorial Hospital
Name: Ellings, Grace			
DOB: 09/02/54			
Room: ICU-2			Physician's
Dr: Audrea Carter, MD			Medication Order

ALLERGY OR SENSITIVITY		DIAGNOSIS shingles,	
NKA		exacerbation of COPD	

DATE	TIME	ORDERS	PHYSICIAN'S SIG.
10/09/2022	0633	Acyclovir 10% ointment 50 g tube	
		Apply 1 g tid utd	
			Audrea Carter, MD

   a. How many grams of acyclovir will be contained in this prescription? Round your answer to the nearest whole gram.

   b. How many doses are contained in this medication order?

Self-check your work in Appendix A.

Review and Assessment

CHAPTER SUMMARY

- Compounding, or the process of using raw ingredients and/or prepared ingredients to create a medication, is a task frequently performed by pharmacy technicians in hospital and compounding pharmacies and, occasionally, in the community pharmacy setting.

- A compounded medication is prepared using a recipe or formula.

- Compounding may require the enlargement or reduction of formulas to meet the needs of the prescriber's order.

- As a pharmacy technician, you must know the current formula, which is the formula in the pharmacy's recipe book, and the desired formula, which is the recipe ordered by a prescriber that alters the various components of the current formula.

- When enlarging or reducing formulas for compounding, you must retain the correct proportion of ingredients from the current formula.

- Compound formulas often include the abbreviation *QSAD*, which means "a quantity sufficient to make."

- The abbreviation *QSAD* almost always refers to an inactive ingredient in a formula and instructs the preparer to use an ingredient up to the specified quantity.

- One way you can reduce or enlarge a formula is to compare the current formula with the desired formula by creating a ratio: desired formula quantity/current formula quantity.

- Once a ratio is created, you can either divide by that amount to reduce a formula or multiply by that amount to enlarge a formula.

- Occasionally, two different strengths of the same active ingredient of a drug or solution are used to make the desired strength.

- An alligation grid is used to assist in the calculations involved in mixing two different strengths to achieve a desired strength.

- When working with an alligation problem, the *desired strength* should be placed in the center square of the alligation grid; the *higher strength* (stronger concentration) should be placed in the upper-left square of the grid; and the *lower strength* (weaker concentration) should be placed in the lower-left square of the grid.

- The weight-in-weight (w/w) formula identifies the number of grams per 100 g of product.

FORMULAS FOR SUCCESS

Enlarging or Reducing a Compounding Formula (Section 7.1)

$$\text{ratio to enlarge or reduce a formula} = \frac{\text{desired formula quantity}}{\text{current formula quantity}}$$

Alligation Grid Template (Section 7.2)

A (higher %)		D (parts of higher %; the difference of B − C)
	B (desired %)	
C (lower %)		E (parts of lower %; the difference of A − B)

KEY

A = higher concentration or strength (stated as a percent [%])
B = desired concentration or strength (stated as a percent [%])
C = lower concentration or strength (stated as a percent [%])
D = parts of higher concentration or strength (difference of B − C)
E = parts of lower concentration or strength (difference of A − B)

Alligation Formulas (Section 7.2)

When using an alligation to determine the amount of each ingredient use the following formulas.

$$\frac{x\text{ mL}}{\text{TV (total volume of desired concentration)}} = \frac{\text{D (higher \% solution)}}{\text{TP (total \# of parts)}}$$

$$\frac{x\text{ mL}}{\text{TV (total volume of desired concentration)}} = \frac{\text{E (lower \% solution)}}{\text{TP (total \# of parts)}}$$

Cross multiply; then divide to solve for x.

Weight-in-Weight Formula (Section 7.3)

$$\text{weight-in-weight (w/w)} = \frac{x\text{ g of medication}}{100\text{ g of product}}$$

Calculation for Percentage Strength of Weight-in-Weight (w/w) Preparations (Section 7.3)

$$\text{percentage strength of w/w preparation} = \frac{x\text{ g of active ingredient}}{100\text{ g of product}} \times 100$$

Take a moment to review what you have learned in this chapter and answer the following questions.

1. The process of using raw or prepared ingredients in the preparation of a drug product for a patient is called
   a. diluting.
   b. reconstituting.
   c. compounding.
   d. dispensing.

2. The term *percentage strength* is commonly used to describe which of the following?
   a. number of grams/mL
   b. number of grams/100 g
   c. number of milligrams/mL
   d. number of milligrams/100 mL

3. A pharmacy's recipe book contains a formula that yields 16 oz total. You want to reduce the recipe to yield 4 oz total. By what number will you divide all the ingredients to make the reduced recipe?
   a. 2
   b. 4
   c. 6
   d. 8

4. The percentage strength of a compounded topical gel is 5%. How do you express this strength in weight?
   a. 5 mg/100 mg
   b. 5 mg/100 g
   c. 5 g/100 mg
   d. 5 g/100 g

5. The percentage strength of a compounded cream is 0.1%. How do you express this strength in weight?
   a. 1 mg/100 mg
   b. 10 mg/100 g
   c. 100 mg/100 g
   d. 1 g/100 g

6. A pharmacy's recipe book contains a formula that yields 1,000 mL total. You want to reduce the recipe to yield 16 oz total. By what number will you multiply all the ingredients to make the recipe?
   a. 0.24
   b. 0.48
   c. 2.4
   d. 4.8

7. With regard to pharmacy compounding, which term has the same meaning as the term *formula*?
   a. *recipe*
   b. *prescription*
   c. *concentration*
   d. *dilution*

8. What method is used when performing calculations for a prescription that requires mixing two different strengths of a drug (a higher-percent strength and a lower-percent strength) to make the desired strength?
   a. alligation
   b. ratio-proportion
   c. dimensional analysis
   d. dilution analysis

9. What is the percentage strength of a solution that contains dextrose 8 g/100 mL?
   a. 0.8%
   b. 8%
   c. 80%
   d. 800%

10. How much $D_{50}W$ and $D_{10}W$ would you need to prepare 2 L of $D_{15}W$?
    a. 1,750 mL of $D_{50}W$; 250 mL of $D_{10}W$
    b. 875 mL of $D_{50}W$; 125 mL of $D_{10}W$
    c. 125 mL of $D_{50}W$; 875 mL of $D_{10}W$
    d. 250 mL of $D_{50}W$; 1,750 mL of $D_{10}W$

FIND SOLUTIONS

Take a moment to consider what you have learned in this chapter and respond thoughtfully to the prompts.

Scenario A: Your pharmacy receives the following prescription. *Note:* The abbreviation *aaa* means "apply to the affected area"; the abbreviation *tid* means "three times daily"; and the abbreviation *prn* means "as needed."

> R̶x̶
>
> Todd Jackson, MD
> Anita Johnson, MD
> Kunal Gupta, MSN, FCNP
> 5730 Congress Avenue
> Boise, ID 83702
> (208) 555-1212 fax (208) 555-1313
>
> DOB *October 18, 1978* DEA# _____
>
> Pt. Name *Lily Nguyen* Date *02/12/2022*
>
> Address   *2934 Anderson Lane*
>   *Boise, ID 83722*
>
> *Mometasone fumarate 0.1% cream*
> *aaa tid prn*
>
> Refill __5__ times (no refill unless indicated)
> _____*Anita Johnson*_____ MD
> _____*N0972*_____ License #

1. How many grams of mometasone fumarate will you need to prepare 100 g of this prescription?

2. How many grams of mometasone fumarate will you need to prepare 30 g of this prescription?

3. How many grams of mometasone fumarate will you need to prepare 15 g of this prescription?

4. If a compounded product contained 2.5 g of mometasone fumarate in 100 g of a cream base, what would its percentage strength be?

5. If a compounded product contained 3 g of mometasone fumarate in 45 g of a cream base, what would its percentage strength be? Round your answer to the nearest tenth of a percent.

Scenario B: A physician prescribes 8 oz of your pharmacy's Magic Mouthwash for a patient. The prescription states that the patient is to swish, gargle, and spit 1–2 teaspoonfuls every six hours as needed for irritation. The pharmacy's recipe book lists a formula to prepare 480 mL total.

Pharmacy's Recipe Book Formula B for Magic Mouthwash (yields 480 mL)	
Viscous lidocaine 2%	80 mL
Mylanta	80 mL
Diphenhydramine 12.5 mg/5 mL elixir	80 mL
Nystatin Oral Suspension 100,000 units	80 mL
Prednisolone 15 mg/5 mL	80 mL
Distilled water	80 mL

6. How many ounces does the pharmacy's current formula make?

7. How many ounces of each ingredient do you need to make 8 oz? Round your answer to the nearest tenth of an ounce.

8. How many milligrams of diphenhydramine are in 8 oz of Magic Mouthwash?

9. How many milligrams of prednisolone are in 8 oz of Magic Mouthwash?

10. Rewrite the administration instructions using the volume measurement in milliliters.

Scenario C: You are instructed to make 454 g of zinc oxide 3% cream. You have in stock zinc oxide 10% cream and zinc oxide 1% cream. Set up your alligation grid using the template below to help you answer the questions below.

A (higher %)		D (parts of higher %; the difference of B − C)
	B (desired %)	
C (lower %)		E (parts of lower %; the difference of A − B)

11. What number belongs in the B square of the grid?

12. What number belongs in the D square of the grid?

13. What number belongs in the E square of the grid?

14. What are the total number of parts (TP)?

15. How much zinc oxide 10% cream and zinc oxide 1% cream are needed to make 454 g of zinc oxide 3% cream? Round your answer to the nearest tenth of a gram.

The online course includes additional review and assessment resources.

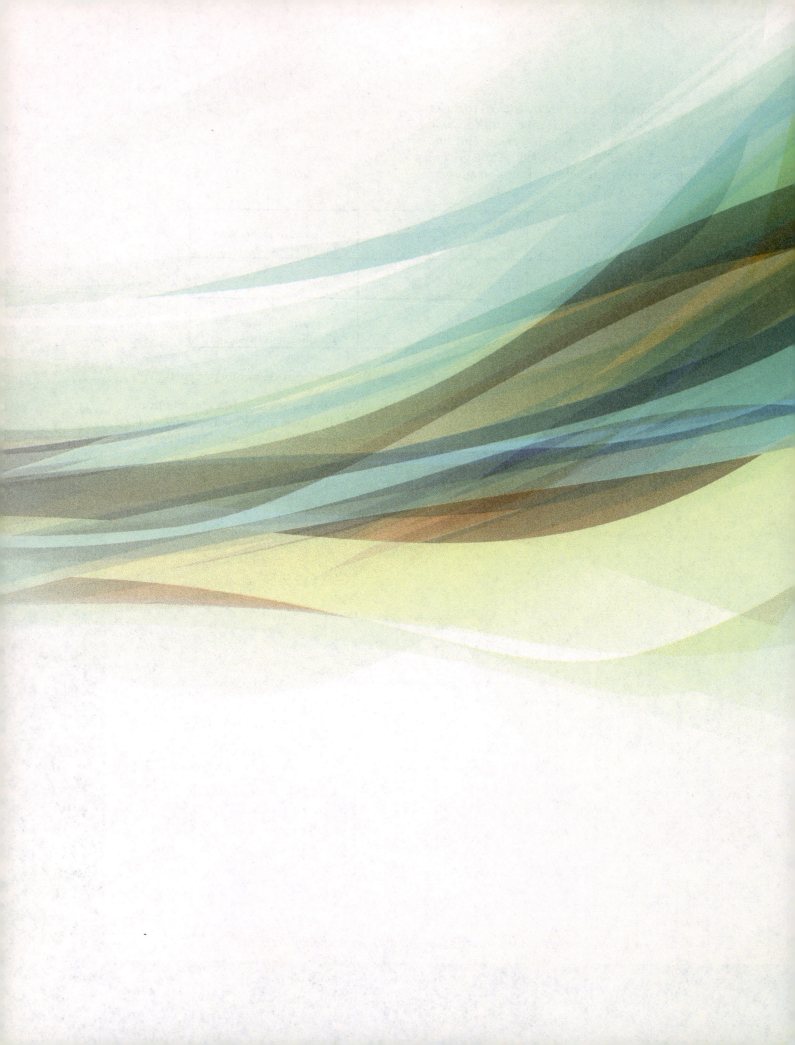

8 Conducting Business Operations

Learning Objectives

1. Describe counting change by using the amount displayed on the cash register's screen and by counting from the purchase price. (Section 8.1)

2. Utilize par level to determine the amount of medication to reorder. (Section 8.2)

3. Define *perpetual inventory record* as it relates to controlled substances. (Section 8.2)

4. Determine number of inventory days' supply and turnover rate. (Section 8.2)

5. Define *depreciation* and calculate annual depreciation in a pharmacy. (Section 8.2)

6. Define *overhead* and calculate overhead cost. (Section 8.3)

7. Compare and contrast base profit, net profit, and gross profit. (Section 8.3)

8. Calculate markup, markup rate, and discounts. (Section 8.3)

9. Describe average wholesale price and utilize it to calculate a pharmacy's medication purchase price. (Section 8.4)

10. Calculate prescription reimbursement. (Section 8.4)

For a key to the body system icons that appear in each chapter of this textbook, refer to the Preface.

ASHP/ACPE Accreditation Standards

To view the *ASHP/ACPE Accreditation Standards* addressed in this chapter, refer to Appendix D.

Business operations are an essential part of community and institutional pharmacy practice. This chapter provides a foundation for calculations related to conducting business operations. Common business-related calculations include accepting payment and counting change, managing pharmacy inventory, determining profit, and understanding insurance reimbursement. Although some topics (such as customer transactions) are more relevant to community pharmacy practice, other topics (such as inventory management and profit) are often used in both the institutional and community pharmacy settings.

8.1 Customer Transactions

In any business, the collection of money occurs. In a community pharmacy, you are responsible for accepting payment for prescriptions or other pharmacy-related items. In these monetary transactions, you must have basic math and point-of-sale cash register skills to calculate the correct costs and, if a customer pays in cash, to count the correct change. For that reason, your ability to count change correctly is a key skill for excellent customer service and pharmacy accounting.

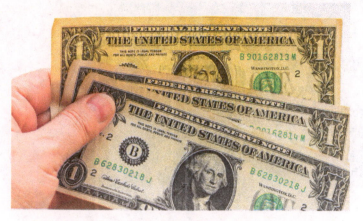

Pharmacy technicians may be required to count change.

Most community pharmacies have a computerized cash register. The cash register's screen displays the amount of change to give the customer if you have properly added all the items to be purchased and entered the correct amount of money the customer has given you. The amount of change should be counted back to the customer to show that you are giving the correct amount. There are two ways you can count change. One method is to simply count the amount displayed on the cash register's screen, and the other method is to count the amount from the purchase price.

Counting Change from the Amount Displayed on the Cash Register's Screen

The easiest method to count change is to count the amount displayed on the cash register's screen. First, confirm the amount of change to be received based on the amount listed on the register. Second, count out the money from largest to smallest bills followed by largest to smallest coins as you place the money in the customer's hand.

Example 8.1.1

A customer purchases a bottle of Tylenol and a bottle of vitamin C for the total purchase price of $10.73. The customer offers you a $50 bill. How would you count out the amount displayed on the cash register's screen as you place the change in the customer's hand?

Step 1. Confirm the amount of change to be received based on the amount displayed on the cash register's screen ($39.27). You can say, "You have *thirty-nine dollars and twenty-seven cents* in change coming." The customer can then tell you if there is a discrepancy.

Step 2. Place the money into the customer's hand, from the largest to the smallest bills, followed by the largest to the smallest coins: one $20 bill, one $10 bill, one $5 bill, four $1 bills, one quarter, and two pennies. As you are returning the change, count out the money to the customer: "*Twenty dollars, thirty, thirty-five, thirty-six, thirty-seven, thirty-eight, thirty-nine, and twenty-five, twenty-six, twenty-seven cents.*"

Although counting the amount displayed on the cash register's screen is the easiest method for you, it is not necessarily the easiest method for the customer to follow. A customer often does not know or pay attention to how much change should be received after a purchase. For that reason, a customer may feel most comfortable having the change counted back by starting at the purchase price and ending with the amount of cash the customer gave you.

Counting Change from the Purchase Price

When counting change from the purchase price, first take the amount of change needed, as noted on the cash register's screen, from the cash drawer. Next, beginning at the purchase price, count out the coins needed to reach the next bill. Then, offer $1 bills to the point where you can use the next highest denomination, which would be a $5 bill. Continue to the next highest denomination until you reach the amount first given to you by the customer.

Example 8.1.2

A woman picks up a prescription with a $15.00 copay. She offers you a $50 bill. How would you count out this customer's change by counting from the purchase price?

Step 1. To begin, take the amount of change needed, as noted on the cash register's screen, from the cash drawer ($35.00).

Step 2. Then state the purchase price ($15.00) and count out $5 bills until you can use the next highest denomination: "*fifteen (purchase price), twenty, ($5 bill), thirty ($10 bill), and fifty ($20 bill).*"

8.1 Problem Set

Read the following scenario and count out the customer's change by using the amount displayed on the cash register's screen.

A customer picks up a prescription with a $5.75 co-pay. The customer offers you a $20 bill. The cash register's screen indicates that the customer should receive $14.25 in change. Your cash register is stocked with pennies, nickels, dimes, quarters, $1 bills, $5 bills, $10 bills, and $20 bills.

1. What coin should you count out to the customer first?

2. What bill should you count out to the customer first?

3. List the type and quantity of coins and bills you will count out to the customer.

Read the following scenario and count out the customer's change by using the amount from the purchase price.

A customer purchases a bottle of over-the-counter (OTC) ibuprofen for $8.49. The customer offers you a $50 bill. The cash register's screen indicates the customer should receive $41.51 in change. Your cash register is stocked with pennies, nickels, dimes, quarters, $1 bills, $5 bills, $10 bills, and $20 bills.

4. What coin should you count out to the customer first?

5. What bill should you count out to the customer first?

6. List the type and quantity of coins and bills you will count out to the customer.

8.2 General Pharmacy and Controlled-Substance Inventories

An **inventory** is a listing of all items that are available for sale in a business. A pharmacy's **inventory value** is the total value of all drugs and other merchandise in stock on a given day. Pharmacy personnel (both in community and institutional settings) must maintain a record of all drugs, supplies, and merchandise purchased and sold to know when to reorder from a wholesaler to restock the pharmacy's shelves. This record allows personnel to continually adjust the pharmacy's inventory levels based on how quickly items are being sold.

Pharmacy personnel must consider shelving design and space as well as available refrigerator and freezer space to maintain adequate inventory. These considerations apply to both the community and institutional pharmacy settings. Keeping medications in stock is a cost to a pharmacy, and a large inventory can hinder cash flow. To minimize the shelf, refrigerator, and freezer space needed and to control inventory costs, pharmacy personnel need to manage their pharmacy's inventory so that medications are readily available when needed, but do not sit unused for an extended period. Pharmacy personnel generally try to manage their pharmacy's inventory so that medications arrive from a wholesaler shortly before they are dispensed and sold. However, there are instances when a pharmacy may need to stock some slow-moving drugs as a service to a small number of patients who require those medications.

Managing General Pharmacy Inventory

In the past, pharmacy personnel kept track of inventory by maintaining handwritten records of all pharmacy purchases and sales. Today, this labor-intensive and time-consuming inventory system has been replaced by computerized inventory records. Whenever drugs, supplies, or other types of merchandise are purchased from a wholesaler and received in a pharmacy, personnel enter the quantity and price into the pharmacy's computer database. As medications are dispensed or used, the computer system automatically adjusts the inventory record for the items purchased. This method of updating the inventory based on purchases is known as *perpetual inventory*.

A pharmacy usually establishes an inventory range for each item, which is sometimes referred to as a *par level*. The par level indicates the minimum and maximum number of units—packages, bottles, boxes, or containers—to have in pharmacy stock for each inventory item. When an inventory item drops to the predetermined minimum par level (sometimes called the *reorder point*), the item is purchased from the wholesaler to restock the pharmacy's supply. The reorder point and reorder quantity for each inventory item are predetermined based on the historical use of the item and the time it takes to get the reorder shipment from the pharmacy's wholesaler.

In general, a reorder quantity is set to replenish the inventory item to a minimum par level. However, it may be more economical to order the maximum par level of an item if a larger package size increases profitability. In addition, there are circumstances that dictate a reorder quantity that exceeds the maximum par level. For example, during cold and flu season, an unusually high number of customers receive prescriptions for the same medications. Consequently, a pharmacy will typically maintain a larger supply of antibiotic, antiviral, and OTC cold remedies in stock than it would at other times of the year.

Calculating the amount needed to bring pharmacy stock to the maximum par level requires subtraction. You subtract the current stock level from the maximum par level.

$$\text{amount needed to bring to maximum par level} = \text{maximum par level} - \text{current stock level}$$

Calculating the amount needed to bring pharmacy stock to the minimum par level also requires subtraction. You subtract the current stock level from the minimum par level.

$$\text{amount needed to bring to minimum par level} = \text{minimum par level} - \text{current stock level}$$

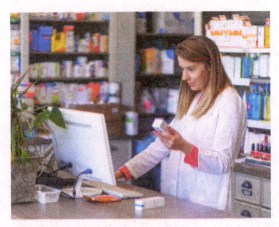

A pharmacy technician is reordering medications that are below par level.

Drug manufacturers typically supply medications in containers that hold various quantities, known as *package sizes*, or *counts*. For example, the antibiotic drug ampicillin, 500 mg capsules, is available in 100-count and 500-count package sizes. The package size that pharmacy personnel order when replenishing inventory depends on how much of the drug the facility is using, how quickly the drug is being used, the package size that is typically ordered, and the price. Often, it is more economical for pharmacy personnel to order a larger package size because both the drug manufacturer and the wholesaler usually offer lower prices on bulk package sizes.

These inventory reorder decisions are typically made by pharmacy personnel who have extensive experience in this area. However, pharmacy technicians should have a basic understanding of the calculations involved in inventory management. The following examples illustrate some of the scenarios encountered in inventory management and their possible solutions.

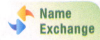

Name Exchange

Protonix is the brand name for the generic drug pantoprazole, which is used to reduce the amount of acid that the stomach produces.

Example 8.2.1

The inventory of pantoprazole 20 mg is to be maintained at a minimum of 240 tablets and at a maximum of 300 tablets. If 15 tablets remain at the end of the day, how many bottles of tablets will be ordered to meet the minimum par level? Pantoprazole 20 mg is commercially available in a bottle containing 90 tablets.

To begin, determine the difference between the minimum par level (240 tablets) and the current stock level (15 tablets).

$$\text{minimum par level} - \text{current stock level} = \text{amount needed to bring to minimum par level}$$

240 tablets − 15 tablets = 225 tablets

Therefore, it will take at least 225 tablets to bring the inventory up to the minimum par level for pantoprazole 20 mg. However, the tablets must be ordered in bottles of 90.

225 tablets ÷ 90 tablets/bottle = 2.5 bottles, rounded up to 3 bottles

Answer: Three bottles of pantoprazole 20 mg must be ordered to meet the minimum par level.

Example 8.2.2

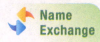
Name Exchange

The generic drug propranolol, a beta blocker, is commonly known as the brand name Inderal LA or Inderal XL.

The inventory of propranolol 10 mg is to be maintained at a minimum of 300 tablets and at a maximum of 1,500 tablets. If 212 tablets remain at the end of the day, how many bottles of propranolol will you order to meet the minimum par level? Propranolol is available in bottles containing 100 tablets, 500 tablets, and 1,000 tablets. You typically order the largest-size bottle.

To begin, determine the difference between the minimum par level (300 tablets) and the current stock level (212 tablets).

$$\frac{\text{minimum}}{\text{par level}} - \frac{\text{current}}{\text{stock level}} = \frac{\text{amount needed to bring}}{\text{to minimum par level}}$$

$$300 \text{ tablets} - 212 \text{ tablets} = 88 \text{ tablets}$$

Answer: Even though it significantly surpasses the minimum, you will order one 1,000-count bottle of propranolol. The resulting inventory will still be within the acceptable range and will not exceed 1,500 tablets.

Example 8.2.3

You would like to replenish the lip balm that is kept on the pharmacy counter by the cash register. The lip balm inventory is to be maintained at a maximum of 30 and at a minimum of 15. If 12 tubes of lip balm remain at the end of the day, how many tubes must be ordered to get as close as possible to the maximum par level? Lip balm wholesale pricing is $10.20/dozen.

To begin, determine the difference between the maximum par level (30 tubes) and the current inventory (12 tubes).

$$\frac{\text{maximum}}{\text{par level}} - \frac{\text{current}}{\text{stock level}} = \frac{\text{amount needed to bring}}{\text{to maximum par level}}$$

$$30 \text{ tubes} - 12 \text{ tubes} = 18 \text{ tubes}$$

Therefore, it will take 18 tubes to bring the inventory up to the maximum par level of 15 tubes.

However, the wholesale pricing for lip balm tubes is only available by the package size of a dozen. Consequently, you will need to order 1 dozen tubes.

Answer: You will need to order 1 dozen tubes of lip balm.

Managing Inventory for Controlled Substances

Controlled substances have different inventory requirements from legend or OTC medications. Federal law dictates inventory requirements for controlled substances based on their schedule. According to the US Drug Enforcement Administration (DEA), inventories for Schedule III, IV, and V controlled substances shall be maintained either separately from all other records of a pharmacy or in such a form that the information required is readily retrievable from ordinary business records of the pharmacy. Federal law, however, dictates that inventories of Schedule II (C–II) controlled substances be maintained separately from all other records in a pharmacy.

In addition to federal laws dictating the management of controlled substances, individual states may have other legal regulations. When federal and state laws differ, pharmacy personnel must follow the stricter inventory requirements.

Because Schedule II controlled-substance inventories must be maintained separately, you need to be familiar with the distinct record-keeping requirements for these medications. Similar to other drugs, C–IIs typically have minimum and maximum par levels. However unlike other medications, the inventory of Schedule II controlled substances must be documented at every step in the process, from purchasing through storage, dispensing, and disposal.

The precise count of each capsule, tablet, patch, liquid, injection, or other dosage form must be closely monitored and documented continually. Consequently, pharmacies have special policies, procedures, and schedules for counting the inventory of C–IIs. To that end, pharmacies maintain an automated or a manual perpetual inventory record to monitor Schedule II controlled-substance inventory.

A **perpetual inventory record** is a method of accounting for all medications on a tablet-by-tablet (or other dosage form) basis. Figure 8.1 shows an example of a printed perpetual inventory record, which documents every Schedule II drug received and dispensed. This inventory record includes the drug name, strength, and dosage form; National Drug Code (NDC) number; manufacturer; date; invoice number; department or unit or prescription number; quantity added or subtracted; inventory balance; initials; and verification initials.

FIGURE 8.1 Sample of a Controlled-Substance Perpetual Inventory Record

Controlled-Substance Perpetual Inventory Record (C-II)

Morphine 25 mg/mL, 1 mL vial (preservative-free)

Drug Name, Strength, and Dosage Form

0000-0000-000   Paradigm Drug Therapies

NDC   **Manufacturer**

	Date	Invoice #	Dept/Unit or Rx #	Qty +/−	Balance	Initials	Verified By
1	7/15/2024	BB888727-9980	n/a	200 vials	200	LMC	P.J., RPh
2	7/16/2024	n/a	5E Floor Stock	− 10	190	LMC	P.J., RPh
3	7/16/2024	n/a	663577	− 10	180	LMC	P.J., RPh
4	7/16/2024	n/a	4W Floor Stock	− 10	170	LMC	P.J., RPh
5	7/17/2024	BB8876392-8873	n/a	100	270	V.V.	L.L., RPh
6	7/17/2024	n/a	887309	− 5	265	V.V.	L.L., RPh
7	7/18/2024	n/a	256663	− 50	215	V.V.	L.L., RPh
8	7/18/2024	n/a	339287	− 30	185	LMC	L.L., RPh
9	7/20/2024	BB267883-9989	n/a	100	285	C.B.	TVG, RPh
10							
11							
12							

In addition, a biennial (every two years) inventory of Schedule II drugs must be taken. Some states (and pharmacies) have even more stringent requirements, such as a yearly inventory. These inventories should closely approximate the perpetual inventory record. For Schedules III, IV, and V substances, an estimated count and/or measure is permitted, unless a container holds more than 1,000 capsules or tablets. If the container has been opened, an exact count is required.

Calculating Unit Price

As part of maintaining inventory, it is important to economize when purchasing stock medications. A pharmacy can often save money by buying in bulk, and it is usually more economical to buy a larger amount of a drug rather than a smaller amount because the per-tablet price is usually lower when the package size or quantity is larger. When purchasing drugs from a wholesaler, pharmacy personnel must balance the optimal inventory level with the replenishment costs of available bulk containers (such as bottles containing 100, 500, or 1,000 tablets).

Unit price is used to determine the cost-effectiveness of medications. **Unit price**, also referred to as *unit cost*, is the price of a single unit of a product. Unit price is calculated by dividing cost by quantity, as shown in the following formula.

$$\text{unit price} = \frac{\text{cost}}{\text{quantity}}$$

Because larger containers typically have a lower unit price, it is usually cost-effective for a pharmacy to purchase these container sizes. However, this rationale may not be the case if the inventory item is used infrequently. If the item is used infrequently, a large bulk container may reach its expiration date before it is used. Because expired medications may not be dispensed and consequently must be destroyed, the pharmacy loses the cost of that inventory. The following examples illustrate calculations commonly performed when comparing bulk pricing and unit pricing.

Example 8.2.4

 An antibiotic is available in the following stock bottle sizes for the prices indicated.

> **100 capsules/bottle, $2.80**
>
> **500 capsules/bottle, $12.10**
>
> **1,000 capsules/bottle, $25.30**

Which container provides the best price per capsule, and what is the price per capsule?

To begin, divide each amount by the number of capsules in the bulk container to determine the unit price.

$$\text{unit price} = \frac{\text{cost}}{\text{quantity}}$$

$$\$2.80 \div 100 \text{ capsules} = \$0.028/\text{capsule}$$

$$\$12.10 \div 500 \text{ capsules} = \$0.0242/\text{capsule}$$

$$\$25.30 \div 1,000 \text{ capsules} = \$0.0253/\text{capsule}$$

Then review the unit price of each capsule to determine which stock bottle size is the most cost-effective for the pharmacy.

Answer: The 500 capsules/bottle size is the best value purchase for this medication at 2.4 cents per capsule.

Example 8.2.5

 In your pharmacy, the maximum par level for amoxicillin 250 mg capsules is 1,000; the minimum par level is 100. At the end of the day, the pharmacy computer's printout provides a list of items that have fallen below the minimum par level and therefore need to be reordered. The printout shows that there are currently 75 amoxicillin 250 mg capsules in the pharmacy stock. Due to a recent increase in the number of amoxicillin prescriptions, the pharmacist has asked you to replenish the stock to the maximum par level for this item. The wholesaler sells amoxicillin 250 mg capsules in the following quantities and prices.

> 1,000-count bottle, $12.55/bottle
>
> 500-count bottle, $8.75/bottle
>
> 250-count bottle, $4.65/bottle
>
> 100-count bottle, $3.60/bottle
>
> 50-count bottle, $2.50/bottle
>
> 25-count bottle, $1.85/bottle

Given the above information, what scenario illustrates the most economical way to replenish the pharmacy's supply of amoxicillin 250 mg capsules?

Step 1. Calculate how many capsules will be needed to replenish this item to at least the maximum par level.

$$\frac{\text{maximum}}{\text{par level}} - \frac{\text{current}}{\text{stock level}} = \frac{\text{amount needed to bring}}{\text{to maximum par level}}$$

1,000 capsules − 75 capsules = 925 capsules

Step 2. Determine the possible ways to replenish this item to the maximum par level.

Solution 1: Order exactly 925 capsules by purchasing one of each of the following:

500-count bottle at	$8.75
250-count bottle at	$4.65
100-count bottle at	$3.60
50-count bottle at	$2.50
+ 25-count bottle at	$1.85
925 capsules	$21.35

In this scenario, the cost to purchase the number of capsules needed is $21.35.

Solution 2: Order enough stock to bring the inventory to at least the maximum par level in the most cost-effective manner, by purchasing the 1,000-count bottle at $12.55. This will bring the stock level to above the maximum. However, there has been a recent increase in the number of amoxicillin prescriptions and this may be allowed.

In this scenario, the cost to purchase the number of capsules needed is $12.55.

Step 3. Determine which scenario is the most cost-effective way to replenish this item.

$$\text{Solution 1 cost} = \$21.35$$
$$\text{Solution 2 cost} = \$12.55$$

Answer: The most cost-effective way to replenish the number of amoxicillin 250 mg capsules to the maximum par level is to purchase a single, 1,000-count bottle for $12.55.

Setting Inventory Goals

Both community and institutional pharmacy settings have inventory. Inventory amounts vary based on factors such as volume of patients served, the number of orders per patient, and seasonal needs. The amount of inventory in the form of drugs and supplies in an institutional pharmacy varies greatly based on the size of the institution and the types of medications stocked. For example, a pharmacy that serves oncology patients may have a much larger dollar value of inventory compared with a general pharmacy because chemotherapy agents are relatively more costly. Today's community pharmacies generally have at least $100,000 of inventory in the form of drugs, supplies, and other merchandise. Regardless of the practice setting, goals are often set to lower the value of inventory and improve cash flow.

Setting inventory goals for a pharmacy requires personnel to attempt to keep the approximate value of inventory, including items on shelves and drugs in the refrigerator and freezer, relatively equal to the cost of all drugs and merchandise sold in a specified period—usually either one week (7 days) or one month (30 days). For example, if a pharmacy manager establishes a goal of "30 days' supply," the pharmacy's goal is to keep the value of its inventory approximately equal to the total cost of the drugs and merchandise utilized by the pharmacy in 30 days.

A pharmacy's computer system typically maintains a record of the value of the inventory currently in the pharmacy. In addition, most computer systems can provide an accurate record of the pharmacy's cost for all products used in the pharmacy in a 24-hour period. Many of these systems can provide printouts of inventory and cost records, as well as average usage and costs for a specified period.

In rare instances, smaller pharmacies may not have ready access to this type of inventory and cost information. In these situations, a pharmacy manager may not know the optimal number of days to use as a goal in calculating costs. However, the manager likely has a good estimate of the current inventory value and can easily calculate average daily cost of items used in the pharmacy (weekly costs/7 days) using the following formula.

Math Morsel

Pharmacy technicians should exercise care not to confuse an *inventory* days' supply with the days' supply that refers to the number of days that a prescription or medication order will last a patient when taken as directed by the patient's prescriber.

$$\text{average daily product cost} = \frac{\text{weekly product cost}}{7 \text{ days}}$$

With this information, the pharmacy manager can then determine how many days it will take (what is referred to as *inventory days' supply*) for the average daily product costs to equal the value of the inventory. The manager can use this information to revise the inventory goal as necessary.

$$\text{number of inventory days' supply} = \frac{\text{value of inventory}}{\text{average daily cost of products used}}$$

Example 8.2.6

Toussaint's Pharmacy has a total inventory value of $103,699. It had sales last week of $37,546, and the cost to the pharmacy of the products sold was $28,837. What is the pharmacy's number of inventory days' supply?

To begin, determine the pharmacy's average daily product cost.

$$\text{average daily product cost} = \frac{\text{weekly product cost}}{\text{7 days}}$$

$$\text{average daily product cost} = \frac{\$28,837}{\text{7 days}} = \$4,119.57$$

Then use the following formula to determine the number of inventory days' supply.

$$\text{number of inventory days' supply} = \frac{\text{value of inventory}}{\text{average daily cost of products used}}$$

$$\text{number of inventory days' supply} = \frac{\$103,699}{\$4,119.57} = 25.17, \text{rounded to 25}$$

Answer: The pharmacy's number of inventory days' supply is 25.

Example 8.2.7

Malaya's Pharmacy has a total inventory value of $176,989. Last week, the pharmacy's sales were $45,813, and the cost to the pharmacy of the products sold was $36,592. The pharmacy's goal for the number of inventory days' supply is 29, but the facility overshot that goal. Determine the number of days that the pharmacy exceeded its inventory days' supply and the cost of the inventory value this represents.

To begin, determine the pharmacy's daily product cost.

$$\text{average daily product cost} = \frac{\text{weekly product cost}}{\text{7 days}}$$

$$\text{average daily product cost} = \frac{\$36,592}{\text{7 days}} = \$5,227.428, \text{rounded to } \$5,227.43$$

Then use the following formula to determine the number of inventory days' supply.

$$\text{number of inventory days' supply} = \frac{\text{value of inventory}}{\text{average daily cost of products used}}$$

$$\text{number of inventory days' supply} = \frac{\$176,989}{\$5,227.43} = 33.9, \text{rounded to 34}$$

Now, subtract the inventory days' supply goal from the current inventory days' supply.

$$34 \text{ days} - 29 \text{ days} = 5 \text{ days}$$

Last, multiply the number of inventory days' supply that the pharmacy is over its goal by the average daily product cost.

$$5 \times \$5,227.43 = \$26,137.15$$

Answer: It takes 34 days for costs to equal the inventory value. In other words, Malaya's Pharmacy is 5 days over its inventory days' supply. If Malaya's Pharmacy can reduce its inventory by $26,137.15, the pharmacy will have met its goal of 29 inventory days' supply.

Calculating Turnover Rate

If a pharmacy does not maintain computerized, or perpetual, inventory, it must perform a physical inventory—or actual count—at specified intervals, usually annually or semiannually. The physical inventory value helps to determine the average annual inventory value as shown by the following formula.

$$\text{average annual inventory value} = \frac{\text{value of initial inventory} + \text{value of current inventory}}{2}$$

Knowing the average annual inventory value allows pharmacy personnel to calculate the number of times the pharmacy's inventory was repurchased during a cycle (typically a year).

Dividing total annual inventory purchases by the average inventory value provides the **turnover rate**, or the number of times the amount of goods in inventory was sold during the year. Turnover rate can be used to determine how quickly a particular item is being utilized. In addition, turnover rate can be applied more broadly to the entire pharmacy inventory, which helps the pharmacy manager know how well the pharmacy is meeting its cash flow goals. Knowing the turnover rate can also help pharmacy personnel determine if the average inventory level should be increased or decreased, as extra costs may be associated with high or low inventories.

$$\text{turnover rate} = \frac{\text{annual inventory purchases}}{\text{average inventory value}}$$

Consider a situation in which a pharmacy has an average inventory value of $25,250 and the cost of its annual inventory purchases is $75,000. Turnover rate can be determined by dividing the annual inventory purchases ($75,000) by the average inventory value ($25,250).

$$\text{turnover rate} = \frac{\$75,000}{\$25,250} = 2.97$$

The inventory will "turn over" 2.97 times, or approximately three times in a year. The following examples offer more practice determining turnover rate.

Example 8.2.8

Pharmacy personnel perform a quarterly inventory and determine that the pharmacy has an average inventory value of $100,000. The pharmacy's annual inventory purchases are $500,000. What is the pharmacy's turnover rate?

$$\text{turnover rate} = \frac{\text{annual inventory purchases}}{\text{average inventory value}}$$

$$\text{turnover rate} = \frac{\$500,000}{\$100,000} = 5$$

Answer: The pharmacy's inventory will "turn over" five times in a year.

Determining Depreciation

An **asset** is a resource owned by a business. Assets can be categorized by their ability to be converted to cash as either fixed assets or current assets. A **fixed asset** (or non-current asset) is an asset that cannot be converted easily into cash. In pharmacy practice, examples of fixed assets include the pharmacy's physical building, equipment such as computers, and furnishings. A **current asset** is an asset that can easily be converted into cash. Medications and OTC products are examples of current assets in the pharmacy setting.

Depreciation is an allowance made to account for the decreasing value of a physical asset over its useful life. Depreciation represents the reduction in value of an asset over the passage of time. Both fixed assets and current assets can depreciate.

Annual depreciation can be calculated by subtracting the **disposal value**, or the value of an item should it be sold or disposed of at the end of its useful life, from the item's total cost, then dividing that difference by the estimated life in years. The following formula is used to calculate annual depreciation.

$$\text{annual depreciation} = \frac{\text{total cost} - \text{disposal value}}{\text{estimated life in years}}$$

Example 8.2.9

Rafael's Pharmacy buys a used, compact car for drug deliveries to local customers. The cost of the car is $9,000. Its estimated useful life is 5 years, and the disposal value is $1,200. What is the annual depreciation of the car?

$$\text{annual depreciation} = \frac{\text{total cost} - \text{disposal value}}{\text{estimated life in years}}$$

$$\text{annual depreciation} = \frac{\$9,000 - \$1,200}{5} = \$1,560$$

Answer: The annual depreciation of the car is $1,560.

8.2 Problem Set

For items 1–9, calculate the number of units that need to be reordered for each drug based on the current inventory and the number of units or packages needed to bring the drug to its minimum par level.

Drug	Count/ Package Size	Minimum Par Level	Maximum Par Level	Current Inventory	Reorder Amount
1. tetracycline 250 mg capsules	500	120	700	80	
2. amoxicillin 500 mg capsules	100	300	400	118	
3. amoxicillin 250 mg capsules	500	240	1,000	180	
4. cefaclor 500 mg tablets	60	20	120	35	
5. cefprozil 250 mg tablets	100	40	150	28	

continues

Drug		Count/ Package Size	Minimum Par Level	Maximum Par Level	Current Inventory	Reorder Amount
6. cefprozil 500 mg tablets		50	20	75	24	
7. metronidazole 500 mg tablets		50	30	120	12	
8. azithromycin 250 mg capsules		30	18	60	36	
9. doxycycline 50 mg capsules		50	30	150	42	

The inventory of topical products, which are often dispensed as "partial containers" (e.g., 1 oz from a 16 oz jar), is checked frequently due to multiple compounding needs, manufacturer back orders, and poor computer tracking of dispensed partial containers of topical products. For these reasons, reordering of topical products must be closely monitored, even with computer-generated orders.

Consider the following scenario:

It is a Friday afternoon and Monday is a holiday. Therefore, the pharmacy is expected to be very busy over the weekend. Because the pharmacy will not be able to get an order from its wholesaler until at least Tuesday, you decide to reorder certain items.

For items 10–14, calculate the reorder amount needed to bring each drug to its maximum par level.

Drug		Count/ Package Size	Minimum Par Level	Maximum Par Level	Current Inventory	Reorder Amount
10. triamcinolone 0.25% cream		15 g	2	4	1	
		80 g	2	4	0	
11. triamcinolone 0.1% ointment		15 g	1	2	1	
		60 g	1	2	1	
		80 g	1	2	0	
12. triamcinolone 0.1% lotion		60 mL	1	2	1	
13. fluocinolone 0.025% cream		15 g	1	2	1	
		60 g	1	2	1	
14. fluocinolone 0.025% ointment		60 g	1	2	0 tubes and 1 order waiting	

For items 15–36, calculate the reorder amount needed to bring each drug to its minimum par level.

Drug		Count/Package Size	Minimum Par Level	Maximum Par Level	Current Inventory	Reorder Amount
15. desoximetasone 0.25% cream		15 g	1	2	0	
		60 g	1	2	0	
		4 oz	1	2	1	
16. desoximetasone 0.05% gel		15 g	1	1	0 on shelf and 1 order waiting	
		60 g	1	1	0	
17. halobetasol 0.05% cream		15 g	1	2	1	
		45 g	1	2	1	
18. fluocinonide 0.05% cream		15 g	1	2	1	
		30 g	2	4	1	
		60 g	2	4	2	
		120 g	1	2	0	
19. fluocinonide 0.05% gel		15 g	1	1	1	
		30 g	1	3	2	
		60 g	1	3	0	
20. fluocinonide 0.05% ointment		15 g	1	2	1	
		30 g	1	2	1	
		60 g	1	2	1 partial	
		120 g	1	2	1	
21. fluocinonide 0.05% solution		20 mL	1	1	0	
		60 mL	1	3	1 partial	
22. ramipril 5 mg capsules		100	120	240	64	
23. verapamil 120 mg SR caplets		100	80	240	52	
24. verapamil 240 mg SR caplets		100	120	360	30	
25. nicardipine 60 mg SR capsules		60	120	240	20	
26. captopril 50 mg tablets		100	150	300	76	
27. furosemide 40 mg tablets		1,000	240	1,500	134	
28. doxazosin 2 mg tablets		100	80	240	83	

continues

Drug		Count/ Package Size	Minimum Par Level	Maximum Par Level	Current Inventory	Reorder Amount
29. atenolol 50 mg tablets		1,000	240	1,500	107	
30. atenolol 100 mg tablets		100	150	300	111	
31. nifedipine 60 mg tablets		300	120	625	12, and two Rx for 60 pending	
32. nifedipine 90 mg tablets		100	120	300	63	
33. lisinopril 5 mg tablets		100	90	260	110	
34. lisinopril 10 mg tablets		1,000	240	1,500	146	
35. lisinopril 20 mg tablets		100	180	250	145	
36. lisinopril 40 mg tablets		100	90	220	152	

37. Review John's Drug Shop inventory below and calculate the reorder amount needed to bring each drug to its maximum par level.

Drug		Count/ Package Size	Minimum Par Level	Maximum Par Level	Current Inventory	Reorder Amount
a. Eucerin cream		100 g	3 jars	10 jars	3 jars	
b. amoxicillin 250 mg capsules		1,000 capsules	1,000 capsules	5,000 capsules	2,400 capsules	
c. NS Nasal Spray		30 mL	12 bottles	24 bottles	4 bottles	
d. NS Nasal Spray		100 mL	3 bottles	12 bottles	1 bottle	
e. Nystatin Oral Suspension		pint bottle (480 mL)	1 bottle	4 bottles	720 mL	

38. Grimm's Pharmacy has a total inventory value of $183,445. Last week, the pharmacy had sales of $47,293, and the cost to the pharmacy for the products sold came to $38,207. The pharmacy's goal is to have an inventory days' supply of 28 days.

    a. How many inventory days' supply does Grimm's Pharmacy have?

    b. How much is the pharmacy over or under its goal in dollars?

39. Corbin's Pharmacy has a total inventory value of $123,490. Last week, the pharmacy had sales of $34,829, and the cost to the pharmacy for the products sold came to $26,504. Corbin's goal is to have an inventory days' supply of 26 days.

    a. How many inventory days' supply does Corbin's Pharmacy have?

    b. How much is the pharmacy over or under its goal in dollars?

40. Singh's Pharmacy has $147,210 in inventory. The pharmacy is currently at its goal of 24 inventory days' supply. What was the approximate cost of products sold last week?

41. Scott's Pharmacy had sales of $51,280 last week. What must the pharmacy's daily sales average be this week in order to make $5,000 more than last week?

42. If a pharmacy's average inventory for the past year was $132,936 and the annual cost total was $1,612,000, what was the turnover rate?

43. If a pharmacy's average inventory for the past year was $156,200 and the annual cost total was $1,768,000, what was the turnover rate?

For items 44–48, calculate the turnover rate for the following drugs sold at Ming's Pharmacy.

Drug		Average Inventory Value	Annual Inventory Purchases	Turnover Rate
44. metformin 500 mg tablets		$520	$20,800	
45. divalproex 250 mg tablets		$178	$5,760	
46. citalopram 40 mg tablets		$360	$7,213	
47. raloxifene 60 mg tablets		$320	$5,060	
48. montelukast 4 mg chewable tablets		$385	$6,000	

49. Nadia's Drug Shop purchases $52,500 of antibiotics annually. The pharmacy does an inventory count twice annually, and its average inventory of antibiotics is $5,000. What is the pharmacy's turnover rate for antibiotics?

50. A pharmacy has a new cash register system. The system costs $8,294 and should last six years. Its disposal value is $2,138. What is its annual depreciation?

51. A hospital pharmacy just purchased two new biological safety cabinets (used for compounding sterile products) at $18,350 each. Each cabinet should last 12 years if maintained properly. The disposal value is $1,567 each. What is the annual depreciation amount for both cabinets?

52. Hydrocodone with acetaminophen 5 mg/325 mg, a Schedule II controlled substance, is available in the following stock bottle sizes for the prices indicated.

 100 tablets/bottle, $9.10
 500 tablets/bottle, $35.30
 1,000 tablets/bottle, $79.80

Which container provides the best price per tablet?

53. The 1,000-tablet bottle of hydrocodone with acetaminophen 5 mg/325 mg was ordered. The perpetual inventory record prior to receipt of the 1,000-tablet bottle is shown below. If the ordered bottle of hydrocodone with acetaminophen 5 mg/325 mg is received by the pharmacy directly after prescription 245709, what is the new cumulative total?

Drug and Dose		Hydrocodone with acetaminophen 5 mg/325 mg			
Record Starting Date		07/16/24			
Record Starting Quantity		600			
Prescription Number	Dispensing Date	Quantity Dispensed	Cumulative Total	Pharmacist Initials	
245699	07/16/22	30	570	LRT	
245709	07/16/22	90	480	LRT	

Self-check your work in Appendix A.

8.3 Business-Related Calculations

Put Down Roots

The word *profit* comes from the Latin word *profectus*, which means "to progress or advance."

Like other types of businesses, pharmacies must perform certain accounting operations on a regular basis. In an institutional pharmacy setting, personnel must closely monitor the inventory of medication and supplies to determine if the facility is staying within its allotted budget. In the community pharmacy setting, it is important for the pharmacy to make a profit. To that end, community pharmacies must effectively manage overhead, income, and base profit; revenue, gross profit and net profit, overall cost, and selling price; profit margin and markup; and discounts. These business concepts and their related calculations are discussed in this section.

Calculating Overhead, Income, and Base Profit

As a pharmacy technician, your role in calculating overhead, income, and base profit depends on your practice setting. In some settings, pharmacy technicians and pharmacists participate in these calculations peripherally. In other settings, pharmacy technicians and pharmacists may take a direct role in performing these business-related calculations.

A pharmacy's **overhead** is its costs related to doing business. This overall cost includes employees' salaries, equipment, and operating expenses such as rent, taxes, utilities, and insurance. Overhead also includes the dollar value of the medications and supply items in the pharmacy inventory.

Income refers to the money or equivalent payments (such as those payments made with credit or debit cards) received from the sale of a medication, supply item, or equipment. **Profit** is the financial gain a business obtains when the income the business earns in a specified period is greater than the costs it incurs to run the business. There are various types of profit. Base profit is calculated based on overhead expenses. In the simplest terms, a pharmacy's **base profit** is determined by subtracting total overhead expenses from total income.

Example 8.3.1

The River City Apothecary Shop has an annual income of $850,000. The pharmacy's annual overhead expenses are listed below. What is the pharmacy's base profit?

salary of pharmacist	$120,000
salaries of two pharmacy technicians ($42,000 each)	$84,000
rent	$34,400
utilities	$5,000
pharmacy software maintenance	$2,200
liability insurance	$3,500
business insurance	$4,000
pharmacy inventory	$550,000
total pharmacy overhead amount	$803,100

Using this information, determine the pharmacy's base profit by subtracting the total pharmacy overhead amount from the pharmacy's annual income.

income	$850,000
overhead	− $803,100
base profit	$46,900

Answer: The base profit of the River City Apothecary Shop is $46,900.

Example 8.3.2

The Willington City Pharmacy has an annual income of $1,250,000. The pharmacy's annual overhead expenses are listed below. What is the pharmacy's base profit?

salaries of two pharmacists ($120,000 each)	$240,000
salary of pharmacy technician	$40,000
salary of pharmacy clerk	$22,500
rent	$36,200
utilities	$7,000
pharmacy software maintenance	$2,900
liability insurance	$4,000
business insurance	$5,000
pharmacy inventory	$625,000
total pharmacy overhead amount	$982,600

Using this information, determine the pharmacy's base profit by subtracting the total pharmacy overhead amount from the pharmacy's annual income.

income	$1,250,000
overhead	– $982,600
base profit	$267,400

Answer: The base profit of the Willington City Pharmacy is $267,400.

A pharmacy manager often sets goals for the pharmacy's annual profit. To determine these goals, the manager begins by finding the current percentage of profit. The **current percentage of profit** is determined by dividing the pharmacy's base profit by its total income and then multiplying that quotient by 100.

$$\text{current percentage of profit} = \frac{\text{base profit}}{\text{annual income}} \times 100$$

The following examples illustrate how to calculate percentage of profit.

Example 8.3.3

Determine the River City Apothecary Shop's current percentage of profit based on the annual income and base profit information calculated in Example 8.3.1. Round to the nearest whole percentage.

To solve this problem, use the current percentage of profit formula.

$$\text{current percentage of profit} = \frac{\text{base profit}}{\text{annual income}} \times 100$$

$$\text{current percentage of profit} = \frac{\$46,900}{\$850,000} \times 100 = 5.52, \text{rounded to } 6$$

Answer: The River City Apothecary Shop has a current percentage of profit of 6%.

Example 8.3.4

Determine the Willington City Pharmacy's current percentage of profit based on the annual income and base profit information calculated in Example 8.3.2. Round to the nearest whole percentage.

To solve this problem, use the current percentage of profit formula.

$$\text{current percentage of profit} = \frac{\text{base profit}}{\text{annual income}} \times 100$$

$$\text{current percentage of profit} = \frac{\$267,400}{\$1,250,000} \times 100 = 21.39, \text{rounded to } 21$$

Answer: The Willington City Pharmacy has a current percentage of profit of 21%.

Once the current percentage of profit is known, the pharmacy manager can determine the desired percentage of profit. The **desired percentage of profit** is the percentage of profit the pharmacy intends to make after the overall cost is subtracted from the selling price.

A related concept is **desired amount of profit**, or the amount of profit the pharmacy intends to make. Desired amount of profit can be calculated using the following formula.

desired amount of profit = overhead × desired percentage of profit

Establishing the desired amount of profit can, in turn, help the pharmacy manager determine the amount of annual income needed to achieve this goal. The **desired income goal** is the amount of income the pharmacy aims to make.

desired income goal = overhead + desired amount of profit

Desired percentage of profit, desired amount of profit, and desired income goal are business calculations that provide the manager with the necessary information to establish a pharmacy's budget and to set sales goals. The following examples illustrate how to calculate desired amount of profit and desired income goal. Note that converting the desired percentage of profit to a decimal allows for easier calculation, but round to the nearest whole percent for your final answer.

Example 8.3.5

The River City Apothecary Shop has set a desired percentage of profit of 25%. Based on the overhead amount of $803,100 provided in Example 8.3.1, what is the pharmacy's desired amount of profit? What is the pharmacy's desired income goal?

To begin, determine the desired amount of profit by finding the product of the overhead and the desired percentage of profit.

desired amount of profit = overhead × desired percentage of profit

desired amount of profit = $803,100 × 0.25 = $200,775

Now calculate the desired income goal by finding the sum of the overhead and desired amount of profit.

desired income goal = overhead + desired amount of profit

desired income goal = $803,100 + $200,775 = $1,003,875

Answer: To meet the desired percentage of profit of 25%, the pharmacy's desired amount of profit is $200,775, and the pharmacy must generate an annual income of $1,003,875.

Example 8.3.6

The Willington City Pharmacy has set a desired percentage of profit of 35%. Based on the overhead amount of $982,600 provided in Example 8.3.2, what is the pharmacy's desired amount of profit? What is the pharmacy's desired income goal?

To begin, determine the desired amount of profit by finding the product of the overhead and the desired percentage of profit.

desired amount of profit = overhead × desired percentage of profit

desired amount of profit = $982,600 × 0.35 = $343,910

Now calculate the desired income goal by finding the sum of the overhead and desired amount of profit.

$$\text{desired income goal} = \text{overhead} + \text{desired amount of profit}$$

$$\text{desired income goal} = \$982{,}600 + \$343{,}910 = \$1{,}326{,}510$$

Answer: To meet the desired percentage of profit of 35%, the pharmacy's desired amount of profit is $343,910, and the pharmacy must generate an annual income of $1,326,510.

Calculating Revenue, Gross Profit, Net Profit, Overall Cost, and Selling Price

Revenue is the total amount of income generated by normal business activities. In a community pharmacy, revenue includes the total amount of income from the sale of prescriptions and OTC medications. Another way to think of revenue is the income generated by typical business operations before expenses are deducted.

Concepts related to revenue are gross profit and net profit. **Gross profit** is the profit a business makes after deducting the costs associated with producing and selling its products or services. It is calculated by finding the difference between revenue and the cost of goods sold, as shown in the following formula.

$$\text{gross profit} = \text{revenue} - \text{cost of goods sold}$$

In pharmacy practice, gross profit may represent the difference between the selling price of a prescription and the pharmacy's purchase price (the price that it costs for the pharmacy to purchase the drug from the manufacturer or drug wholesaler). This relationship between the selling price and the purchase price does not take into account the cost of preparing and dispensing the drug. Therefore, the gross profit is always more than the net profit.

Net profit is the amount of income remaining after accounting for business expenses. Another way to think of net profit is the difference between the amount earned and the amount spent in buying, operating, or producing an item. In the pharmacy practice setting, net profit could be the difference between the sales of all medications and the costs of purchasing the medications, running the pharmacy, and paying taxes. This relationship is shown in the following formula.

$$\text{net profit} = \text{revenue} - \text{expenses}$$

Net profit can be calculated for individual business transactions in the pharmacy setting. In these instances, net profit is the difference between the selling price of a medication and its overall cost. The **selling price** is the amount received when a pharmacy product is sold. This price is often called the *retail price*. Simply put, the selling price determines the amount due from a customer to the pharmacy for the sale of drugs and other products and the overall cost of the medication. The following formula is used to calculate net profit for a prescription.

$$\text{net profit for a prescription} = \text{selling price of the prescription} - \text{overall cost}$$

The **overall cost** is the sum of the cost to purchase the drug from the wholesaler or manufacturer (known as the pharmacy's *purchase price*) and the dispensing cost. The **dispensing cost** covers all costs beyond the drug's purchase price that are related to filling a prescription, such as pharmacy overhead, professional handling, prescription processing and recording, and patient consultation and counseling. The **dispensing fee** is the amount the pharmacy charges for a medication that is over and above the price it pays for the medication. The dispensing fee may be more, less, or the same as the dispensing cost. The formula below is used to calculate overall cost of an item.

$$\text{overall cost} = \text{pharmacy's purchase price} + \text{dispensing cost}$$

When calculating profit on an individual prescription, the overall cost of the medication (pharmacy's purchase price plus dispensing cost) is compared with the amount the pharmacy receives for the dispensed drug.

Based on its desired percentage of profit, a pharmacy will decide on a selling price for a medication or supply item. As mentioned earlier, the desired percentage of profit is the percentage of profit the pharmacy intends to make on the product after the overall cost is subtracted from the selling price. To easily calculate the selling price, convert the desired percentage of profit to a decimal. If the pharmacy has correctly set the selling price, the net profit should yield the desired percentage of profit.

$$\text{selling price} = (\text{overall cost} \times \text{desired percentage of profit}) + \text{overall cost}$$

The following examples show how to calculate net profit, overall cost, and selling price.

 Example 8.3.7

A pharmacy's purchase price of a pint bottle of Nystatin Oral Suspension is $20.25. After considering the various factors that influence pharmacy costs, the pharmacy manager determines that the pharmacy's cost to dispense this medication is $5.10. Determine the overall cost for this medication. If the pharmacy has a desired percentage of profit of 20% for this medication, what should the selling price be? What is the pharmacy's net profit?

To begin, determine the overall cost by finding the sum of the pharmacy's purchase price and dispensing cost.

overall cost = pharmacy's purchase price + dispensing cost

overall cost = $20.25 + $5.10 = $25.35

Then use the following formula to determine the selling price.

selling price = (overall cost × desired percentage of profit) + overall cost

selling price = ($25.35 × 0.20) + $25.35 = $30.42

Last, determine the net profit by finding the difference between the selling price and the overall cost.

net profit = selling price − overall cost

net profit = $30.42 − $25.35 = $5.07

Answer: The overall cost for a pint bottle of Nystatin Oral Suspension is $25.35. To yield a desired percentage of profit of $5.07, or 20%, the selling price of the item must be $30.42.

Example 8.3.8

 A pharmacy purchased a 30-count bottle of propranolol 10 mg tablets at a price of $1.20. A customer presents a prescription that requires you to dispense a total of 30 tablets. The pharmacy's dispensing cost is $4.25 for each prescription it fills. The total charge to the customer for this prescription is $8.59. Calculate the net profit that the pharmacy made on the sale of this prescription.

To begin, calculate the overall cost by finding the sum of the pharmacy's purchasing price of the prescription and the dispensing cost.

overall cost = pharmacy's purchase price of the prescription + dispensing cost

overall cost = $1.20 + $4.25 = $5.45

Then determine the net profit by finding the difference between the selling price and the overall cost.

net profit = selling price − overall cost

net profit = $8.59 − $5.45 = $3.14

Answer: The pharmacy made a net profit of $3.14 on the sale of this prescription.

Determining Profit Margin and Markup

Profit margin is another way to express profit. Profit margin relates profit to revenue. **Gross profit margin**, often expressed as a percentage, is the quotient of gross profit and revenue times 100, as shown in the following formula.

$$\text{gross profit margin (\%)} = \frac{\text{gross profit}}{\text{revenue}} \times 100$$

Consider an example in which a pharmacy sells a medication to a patient for $30. The cost to the pharmacy for that medication was $10. In this instance, the gross profit would be $20. The gross profit margin would be 66.6% and would be calculated by dividing the gross profit ($20) by the revenue ($30).

Net profit margin, often expressed as a percentage is the quotient of net profit and revenue times 100, as reflected in the following formula.

$$\text{net profit margin (\%)} = \frac{\text{net profit}}{\text{revenue}} \times 100$$

Consider the previous example in which a pharmacy sells a medication to a patient for $30. Recall that net profit is the difference between the selling price of a prescription and the overall cost to the pharmacy for that medication. If the overall cost to the pharmacy for that medication is $15, the net profit is $15 ($30 − $15). The net profit margin would be 50% and is calculated by dividing the net profit ($15) by the revenue ($30). This example resulted in a positive profit margin, called a *gain*. A loss—sometimes called a *negative profit*—occurs when the selling price of a product is less than the cost.

Example 8.3.9

A pharmacy sells a prescription medication to a patient for $100. The cost of the pharmacy to obtain that medication was $60. The overall cost to the pharmacy for that same medication was $80. Calculate the pharmacy's gross profit margin and net profit margin for the prescription.

To begin, calculate the gross profit. Gross profit is the difference between revenue ($100) and the cost of goods sold ($60).

$$\text{gross profit} = \$100 - \$60 = \$40$$

Next, use the following formula to determine the gross profit margin.

$$\text{gross profit margin} = \frac{\text{gross profit}}{\text{revenue}} \times 100$$

$$\text{gross profit margin} = \frac{\$40}{\$100} \times 100 = 40\%$$

Now, calculate the net profit by using the following formula.

$$\text{net profit} = \text{selling price} - \text{overall cost}$$

$$\text{net profit} = \$100 - \$80 = \$20$$

Last, calculate the net profit margin by using the following formula.

$$\text{net profit margin} = \frac{\text{net profit}}{\text{revenue}} \times 100$$

$$\text{net profit margin} = \frac{\$20}{\$100} \times 100 = 20\%$$

Answer: For this prescription, the pharmacy's gross profit margin is 40%, and its net profit margin is 20%.

Markup is the amount the cost of a product is increased to the selling price. Markup can be expressed as an amount or a percent. **Markup amount** is the difference between the selling price and the cost of obtaining the product, as shown in the following formula.

$$\text{markup amount} = \text{selling price} - \text{obtaining cost}$$

In the pharmacy practice setting, markup could be the difference in the cost to the pharmacy of obtaining a bottle of acetaminophen and the price at which the pharmacy sells that same bottle. Markup could also be the cost of obtaining a prescription medication and the amount that a patient is charged for that same prescription medication.

As mentioned earlier, markup can also be expressed as a percent. **Markup percentage** (also called *markup rate*) is the markup amount (or the difference between the selling price and obtaining cost) divided by the cost of obtaining the medication.

$$\text{markup percentage} = \frac{\text{markup amount}}{\text{obtaining cost}} \times 100$$

$$= \frac{\text{selling price} - \text{obtaining cost}}{\text{cost}} \times 100$$

The following example calculates markup amount and rate.

Example 8.3.10

Name Exchange

The generic drug metformin, commonly used to treat diabetes, is also known by the brand name Glucophage.

A 30-day supply of the diabetes medication metformin has a selling price of $45. The pharmacy's purchase price is $30. What is the markup amount? What is the markup percentage?

To begin, determine the markup amount by finding the difference between the selling price and the pharmacy's purchase price.

$$\text{markup amount} = \text{selling price} - \text{obtaining price}$$

$$\text{markup amount} = \$45 - \$30 = \$15$$

Now, use the markup percentage formula to calculate the percentage markup.

$$\text{markup rate} = \frac{\text{markup amount}}{\text{obtaining cost}} \times 100$$

$$\text{markup rate} = \frac{\$15}{\$30} \times 100 = 50\%$$

Answer: The markup amount on a 30-day supply of metformin is $15. The markup rate is 50%.

Markup rates on brand-name drugs are typically lower than markup rates on generic drugs. Although the markup rates on generic medications are typically higher, the selling prices of generic drugs are typically lower than brand-name drugs.

As a result of these markup practices, the percentage of profit from selling generic drugs may be higher than the percentage of profit for the corresponding brand-name products. For example, a pharmacy may have a purchase price of $15 for a generic drug and a markup of 33%, which would result in a selling price of $19.95 and a $4.95 profit for the pharmacy. The corresponding brand-name drug may have a purchase price of $30 and a markup of 5%, which would result in a selling price of $31.50 and a $1.50 profit for the pharmacy.

In general, both the patient and the pharmacy benefit financially from using generic medications. The patient purchases the medication at a lower cost, and the pharmacy receives a larger profit. Although the pharmacy's percentage of profit from selling a generic drug is generally higher than the percentage of profit for the corresponding brand-name drug, the pharmacy may not make a huge profit from the sale of an individual drug due to a relatively low selling price of the generic drug.

A growing trend in community pharmacies is to sell generic drugs to customers at a flat dollar rate, such as $4 or $7, regardless of the cost of the drugs, which fluctuates over time. A **flat rate medication price** is a low pharmacy selling price for a certain amount of medication designed to last a specific number of days—for example, a 30-day or 90-day supply. The types of medications that are available to customers at a flat rate are typically generic medications with low pharmacy purchase prices. Because the medications are inexpensive for pharmacies to purchase, the pharmacies are still able to make a profit on the drugs while generating additional sales from nonpharmacy sales, OTC products, or other prescriptions that patients may purchase at the same time. Table 8.1 lists examples of medications that are often sold at a flat rate.

TABLE 8.1 Common Flat-Rate Medications

Medication	Indication
amoxicillin	bacterial infections
atenolol	hypertension or heart conditions
estradiol	estrogen deficiency
fluoxetine	depression
levothyroxine	thyroid disorders
lisinopril	hypertension
loratadine	allergies
metformin	diabetes
naproxen	pain and inflammation

The following example applies the formulas for markup amount and markup rate to a flat-rate prescription to illustrate how profitable such sales can be for a pharmacy.

Example 8.3.11

 A community pharmacy that has advertised a $4.00 flat-rate price for generic prescriptions receives a prescription for #30 amoxicillin 250 mg capsules. If the pharmacy's purchase price for these #30 capsules is $1.20, what is the percentage of profit on this prescription when it is sold for the flat-rate price?

To begin, find the markup amount by calculating the difference between the selling price and the pharmacy's purchase price.

$$\text{markup amount} = \text{selling price} - \text{obtaining price}$$

$$\text{markup amount} = \$4.00 - \$1.20 = \$2.80$$

Then find the markup rate by using the following formula.

$$\text{markup rate} = \frac{\text{markup amount}}{\text{obtaining cost}} \times 100$$

$$\text{markup rate} = \frac{\$2.80}{\$1.20} \times 100 = 233\%$$

Answer: The percentage of profit on amoxicillin sold for the flat rate of $4.00 is 233%. Note that although the markup rate is high, the profit is still relatively low due to the drug's low cost.

Working with Discounts

Sometimes, a manufacturer or supplier offers an item at a lower price to a pharmacy. The amount by which the price is reduced is the **discount**. Similarly, a pharmacy may offer consumers a discount, or a reduction from what is typically charged, as an incentive to purchase an item. The **discount rate** is the percent by which the price is reduced from the regular selling price. When working with percents, it is helpful to change the discount rate from a percent to a decimal.

$$\text{discount amount} = \text{regular selling price} \times \text{discount rate}$$

The **sale price** is the difference between the regular selling price and the discount amount.

sale price = regular selling price − discount amount

 Math Morsel

When working with percents, pharmacy technicians should change the discount rate from a percent to a decimal.

Therefore, to determine a discount, you would first calculate the discount amount, and then you would subtract that amount from the regular selling price.

You are likely familiar with the concept of discounts based on your experience buying items on sale. For example, a sale that offers a 50% discount means that a sale item may be purchased at one-half of the regular selling price. In such a scenario, the discount amount (also known as the *discounted selling price*) is calculated by multiplying the regular price by 0.50 (50% = 0.50). In this example, the sale price may also be calculated by dividing the regular selling price by two.

 # WORKPLACE WISDOM

The approach you just learned to determine the sale price of an item was to calculate the discount amount first (regular selling price × discount rate = discount amount) and then subtract the discount amount from the regular selling price (regular selling price − discount price = sale price). Consequently, this method focuses on the discount rate.

Although the described approach provides an accurate way to calculate sale price, there is another commonly used method that pharmacy personnel may use. The alternative method calculates the sale price directly by focusing on the percent of the regular selling price that will be paid. To that end, you would subtract the discount rate from 100% to determine the selling price.

For example, consider calculating the sale price of a medication that costs $100 and is discounted by 10%. Using the method described in this chapter, you would first calculate the discount amount.

discount amount = regular selling price × discount rate

discount amount = $100 × 0.10 = $10

Then you would subtract this discount amount from the selling price to determine the sale price.

sale price = regular selling price − discount amount

sale price = $100 − $10 = $90

The alternative method focuses on the fact the sale price is 90% of the regular price. This price is determined by subtracting the discount rate from 100%.

100% − 10% = 90%

To calculate the sale price, you can simply multiply the regular selling price by 90% (0.90).

$100 × 0.90 = $90

The following example demonstrates how to calculate discount amount and determine sale price on pharmacy items.

Example 8.3.12

 A community pharmacy has announced a 40% off sale on all headache products during the two weeks leading up to the tax-filing deadline. The following products are on sale:

Tylenol 325 mg tablets, 100 count, regular selling price of $6.99

Excedrin Migraine tablets, 100 count, regular selling price of $7.89

Advil 250 mg tablets, 100 count, regular selling price of $7.29

If a customer purchases one bottle of each item at the sale price, how much will the customer pay for each drug? How much will the customer pay for the entire purchase?

To begin, calculate the discount amount for each medication using the following formula.

discount amount = regular selling price × discount rate

Tylenol: $6.99 × 0.40 = $2.796, rounded to $2.80

Excedrin Migraine: $7.89 × 0.40 = $3.156, rounded to $3.16

Advil: $7.29 × 0.40 = $2.916, rounded to $2.92

Now determine the sale price for each medication using the following formula.

sale price = regular selling price − discount amount

Tylenol: $6.99 − $2.80 = $4.19

Excedrin Migraine: $7.89 − $3.16 = $4.73

Advil: $7.29 − $2.92 = $4.37

Last, calculate the amount the customer will pay for the entire purchase by adding the sale price of each item.

$4.19 + $4.73 + $4.37 = $13.29

Answer: The customer will pay $4.19 for Tylenol, $4.73 for Excedrin Migraine, and $4.37 for Advil. For the entire purchase, the customer will pay $13.29.

The previous example showed how a pharmacy may discount an OTC product for customers. However, a pharmacy can also receive discounts from wholesalers. The following example shows this situation.

Example 8.3.13

 A community pharmacy purchases five cases of hydrocortisone cream at $100 per case. If the account is paid in full within 30 days, the wholesaler will give a 15% discount on the purchase. How much money will the pharmacy save if it pays the account in full within 30 days? What will be the sale price for the five cases?

To begin, calculate the pharmacy's purchase price of five cases at the regular selling price. You can complete this calculation by using the ratio-proportion method or by using the dimensional analysis method.

Ratio-Proportion Method

$$\frac{\$ x}{5 \text{ cases}} = \frac{\$100}{1 \text{ case}}$$

$$\$ x \, (1 \text{ case}) = \$100 \, (5 \text{ cases})$$

$$x = \$500$$

Dimensional Analysis Method

$$\frac{5 \text{ cases}}{1} \times \frac{\$100}{1 \text{ case}} = \$500$$

Now determine the discount amount by using the following formula.

$$\text{discount amount} = \text{regular selling price} \times \text{discount rate}$$

$$\text{discount amount} = \$500 \times 0.15 = \$75$$

Last, calculate the discounted sale price.

$$\text{sale price} = \text{regular selling price} - \text{discount amount}$$

$$\$500 - \$75 = \$425$$

Answer: If the pharmacy pays the account in full within 30 days, it will save $75 off of the regular selling price. The sale price for the five cases is $425.

8.3 Problem Set

Birch Lake Pharmacy has the following overhead expenses. Use this information to answer questions 1–3.

salary of pharmacist	$135,000
salary of pharmacy technician	$52,000
rent	$23,000
utilities	$6,000
computer maintenance	$4,000
software subscriptions	$2,000
liability insurance	$4,000
business insurance	$4,000
pharmacy inventory	$750,000
total pharmacy overhead amount	$980,000

1. If an 18% profit is desirable, what must the pharmacy's income be to meet this goal?

2. If the pharmacy's income is $1,401,489, what is its percentage of profit?

3. If the pharmacy's income is $1,191,692, what is its percentage of profit?

Summit Avenue Pharmacy has the following overhead expenses. Use this information to answer questions 4–6.

salary of pharmacist	$72,000
salary of pharmacy technician	$52,000
rent	$13,000
utilities	$5,500
computer maintenance	$2,000
software subscriptions	$1,500
liability insurance	$4,000
business insurance	$3,500
pharmacy inventory	$50,000
total pharmacy overhead amount	$203,500

4. If a 20% profit is desirable, what must the pharmacy's income be to meet this goal?

5. If the pharmacy's income is $991,982, what is its percentage of profit?

6. If the pharmacy's income is $1,248,301, what is its percentage of profit?

7. A pharmacy determines that its income for the week was $54,617.53 and that the net profit was $3,700.83. What was the overhead for the week?

8. Martelli's Pharmacy has a weekly overhead of $13,033.06. If this pharmacy is to make a 22% profit, what must its sales of goods and services amount to each week?

For items 9–13, calculate the dollar amount of net profit for the following prescription drug items and round your answer to the nearest whole percent. Note that the pharmacy's dispensing cost is $4.25 for each prescription.

9. Medication: propranolol 10 mg
Pharmacy's purchase price: $3.96
Count: 100 tablets
Amount dispensed: 50 tablets
Pharmacy's selling price: $8.59

10. Medication: amoxicillin 250 mg
Pharmacy's purchase price: $8.50
Count: 500 capsules
Amount dispensed: 30 capsules
Pharmacy's selling price: $14.80

11. Medication: paroxetine 20 mg
Pharmacy's purchase price: $118.50
Count: 100 tablets
Amount dispensed: 30 tablets
Pharmacy's selling price: $45.50

12. Medication: furosemide 40 mg
Pharmacy's purchase price: $83.50
Count: 500 tablets
Amount dispensed: 100 tablets
Pharmacy's selling price: $23.16

13. Medication: levothyroxine 100 mcg
Pharmacy's purchase price: $41.20
Count: 100 tablets
Amount dispensed: 90 tablets
Pharmacy's selling price: $41.70

For items 14 and 15, calculate the markup amount and markup rate for each prescription. Round the markup amount to the nearest cent, and round the markup rate to the nearest tenth of a percent.

14. Medication: promethazine cough syrup
Pharmacy's purchase price: $17.50
Pharmacy's selling price: $25.34

15. Medication: Loestrin oral contraceptive 28-day pack
Pharmacy's purchase price: $12.30
Pharmacy's selling price: $17.90

A pharmacy is selling the products listed in items 16–23 at a discount this week. Calculate the sale price for each product. Round your answers to the nearest cent.

16. cough syrup: regular selling price, $5.89; discounted 20%

17. facial tissues: regular selling price, $1.19; discounted 15%

18. hair color kit: regular selling price, $7.29; discounted 30%

19. body lotion: regular selling price, $5.69; discounted 15%

20. baby shampoo: regular selling price, $3.89; discounted 25%

21. antacid liquid: regular selling price, $4.26; discounted 30%

22. acetaminophen tablets: regular selling price, $8.70; discounted 50%

23. toothpaste: regular selling price, $2.99; discounted 40%

For questions 24–29, perform the necessary calculations and state the answer in dollars (rounded to the nearest cent) or percentages (rounded to the nearest whole percent) as indicated.

24. Antiviral ointment costs a pharmacy $12.50 per tube. The standard markup is 30%. What is the total selling price of a box of 12 tubes?

25. Eyedrops with antihistamine are purchased from the manufacturer in cases of 36 drop-dispenser bottles. The pharmacy desires a markup of $1.75 per bottle. The pharmacy's purchase price is $111.60 per case. What is the selling price per bottle?

26. Identify the markup amount and the selling price of an oral antibiotic suspension that costs the pharmacy $15.60 per bottle if the markup rate is 25%.

27. Asthma tablets cost the pharmacy $24.80 for a month's supply, and the selling price is $30.75. Calculate the markup rate.

28. Calculate the gross profit from a medication that costs the pharmacy $520 for 1,000 tablets and sells for $650.

29. The cost of dispensing the medication in item 28 is $2.05 per 100 tablets. Calculate the net profit for selling one tablet.

The pharmacy where you work has received a shipment of medications and supplies from its wholesaler. Calculate the pharmacy's markup amount and selling price for each item listed in questions 30–36.

Drug	Count/ Quantity	Pharmacy's Purchase Price	Markup Rate	Markup Amount	Selling Price
30. Augmentin oral solution	1,200 mL	$120.50	25%		
31. triamcinolone foot powder	12 containers	$24.00	15%		
32. ibuprofen	2,000 tablets	$200.00	27%		
33. Band-Aids	10 boxes	$27.50	21%		
34. Neosporin antibiotic ointment	18 tubes	$67.50	18%		
35. birth control 28-day packs	24 packs	$840.00	32%		
36. DiaBeta	600 tablets	$550.00	30%		

37. Calculate the total amount that the pharmacy spent on the shipment above. Then determine the total amount the pharmacy made upon selling all of the items. Finally, calculate the overall markup rate for the entire shipment.

Self-check your work in Appendix A.

8.4 Insurance Reimbursements for Prescriptions

Put Down Roots

The term *reimbursement* has its roots in Latin. The root *re* means "back"; the root *imburse* means "put into a purse." Consequently, the word *reimbursement* literally means "to put back into a purse," or to receive a refund of personal monies from an individual or an institution.

Reimbursement for prescription and pharmacy services is largely controlled by contracts with insurance companies and is often brokered through a large prescription processing service called a **pharmacy benefits manager (PBM)**. PBMs use a pharmacy benefits management system that determines the amount of money that will be paid to pharmacies in insurance reimbursement for prescriptions.

Prescription reimbursement may be calculated based on a pharmacy's purchase price or the wholesale price of a medication. Prescription reimbursement may also be established by a set contract for an approved list of preferred drugs. The amount of money paid by a PBM for a particular prescription is calculated and approved by the PBM's computer system. This cost is not typically calculated by personnel in the pharmacy. Nevertheless, it is helpful to understand the reimbursement process and the methods used to calculate the reimbursement amount for medications. Patients are likely to ask questions about charges and reimbursements, so having a basic understanding of this process, which is sometimes called *reconciliation*, is essential.

Although some prescription claims will be reconciled by an individual pharmacy, most prescription claims will pass electronically through a PBM or similar type of clearinghouse that is responsible for processing and settling insurance claims. These businesses bill the insurance companies under contract and then reimburse the pharmacy periodically for a batch of prescriptions. Batch reimbursements may be made daily, weekly, or monthly. Some chain pharmacies may receive a single reimbursement payment that covers a large number of stores. In these instances, the individual store does not receive a check from the PBM, but rather an invoice or a memo indicating the amount of money that the company is being reimbursed.

One of the most challenging aspects of working in a community pharmacy is relaying the rejection or denial of prescription drug charges to patients and handling their subsequent reactions to this information. In such instances, the customers must pay out-of-pocket costs for the prescriptions. Because of the costs of the prescriptions, some customers may be unable to pay for the medications and, therefore, become upset with pharmacy personnel.

Using Average Wholesale Pricing

A pharmacy may potentially receive payment from several different sources. Historically, patients were responsible for paying for their own medications. However, beginning in the mid-1970s, health maintenance organizations (HMOs) and health insurers began to assume a portion of the responsibility for healthcare costs, including patient medications. More recently, HMOs and health insurers have become major players in determining the cost of health care, including the cost of prescriptions.

The **average wholesale price (AWP)** of a drug refers to an average price at which a drug is purchased at the wholesale level, or the average value at which wholesalers sell a particular drug to pharmacies.

Pharmacies often purchase medications from suppliers at a price based on AWP. For example, a pharmacy may purchase a medication as a percentage or at a markup rate (which may be positive or negative, depending on the agreement) of AWP. Wholesalers may sell drugs below AWP in some situations, such as when volume discounts, contract prices, or rebates from drug manufacturers are available.

medication purchase price based on AWP = AWP ± (AWP × markup rate)

The following example illustrates how to use this formula.

Example 8.4.1

The AWP for 90 g of tretinoin 0.1% cream is $100. A community pharmacy has an agreement with its wholesale supplier to purchase this medication at AWP minus 10%. How much will the pharmacy pay for 90 g of tretinoin 0.1% cream?

Use the following formula to calculate the pharmacy's purchase price. Because the pharmacy's agreement is AWP minus 10%, you *subtract* the product of AWP and the markup rate from the AWP.

medication purchase price based on AWP = AWP ± (AWP × markup rate)

medication purchase price based on AWP = $100 − ($100 × 0.10)

$$\$100 - \$10 = \$90$$

Answer: The pharmacy will pay $90 for 90 g of tretinoin 0.1% cream.

Third parties, such as PBMs, typically reimburse a pharmacy based on a percentage of the AWP. Therefore, the pharmacy has an incentive to purchase a drug below its AWP whenever possible.

Each third-party reimbursement system (insurance company or PBM) has a predetermined prescription reimbursement amount for each drug. The formula that determines the amount of prescription reimbursement varies depending on the current AWP for that drug, the percentage or markup rate (which may be either positive or negative depending on the agreement with the third party), and the individual pharmacy's dispensing fee. In practice, you will often hear phrases such as *AWP plus 10%* or *AWP less 15%.* Note that when the phrase *AWP less* is used, it has the same meaning as *AWP minus the given percent.* When the phrase *AWP plus* is used, it has the same meaning as *AWP plus the given percent.* The following formula calculates prescription reimbursement based on AWP.

$$\frac{\text{prescription}}{\text{reimbursement}} = \text{AWP} \pm \frac{(\text{AWP} \times \text{reimbursement}}{\text{percentage of AWP})} + \frac{\text{dispensing}}{\text{fee}}$$

The amount that an insurance company or patient is charged for a prescription is typically predetermined by PBMs and is calculated automatically through the pharmacy's computer system. Pricing information is preloaded into the PBM's computer system based on the insurance company contracts with the pharmacy. Pharmacy personnel can then access that pricing information online. The following examples illustrate one of the methods used to calculate the amount billed, which is similar to the calculation for prescription reimbursement shown above.

Example 8.4.2

A pharmacy has three drugs with the following AWPs:

> **Drug A, AWP $120.00**
>
> **Drug B, AWP $80.00**
>
> **Drug C, AWP $25.00**

The pharmacy has a markup rate of 5% and a dispensing fee of $4.00 for each of these drugs. If a patient presents a prescription for each of these drugs, what will be the total billed to the patient?

Step 1. Begin by calculating the amount billed to the patient for each of the individual drugs.

Drug A

$$\frac{\text{prescription}}{\text{reimbursement}} = \text{AWP} \pm \frac{(\text{AWP} \times \text{reimbursement}}{\text{percentage of AWP})} + \frac{\text{dispensing}}{\text{fee}}$$

prescription reimbursement = $120.00 + ($120.00 \times 0.05) + $4.00

$120.00 + $6.00 + $4.00 = $130.00

Drug B

$$\frac{\text{prescription}}{\text{reimbursement}} = \text{AWP} \pm \frac{(\text{AWP} \times \text{reimbursement}}{\text{percentage of AWP})} + \frac{\text{dispensing}}{\text{fee}}$$

prescription reimbursement = $80.00 + ($80.00 \times 0.05) + $4.00

$80.00 + $4.00 + $4.00 = $88.00

Drug C

$$\frac{\text{prescription}}{\text{reimbursement}} = \text{AWP} \pm \frac{(\text{AWP} \times \text{reimbursement}}{\text{percentage of AWP})} + \frac{\text{dispensing}}{\text{fee}}$$

prescription reimbursement = $25.00 + ($25.00 \times 0.05) + $4.00

$25.00 + $1.25 + $4.00 = $30.25

Step 2. Determine the total amount billed by adding the amounts billed for the three drugs.

$130.00 + $88.00 + $30.25 = $248.25

Answer: The total billed to the patient for prescription reimbursement is $248.25.

Pharmacy personnel may be required to calculate profit as applied to prescription reimbursement. In the following examples, gross profit will be determined. Recall that gross profit is the difference between revenue and the cost of goods sold. Gross profit can be positive or negative. Negative gross profit may be referred to as a *loss*. When applied to prescription reimbursement, gross profit is the difference between the pharmacy's reimbursement for a medication (revenue) and the cost of obtaining the medication (cost of goods sold).

Example 8.4.3

A medication is packaged in a quantity of 60 tablets and has an AWP of $100.00. A pharmacy has an agreement with its wholesale supplier to purchase the drug at AWP minus 15%. The insurer is willing to pay AWP plus 5% plus a $2.00 dispensing fee. What is the pharmacy's gross profit for this prescription?

To begin, calculate the amount the pharmacy will pay for the medication from its wholesale supplier. To do so, use the formula below.

medication purchase price based on AWP = AWP $\pm$ (AWP $\times$ markup rate)

medication purchase price based on AWP = $100.00 - ($100.00 \times 0.15)

$100.00 - $15.00 = $85.00

Therefore, the pharmacy can purchase this drug at $85.00 per 60 tablets.

Next, determine the amount the insurer is willing to pay for 60 tablets. You know the insurance company will pay the pharmacy AWP plus 5% plus a dispensing fee of $2.00. To calculate this reimbursement, use the following formula.

$$\text{prescription reimbursement} = \text{AWP} \pm \left(\text{AWP} \times \text{reimbursement percentage of AWP}\right) + \text{dispensing fee}$$

prescription reimbursement = $100.00 + ($100.00 × 0.05) + $2.00

$100.00 + $5.00 + $2.00 = $107.00

Finally, calculate the pharmacy's profit on 60 tablets. This amount is obtained by subtracting the pharmacy's purchase price from the insurer's reimbursement.

$107.00 − $85.00 = $22.00

Answer: The pharmacy's gross profit for this prescription is $22.00.

Example 8.4.4

The patient in Example 8.4.3 would prefer to receive 30 tablets of the medication instead of 60 tablets. What is the pharmacy's gross profit for this prescription?

You can solve this problem by using the ratio-proportion method or by using the dimensional analysis method. For this example, only the ratio-proportion method will be shown.

To begin, determine the pharmacy's cost for 30 tablets. You know the pharmacy paid $85.00 for 60 tablets. Set up a proportion by placing the unknown variable *x* dollars (cost of 30 tablets) over the number of patient-requested tablets on the left side of the equation and the pharmacy's cost for 60 tablets on the right side of the equation. Be sure that the units in the numerators and in the denominators match. Then cross multiply, cancel like units, and divide to solve for *x*.

$$\frac{x}{30\ \text{tablets}} = \frac{\$85.00}{60\ \text{tablets}}$$

$$x\ (60\ \text{tablets}) = \$85.00\ (30\ \text{tablets})$$

$$x = \$42.50$$

Next, determine the amount the insurer is willing to pay for 30 tablets. To do so, calculate the AWP for 30 tablets. Set up a proportion by placing the unknown variable *x* dollars (cost of 30 tablets) over the number of patient-requested tablets on the left side of the equation and the AWP for 60 tablets on the right side of the equation. Be sure that the units in the numerators and denominators match. Then cross multiply, cancel like units, and divide to solve for *x*.

$$\frac{x}{30\ \text{tablets}} = \frac{\$100.00}{60\ \text{tablets}}$$

$$x\ (60\ \text{tablets}) = \$100.00\ (30\ \text{tablets})$$

$$x = \$50.00$$

Now, use this information to determine the prescription reimbursement for 30 tablets. You know the insurer will pay the pharmacy AWP plus 5% plus a dispensing fee of $2.00. With that in mind, use the following formula.

$$\text{prescription reimbursement} = \text{AWP} \pm \left(\text{AWP} \times \text{reimbursement percentage of AWP}\right) + \text{dispensing fee}$$

prescription reimbursement = $50.00 + ($50.00 × 0.05) + $2.00

$$\$50.00 + \$2.50 + \$2.00 = \$54.50$$

Finally, find the pharmacy's gross profit on 30 tablets. This amount is obtained by subtracting the pharmacy's purchase price from the insurer's reimbursement.

$$\$54.50 - \$42.50 = \$12.00$$

Answer: The pharmacy's gross profit for 30 tablets of this medication is $12.00.

Example 8.4.5

A community pharmacy purchased a 250-count bottle of esomeprazole 40 mg capsules at AWP. The insurance plan reimburses at AWP plus 4% and allows a $5.00 dispensing fee on this prescription. If the AWP is $82.00 and the patient receives a prescription for 90 capsules, what is the amount that the pharmacy will submit for reimbursement? What is the pharmacy's gross profit on this prescription? Round your answer to the nearest cent.

You can solve this problem by using the ratio-proportion method or by using the dimensional analysis method. For this example, only the dimensional analysis method will be shown.

To begin, determine the pharmacy's purchase price for 90 capsules.

$$\frac{\$82.00}{250 \text{ capsules}} \times \frac{90 \text{ capsules}}{1} = \$29.52$$

Next, use this information to determine the prescription reimbursement for 90 capsules. You know the insurer will pay the pharmacy AWP plus 4% plus a dispensing fee of $5.00. Use the following formula to calculate this reimbursement.

$$\frac{\text{prescription}}{\text{reimbursement}} = \text{AWP} \pm \frac{(\text{AWP} \times \text{reimbursement}}{\text{percentage of AWP})} + \frac{\text{dispensing}}{\text{fee}}$$

$$\text{prescription reimbursement} = \$29.52 + (\$29.52 \times 0.04) + \$5.00$$

$$\$29.52 + \$1.18 + \$5.00 = \$35.70$$

Last, calculate the gross profit by finding the difference between the prescription reimbursement and the pharmacy's purchase price.

$$\$35.70 - \$29.52 = \$6.18$$

Answer: The pharmacy will submit $35.70 for reimbursement. The pharmacy's gross profit on this prescription is $6.18.

Some insurance plans do not allow pharmacies to charge a dispensing fee. In these cases, prescription reimbursement is calculated by adding AWP to the markup *without* adding a dispensing fee.

Example 8.4.6

A pharmacy purchased a 100-count bottle of amlodipine 10 mg tablets at the AWP of $118.00. A patient presents a prescription that requires you to dispense 30 tablets. The patient's insurance plan does not allow the pharmacy to charge a dispensing fee. If the plan calls for the pharmacy to be reimbursed at AWP less 10%, what is the pharmacy's reimbursement on this prescription? What is the pharmacy's gross profit on this prescription?

You can solve this problem by using the ratio-proportion method or by using the dimensional analysis method. For this example, only the dimensional analysis method will be shown.

To begin, you know the pharmacy's cost for 100 amlodipine tablets. Therefore, you can determine the cost for 30 tablets.

$$\frac{\$118.00}{100 \text{ tablets}} \times \frac{30 \text{ tablets}}{1} = \$35.40$$

Next, determine the prescription reimbursement, which is AWP less 10%. Remember that the insurance plan does not allow the pharmacy to charge a dispensing fee. Use the formula below to calculate this reimbursement.

$$\text{prescription reimbursement} = \text{AWP} \pm (\text{AWP} \times \text{reimbursement percentage of AWP}) + \text{dispensing fee}$$

$$\text{prescription reimbursement} = \$35.40 - (\$35.40 \times 0.10) + \$0.00$$

$$\$35.40 - \$3.54 + \$0.00 = \$31.86$$

Last, determine the gross profit. This amount is obtained by subtracting the pharmacy's purchase price from the insurer's reimbursement.

$$\$31.86 - \$35.40 = -\$3.54$$

Answer: The pharmacy's reimbursement on this prescription is $31.86. The pharmacy's gross profit is −$3.54 (otherwise known as a loss of $3.54).

The previous examples calculated pharmacy cost and gross profit per prescription. However, both pharmacy cost and gross profit can be calculated per medication unit (for example, per capsule or tablet for solid dosage forms or per milliliter or ounce for liquid dosage forms). The following example calculates pharmacy cost and gross profit per capsule.

Example 8.4.7

A community pharmacy purchased 200 capsules from its wholesale supplier at an AWP of $125.00 minus 20%. The insurer allows a charge of AWP plus 3% per 200 capsules. The insurer does not allow a dispensing fee. How much does one capsule cost the pharmacy to purchase? What is the reimbursement per capsule? What is the pharmacy's gross profit per capsule? Round your answer to the nearest cent.

To begin, determine the amount the pharmacy will pay for 200 capsules of medication from its wholesale supplier. Use the following formula to make this determination.

$$\text{medication purchase price based on AWP} = \text{AWP} \pm (\text{AWP} \times \text{markup rate})$$

$$\text{medication purchase price based on AWP} = \$125.00 - (\$125.00 \times 0.20)$$

$$\$125.00 - \$25.00 = \$100.00$$

Next, calculate the pharmacy's purchase price per capsule by dividing the medication purchase price by the number of capsules.

$$\frac{\$100.00}{200 \text{ capsules}} = \$0.50/\text{capsule}$$

Now, determine the prescription reimbursement, which is AWP plus 3%. Remember that the insurance plan does not allow the pharmacy to charge a dispensing fee. Use the formula below.

$$\frac{\text{prescription}}{\text{reimbursement}} = \text{AWP} \pm \frac{(\text{AWP} \times \text{reimbursement}}{\text{percentage of AWP})} + \frac{\text{dispensing}}{\text{fee}}$$

prescription reimbursement = $125.00 + ($125.00 × 0.03) + $0.00

$125.00 + $3.75 + $0.00 = $128.75

Then calculate the reimbursement per capsule by dividing the prescription reimbursement by the number of capsules.

$$\frac{\$128.75}{200 \text{ capsules}} = \$0.64375/\text{capsule, rounded to } \$0.64/\text{capsule}$$

Last, determine the pharmacy's gross profit per capsule by subtracting the pharmacy's cost per capsule from the reimbursement per capsule.

$0.64/capsule − $0.50/capsule = $0.14/capsule

Answer: The pharmacy's cost is $0.50/capsule, and the reimbursement is $0.64/capsule. The pharmacy's gross profit per capsule is $0.14.

Figuring Capitation Fees

Some insurers use a prescription reimbursement plan in which the pharmacy is paid a monthly fee, called a *capitation fee*, for some patients. The insurer pays the pharmacy the monthly fee whether or not the patients on the plan receive prescriptions during that month. Under this type of plan, the pharmacy must dispense the patients' prescriptions, even if the pharmacy's purchase price of the medications and the dispensing fees are more than the monthly reimbursement amount. Under plans that use capitation fees, pharmacies are not allowed to charge a dispensing fee unless the contract between the pharmacy and the third-party payer specifically states that a dispensing fee is allowed. To determine profit margin for a patient with prescription insurance that utilizes a capitation fee, you must subtract the cost of prescriptions filled from the agreed-upon capitation fee. The following examples highlight this process.

Example 8.4.8

O'Rourke's Drug Store receives a monthly capitation fee of $250.00 for Paul Arcand. During April, Paul fills three prescriptions totaling $198.75, which includes the dispensing fee. How much profit does the capitation fee provide?

In this case, the monthly fee exceeds the total of the pharmacy's purchase price, yielding a profit for the pharmacy.

$250.00 − $198.75 = $51.25

Answer: The capitation fee provides O'Rourke's Drug Store with a profit of $51.25.

Example 8.4.9

Cindy Carver has the same insurance plan as Paul Arcand, with the same capitation fee, $250.00 per month. During April, Cindy fills four prescriptions at the Willow Creek Pharmacy for a total of $301.25. What is the profit margin?

In this case, the pharmacy's purchase price of the prescriptions exceeds the monthly capitation fee. The pharmacy loses money, so the profit is expressed as a negative number.

$$\$250.00 - \$301.25 = -\$51.25$$

Answer: The Willow Creek Pharmacy has a negative profit (or loss) of $51.25.

8.4 Problem Set

For items 1–3, calculate the reimbursement for each prescription based on AWP less 13%. The pharmacy is not permitted to charge a dispensing fee on these prescriptions. Round your answers to the nearest hundredth.

1. AWP $48.90 per 60 tablets; dispense 20 tablets

2. AWP $84.07 per 100 tablets; dispense 30 tablets

3. AWP $30.25 per 1,000 tablets; dispense 100 tablets

For items 4–6, calculate the reimbursement for each prescription based on AWP plus 4%. The pharmacy charges a $6.25 dispensing fee for each prescription. Round your answers to the nearest hundredth.

4. AWP $120.68 per 500 tablets; dispense 30 tablets

5. AWP $39.78 per 100 capsules; dispense 60 capsules

6. AWP $317.50 per 30 tablets; dispense 20 tablets

For problems 7–10, round your answers to the nearest hundredth.

7. A pharmacy purchased 100 tablets at an AWP of $71.35. The insurer will pay AWP plus 3.5% and a $4.50 dispensing fee.

a. If the pharmacy dispenses a prescription of 50 tablets, what is the pharmacy's medication cost?

b. What is the reimbursement for this prescription?

c. What is the gross profit for this prescription?

8. A pharmacy purchased five albuterol metered-dose inhalers (MDIs) at a cost of AWP less 3%. The third-party payer will reimburse at AWP plus 5% and does not allow a dispensing fee. The AWP is $36.35 per inhaler.

a. If the pharmacy dispenses a single prescription of two MDIs, what is the pharmacy's cost of the prescription?

b. What is the reimbursement for this prescription?

c. What is the gross profit for this prescription?

9. A pharmacy purchased a 30-count bottle of tadalafil (Cialis) tablets at an AWP of $302.35. The PBM will pay AWP less 3% and allows a $7.00 dispensing fee per prescription.

a. If the pharmacy dispenses a prescription for 10 tablets, what is the pharmacy's cost of the prescription?

b. What is the reimbursement for this prescription?

c. What is the gross profit for this prescription?

10. A pharmacy purchased 50 tablets of atorvastatin (Lipitor) at an AWP of $117.35. The insurance company will reimburse at AWP plus 3% and a $4.00 dispensing fee.

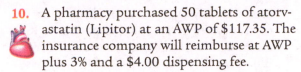

   a. If the pharmacy dispenses 30 tablets, what is the pharmacy's cost of the prescription?

   b. What is the reimbursement for this prescription?

   c. What is the gross profit for this prescription?

11. A pharmacy purchased an 80 g bulk jar of triamcinolone cream at an AWP of $85.35. The PBM will reimburse at AWP plus 4.5% but does not allow a dispensing fee.

   a. If the pharmacy dispenses a prescription for 15 g of the cream, what is the pharmacy's cost of the prescription?

   b. What is the reimbursement for this prescription?

   c. What is the gross profit for this prescription?

12. Mountain HMO pays a monthly patient capitation fee of $310.00 per patient. Six patients on this plan have prescriptions filled in July. The pharmacy's purchase price for the prescriptions are as follows:

   Patient A: $15.75, $106.50, $27.80
   Patient B: $210.00
   Patient C: $47.50, $105.25, $160.00, $52.00
   Patient D: $150.00, $210.00, $76.00
   Patient E: $10.50, $28.00, $62.50
   Patient F: $210.00, $210.00, $17.00

   a. What total amount of capitation fees was reimbursed from the HMO to the pharmacy?

   b. What is the pharmacy's purchase price for all of the prescriptions on this plan?

   c. Did the pharmacy make a profit or lose money?

   d. What is the gross profit for these prescriptions?

13. Valley HMO pays AWP plus 3% and a $2.00 dispensing fee for each prescription dispensed. Six patients on this plan have prescriptions filled in July. The pharmacy paid AWP purchase prices for the prescriptions as follows:

   Patient A: $15.75, $106.50, $27.80
   Patient B: $210.00
   Patient C: $47.50, $105.25, $160.00, $52.00
   Patient D: $150.00, $210.00, $76.00
   Patient E: $10.50, $28.00, $62.50
   Patient F: $210.00, $210.00, $17.00

   a. What is the pharmacy's purchase price for all of the prescriptions on this plan?

   b. What is the amount that the pharmacy will submit for insurance reimbursement on this plan?

   c. Did the pharmacy make a profit or lose money?

   d. What is the gross profit for these prescriptions?

   e. Compare your answers for question 13 with your answers for question 12. Did the pharmacy make more money under the Mountain HMO's capitation plan, or under the Valley HMO's plan? How much more?

14. Jackson HMO pays a monthly patient capitation fee of $275.00 per patient to Healthy Pharmacy. Healthy Pharmacy contracts with Jackson HMO to serve 10 of Jackson's clients. Five of the Jackson HMO clients have prescriptions filled during the month of June; the other five patients do not have any prescriptions filled in June. The pharmacy's purchase prices for these prescriptions are as follows:

   Patient A: $89.63
   Patient B: $126.54 (total cost for two prescriptions)
   Patient C: $420.45 (total cost for five prescriptions)
   Patient D: $117.50
   Patient E: $46.75

a. What total amount of capitation fees was reimbursed from the HMO to the pharmacy?

b. What is the pharmacy's medication cost for all of the prescriptions on this plan?

c. Did the pharmacy make a profit or lose money?

d. What is the amount of the pharmacy's profit or loss?

15. Baker HMO pays a monthly patient capitation fee of $275.00 per patient to Healthy Pharmacy. Healthy Pharmacy contracts with Baker HMO to serve 12 of Baker's clients. Five of the Baker HMO clients have prescriptions filled during the month of May; the other seven clients did not have any prescriptions filled in May. The pharmacy's purchase prices for these prescriptions are as follows:

Patient A: $78.26, $75.23, $25.48
Patient B: $128.46, $21.86
Patient C: $61.89, $41.20
Patient D: $16.59, $5.80, $3.87, $21.67
Patient E: $58.24

a. What total amount of capitation fees was reimbursed from the HMO to the pharmacy?

b. What is the pharmacy's medication cost for all of the prescriptions on this plan?

c. Did the pharmacy make a profit or lose money?

d. What is the amount of the pharmacy's gross profit or loss?

16. Blue Care HMO pays a monthly patient capitation fee of $225.00 per patient to Key Pharmacy. Key Pharmacy contracts with Blue Care HMO to serve 40 of Blue Care's clients. Twelve of the Blue Care HMO clients have prescriptions filled during the month of August; the other 28 clients did not have any prescriptions filled in August. The pharmacy's purchase price for all of the Blue Care prescriptions filled in August is $1,867.50. The contract with Blue Care HMO allows the pharmacy to bill for a single charge of $60.00 for dispensing fees for the month.

a. Taking into consideration the allowable dispensing fees, what total amount was reimbursed from the HMO to the pharmacy for the month of August?

b. Did the pharmacy make a profit or lose money?

c. What is the amount of the pharmacy's profit or loss?

17. Wellness Insurance Company pays a monthly patient capitation fee of $210.00 per patient to Apple Pharmacy. Apple Pharmacy contracts with Wellness to serve 42 of the Wellness Insurance Company's clients. During the month of September, 39 of the Wellness Insurance Company's clients had a total of 54 prescriptions filled. Apple Pharmacy's drug costs for all of the Wellness Insurance Company prescriptions filled in September are $9,634.73. The contract with Wellness Insurance Company allows the pharmacy to bill $4.25 in dispensing fees for each filled prescription.

a. Taking into consideration the allowable dispensing fees, what total amount was reimbursed from the insurance company to the pharmacy for the month of September?

b. Did the pharmacy make a profit or lose money?

c. What is the amount of the pharmacy's profit or loss?

Self-check your work in Appendix A.

Review and Assessment

CHAPTER SUMMARY

- As a pharmacy technician working in a community pharmacy, you are responsible for accepting payment for prescriptions and other pharmacy-related items.

- Counting change can be done by counting the amount displayed on the cash register's screen or by counting the amount from the purchase price.

- As a pharmacy technician, you are actively involved in managing pharmacy inventory, determining inventory days' supply, establishing the turnover rate, and replenishing stock to the desired par level.

- Schedule II controlled substances require a perpetual inventory record.

- Pharmacies must consider both income and overhead when calculating profit and when setting goals for desired percentage of profit.

- The net profit is the amount of income remaining after accounting for business expenses. In the pharmacy practice setting, net profit could be the difference between the sales of all medications and the cost of purchasing the medications, operating the pharmacy, and paying taxes.

- Pharmacies have contracts with wholesalers who provide drugs and supply items from the manufacturers to the pharmacies.

- Pharmacies have contracts with pharmacy benefits managers (PBMs) who broker insurance reimbursement claims.

- Pharmacy personnel must be familiar with the average wholesale price and capitation fees that affect the profitability of their facilities.

FORMULAS FOR SUCCESS

Inventory Formulas (Section 8.2)

amount needed to bring to maximum par level = maximum par level − current stock level

amount needed to bring to minimum par level = minimum par level − current stock level

$$\text{unit price} = \frac{\text{cost}}{\text{quantity}}$$

$$\text{average daily product cost} = \frac{\text{weekly product cost}}{7 \text{ days}}$$

$$\text{number of inventory days' supply} = \frac{\text{value of inventory}}{\text{average daily cost of products used}}$$

$$\text{average annual inventory value} = \frac{\text{value of initial inventory} + \text{value of current inventory}}{2}$$

$$\text{turnover rate} = \frac{\text{annual inventory purchases}}{\text{average inventory value}}$$

$$\text{annual depreciation} = \frac{\text{total cost} - \text{disposal value}}{\text{estimated life in years}}$$

Business-Related Formulas (Section 8.3)

$$\text{current percentage of profit} = \frac{\text{base profit}}{\text{annual income}} \times 100$$

desired amount of profit = overhead × desired percentage of profit

desired income goal = overhead + desired amount of profit

gross profit = revenue − cost of goods sold

net profit = revenue − expenses

net profit for a prescription = selling price of the prescription − overall cost

overall cost = pharmacy's purchase price + dispensing cost

selling price = (overall cost × desired percentage of profit) + overall cost

$$\text{gross profit margin (\%)} = \frac{\text{gross profit}}{\text{revenue}} \times 100$$

$$\text{net profit margin (\%)} = \frac{\text{net profit}}{\text{revenue}} \times 100$$

markup amount = selling price − obtaining cost

$$\text{markup percentage} = \frac{\text{markup amount}}{\text{obtaining cost}} \times 100 = \frac{\text{selling price} - \text{obtaining cost}}{\text{obtaining cost}} \times 100$$

discount amount = regular selling price × discount rate

sale price = regular selling price − discount amount

Prescription Insurance Reimbursement Formulas (Section 8.4)

medication purchase price based on AWP = AWP ± (AWP × markup rate)

prescription reimbursement = AWP ± (AWP × reimbursement percentage of AWP) + dispensing fee

CHECK YOUR UNDERSTANDING

Take a moment to review what you have learned in this chapter and answer the following questions.

1. Which term refers to the money or equivalent received from the sale of a medication, supply item, or equipment?
   a. overhead
   b. profit
   c. net profit
   d. income

2. Which term is used to describe the difference between the selling price and the overall cost?
   a. profit
   b. net profit
   c. gross profit
   d. percentage of profit

3. Which term describes all of the drugs, supply items, and merchandise on hand in a pharmacy?
   a. pharmacy stock
   b. pharmacy overhead
   c. pharmacy inventory
   d. pharmacy supply

4. Which term is used to describe the minimum and maximum inventory range for a pharmacy item?
   a. markup level
   b. PBM level
   c. AWP level
   d. par level

5. Which term is used to describe the number of times the amount of goods in inventory was sold during the year?
   a. flat rate
   b. discount rate
   c. turnover rate
   d. markup rate

6. What is the percentage of profit if a pharmacy has a base profit of $110,000 and an annual income of $500,000?
   a. 0.22%
   b. 2.2%
   c. 22%
   d. 220%

7. What should the selling price be for an item that a pharmacy purchased for $25 and that costs the pharmacy $5 to dispense if the pharmacy desires a 20% profit?
   a. $24
   b. $25
   c. $36
   d. $37

8. A pharmacy purchased a 100-count bottle of medication at a price of $7.50. You dispense a prescription for 30 tablets to a customer, who paid $12.53 for the prescription. The pharmacy's dispensing cost is $3.50. What is the net profit on this sale?
   a. $0.92
   b. $9.23
   c. $0.68
   d. $6.78

9. Calculate the markup amount and the markup rate using the following information. Round the markup rate to the nearest whole percent.

Propranolol 10 mg tablets
Pharmacy's purchase price: $3.96
Pharmacy's selling price: $8.59

a. $4.63; 117%
b. $4.63; 463%
c. $12.55; 396%
d. $12.55; 859%

10. Calculate the markup amount and the markup rate using the following information. Round the markup rate to the nearest whole percent.

Amoxicillin 250 mg
Pharmacy's purchase price: $8.50
Pharmacy's selling price: $14.80

a. $6.30; 63%
b. $6.30; 74%
c. $23.30; 27.4%
d. $23.40; 274%

FIND SOLUTIONS

Take a moment to consider what you have learned in this chapter and respond thoughtfully to the prompts.

Note: *To indicate your answers for Scenario A (questions 1–3) and Scenario B (questions 4–7), ask your instructor for the corresponding handouts.*

 Scenario A: In your pharmacy, the minimum par level for amoxicillin 250 mg capsules is 500; the maximum par level is 2,000. At the end of the day, the pharmacy computer provides a printed list of items that have fallen below the minimum par level and, therefore, need to be reordered. The printout indicates that there are currently 350 amoxicillin 250 mg capsules in the pharmacy stock. Given the information below, determine the most economical way to replenish the pharmacy's supply of amoxicillin 250 mg capsules to the minimum par level.

The wholesaler sells amoxicillin 250 mg capsules in the quantities and prices listed below.

Amoxicillin 250 mg capsules; 1,000-count bottle; $10.00 per bottle

Amoxicillin 250 mg capsules; 500-count bottle; $8.75 per bottle

Amoxicillin 250 mg capsules; 250-count bottle; $4.65 per bottle

Amoxicillin 250 mg capsules; 100-count bottle; $3.60 per bottle

Amoxicillin 250 mg capsules; 50-count bottle; $2.50 per bottle

Amoxicillin 250 mg capsules; 25-count bottle; $1.85 per bottle

For questions 1–3, record your answers on the handout that you obtained from your instructor.

1. What size/quantity bottle(s) will you order?

2. How many of each bottle will you order?

3. What will the final cost be for this order?

Scenario B: Beneficial HMO pays a per-client capitation fee of $149.00 per month to the Georgetown Pharmacy. The pharmacy is contracted to serve 127 of the HMO's clients and their families. During the month of December, 21 of these clients or their family members had a total of 52 prescriptions filled at the pharmacy. The pharmacy's total drug cost for these prescriptions was $6,283.24. The contract allows the pharmacy to bill a $3.50 dispensing fee for each filled prescription.

For questions 4–7, record your answers on the handout that you obtained from your instructor.

4. What is the total amount that the HMO reimbursed the pharmacy for capitation fees?

5. What is the pharmacy's drug cost for all of the prescriptions on this plan?

6. Did the pharmacy make a profit or lose money?

7. What is the amount of the pharmacy's profit or loss?

Sixth Avenue Pharmacy has the following overhead expenses. Use this information to answer questions 8–15.

pharmacist salary	$235,000
pharmacy technician salary	$152,000
rent	$23,000
utilities	$6,000
computer maintenance	$6,000
software subscriptions	$2,000
liability insurance	$12,000
business insurance	$4,000
drug purchases	$750,000

8. What is the pharmacy's total annual overhead expenses?

9. If an 18% profit is desirable, what must the pharmacy's income be to meet this goal?

10. If a 33% profit is desirable, what must the pharmacy's income be to meet this goal?

11. If the average inventory value is $238,000, what is the pharmacy's turnover rate?

12. If the pharmacy's annual income is $1,601,489, what is its percentage of profit? Round your answer to the nearest tenth of a percent.

13. If the pharmacy's income is $1,891,692, what is its percentage of profit?

14. Sixth Avenue Pharmacy purchases a new set of graduated cylinders for $200. The estimated life of the graduated cylinders is 10 years, at which time the disposal value is $12. What is the annual depreciation of the graduated cylinders?

15. Sixth Avenue Pharmacy purchases a new filing cabinet for $50. The estimated life of the cabinet is 7 years, at which time the disposal value is $15. What is the annual depreciation of the filing cabinet?

 The online course includes additional review and assessment resources.

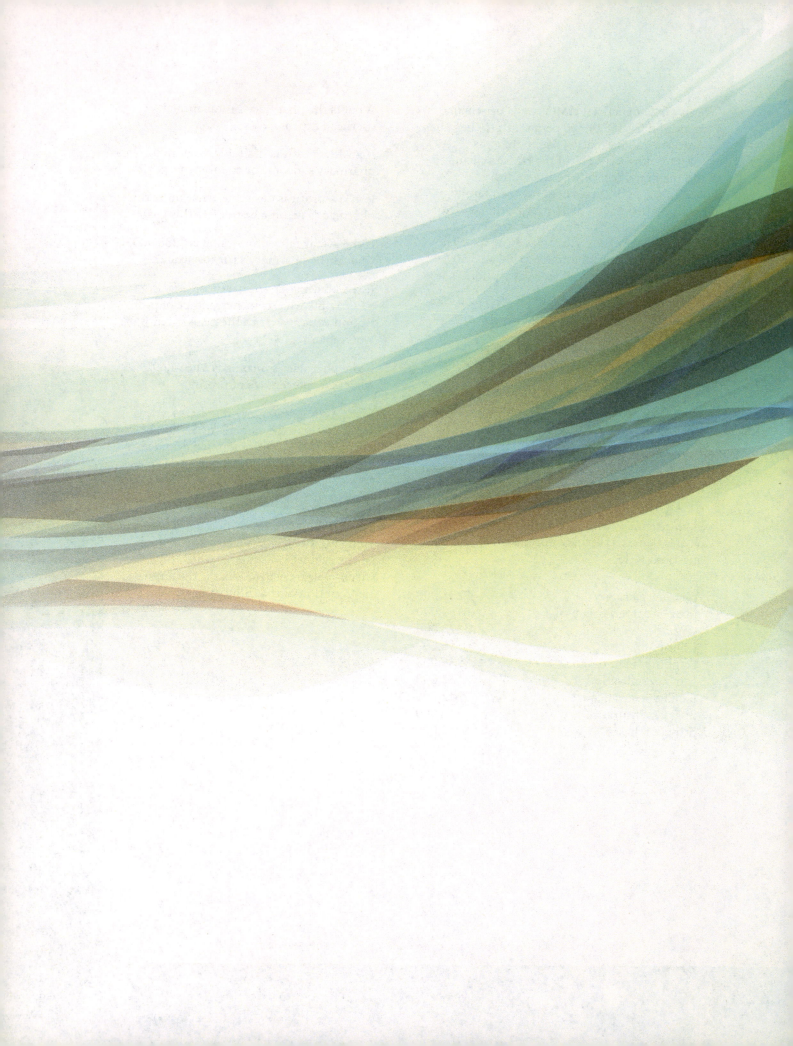

Performing Calculations for Sterile Parenteral Solutions

9

Learning Objectives

1 Express weight-in-volume and volume-in-volume solutions as ratio strengths. (Sections 9.1, 9.2)

2 Express weight-in-volume and volume-in-volume solutions as percentage strength. (Sections 9.1, 9.2)

3 Calculate weight and percentage strength for weight-in-volume and volume-in-volume solutions. (Sections 9.1, 9.2)

4 Compute flow rate, total volume, and infusion time. (Section 9.3)

5 Determine the number of intravenous bags needed for a 24-hour period. (Section 9.3)

For a key to the body system icons that appear in each chapter of this textbook, refer to the Preface.

6 Express flow rate in milliliters per hour, milligrams per hour, milliequivalents per hour, units per hour, drops per minute, and milligrams per drop. (Sections 9.3, 9.4)

7 Define the term *drop factor*. (Section 9.4)

8 Calculate the volume of concentrated solution and diluent needed to compound a special dilution. (Section 9.5)

9 Determine the volume of base solution and additives needed to compound parenteral nutrition. (Section 9.5)

ASHP/ACPE Accreditation Standards

To view the *ASHP/ACPE Accreditation Standards* addressed in this chapter, refer to Appendix D.

Chapter 6 introduced you to calculations related to sterile compounding. The concepts of measuring injections, calculating the volume needed of an injectable solution or the quantity contained in a given volume of an injectable solution, and determining ratio strength were discussed. This chapter will advance your learning in calculations for sterile compounding. Weight-in-volume and volume-in-volume calculations will be addressed. In addition, the concepts of intravenous (IV) flow rate and drop factor calculations will be introduced. Last, you will be exposed to special dilution calculations.

9.1 Weight-in-Volume Calculations

Sterile compounding typically involves the use of solutions. As you learned in Chapter 5, a solution is a mixture of one or more solutes dissolved in a solvent. A solvent is the substance in which a solute dissolves. A solute is the substance that dissolves in a solvent. Consider the solution created by combining table salt (NaCl) and a glass of hot water. In this example, the solvent is the hot water and the solutes are sodium and chloride.

In general, when comparing two solutions that contain the same components, the solution containing the smaller amount of solute is considered **dilute**. The solution containing the larger amount of solute is considered **concentrated**.

Solutions may contain any of the three states of matter: gas, liquid, or solid. However, in the preparation of sterile parenteral products, the most common solutions are comprised of a solid in a liquid (such as sugar or dextrose in water) or a liquid in a liquid (such as vinegar in water). This section will discuss calculations related to **solid-in-liquid solutions**, or solutions that are comprised of a solid solute and a liquid solvent. This type of solution is commonly known as a *weight-in-volume (w/v) solution*.

Expressing Weight-in-Volume Solutions

Quick Study

Pharmacy technicians should know that the term *percentage means* "per 100." Therefore, the term *percentage strength* means "parts per 100."

As discussed in Chapters 2 and 6, the concentration of one substance dissolved in another substance may be expressed as either a ratio strength (such as 25/100 or 1:4) or a percentage strength (such as 25%). The ratio strength of a w/v solution refers to the number of grams of solute per 100 milliliters (mL) of solution.

$$\text{ratio strength of a weight-in-volume (w/v) solution} = \frac{x \text{ g of solute}}{100 \text{ mL of solution}}$$

The percentage strength of a w/v solution is expressed as the grams (g) of solute per 100 mL of solution multiplied by 100.

$$\text{percentage strength of a weight-in-volume (w/v) solution} = \frac{x \text{ g of solute}}{100 \text{ mL of solution}} \times 100$$

The following examples demonstrate how to express components of w/v solutions.

Example 9.1.1

Your pharmacy stocks a 10% solution of dextrose in water. Express this percentage strength as a ratio strength of a w/v solution.

A w/v solution, by definition, is expressed as grams of solute per 100 mL of solution. Another way to express this same concept is to say that an IV solution with a concentration of 10% dextrose provides 10 g of dextrose for every 100 mL of fluid that is administered to the patient.

$$\frac{10 \text{ g of dextrose}}{100 \text{ mL of solution}} = \frac{10 \text{ g}}{100 \text{ mL}}$$

Answer: A 10% solution of dextrose in water is 10 g of dextrose per 100 mL of solution.

WORKPLACE WISDOM

Containers of commercially available IV solutions are labeled with the following volumes: 25 mL, 50 mL, 100 mL, 250 mL, 500 mL, or 1,000 mL. However, the actual volumes in these containers are greater than the labeled amounts. Manufacturers of IV solutions purposefully overfill IV solution containers to protect against potential volume loss due to product evaporation. As a result, variability in the actual volumes of IV solution containers occurs. For example, an IV solution of normal saline may be labeled as containing 100 mL. However, the actual volume in the container is likely greater than 100 mL. In clinical practice, there are many circumstances in which the additional volume is considered negligible. In these cases, the overfill volume is ignored. However, there are other instances in which overfill volume must be taken into account. When overfill volume must be accounted for, a specific volume will be removed from an overfilled container. For the purposes of calculations in this chapter, assume that volumes of IV solutions are accurate and that any overfill is negligible.

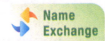

Name Exchange

A 0.9% sodium chloride (NaCl) solution may be referred to as *normal saline* or *NS* by healthcare personnel.

Example 9.1.2

Express the components of a 0.9% solution of sodium chloride (NaCl) in the form of a w/v solution.

A 0.9% NaCl solution contains 0.9 g of NaCl in each 100 mL of fluid. Another way to express this same concept is to say that an IV solution with a concentration of 0.9% NaCl provides 0.9 g of NaCl for every 100 mL of fluid that is administered to the patient.

$$\frac{0.9 \text{ g of NaCl}}{100 \text{ mL of solution}} \quad \text{or} \quad \frac{0.9 \text{ g}}{100 \text{ mL}}$$

Answer: A 0.9% solution of NaCl is 0.9 g of NaCl per 100 mL of solution.

Calculating Weights Based on Percentage Strength

The amount of medication in a w/v solution is not always explicitly given. For instance, IV solutions that are administered in large volumes are labeled as a percentage strength, such as dextrose 5% in water (D_5W). Normal saline (NS) is a solution of water and sodium chloride at 0.9% concentration. Both examples list percentage strength instead of weight of solute per volume of solution. However, the weight of solute can be calculated from percentage strength, as shown in the following example.

Example 9.1.3

How many grams of dextrose are in 1 liter (L) of D$_s$W?

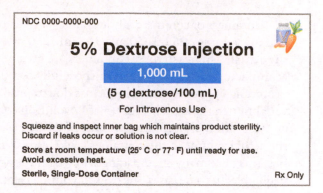

NDC 0000-0000-000

5% Dextrose Injection

1,000 mL

(5 g dextrose/100 mL)

For Intravenous Use

Squeeze and inspect inner bag which maintains product sterility.
Discard if leaks occur or solution is not clear.

Store at room temperature (25° C or 77° F) until ready for use.
Avoid excessive heat.

Sterile, Single-Dose Container   Rx Only

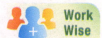

Remember that D$_s$W means dextrose 5% in water, or a concentration of 5 g/100 mL.

You can solve this problem by using the ratio-proportion method or by using the dimensional analysis method.

Ratio-Proportion Method

To begin, convert 1 L to 1,000 mL.

Then set up a proportion by placing the unknown amount (*x* g) over the conversion on the left side and the known amount (5 g/100 mL) on the right side of the proportion. Be sure that the units in the numerators and in the denominators match. Then cross multiply, cancel similar units (like terms), and divide to solve for *x*.

$$\frac{x \text{ g}}{1,000 \text{ mL}} = \frac{5 \text{ g}}{100 \text{ mL}}$$

$$x \text{ g} (100 \text{ mL}) = 5 \text{ g} (1,000 \text{ mL})$$

$$x = 50 \text{ g}$$

Dimensional Analysis Method

$$\frac{1 \text{ L}}{1} \times \frac{1,000 \text{ mL}}{1 \text{ L}} \times \frac{5 \text{ g}}{100 \text{ mL}} = 50 \text{ g}$$

Answer: There are 50 g of dextrose in 1 L of D$_s$W.

Example 9.1.4

How many grams of sodium chloride (NaCl) are in 1 L of 0.9% sodium chloride solution, also known as *normal saline (NS) solution*?

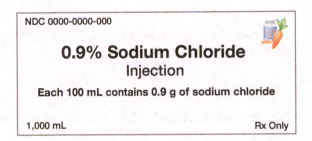

NDC 0000-0000-000

0.9% Sodium Chloride
Injection

Each 100 mL contains 0.9 g of sodium chloride

1,000 mL   Rx Only

You can solve this problem by using the ratio-proportion method or by using the dimensional analysis method.

Ratio-Proportion Method

To begin, convert 1 L to 1,000 mL.

Then set up a proportion by placing the unknown amount (x g) over the conversion on the left side and the known amount (0.9 g/100 mL) on the right side of the proportion. Be sure that the units in the numerators and in the denominators match. Then cross multiply, cancel similar units (like terms), and divide to solve for x.

$$\frac{x \text{ g}}{1,000 \text{ mL}} = \frac{0.9 \text{ g}}{100 \text{ mL}}$$

$$x \text{ g} (100 \text{ mL}) = 0.9 \text{ g} (1,000 \text{ mL})$$

$$x = 9 \text{ g}$$

Dimensional Analysis Method

$$\frac{1 \text{ L}}{1} \times \frac{1,000 \text{ mL}}{1 \text{ L}} \times \frac{0.9 \text{ g}}{100 \text{ mL}} = 9 \text{ g}$$

Answer: There are 9 g of NaCl in 1 L of NS.

Calculating Percentage Strength

When the amount of solute and the total volume of the final solution are known, you can calculate the percentage strength. This can be calculated several ways. One way is to express the strength as grams of solute per 100 mL of solution. For example, consider a 4 mL solution that contains 2 g of solute. To determine the percentage strength, you would set up a proportion by placing the unknown amount (x g) over 100 mL on the left side and the known amount (2 g/4 mL) on the right side of the equation.

$$\frac{x \text{ g}}{100 \text{ mL}} = \frac{2 \text{ g}}{4 \text{ mL}}$$

You would then cross multiply, cancel similar units (like terms), and divide to solve for x.

$$x \text{ g (4 mL)} = 2 \text{ g (100mL)}$$

$$x = 50 \text{ g}$$

Then you would rewrite the fraction that contained the unknown amount and multiply by 100 to find the percentage strength.

$$\frac{50 \text{ g}}{100 \text{ mL}} \times 100 = 50\%$$

The percentage strength of the solution containing 2 g of solute and 4 mL of solution is 50%.

Another way to determine percentage strength of a w/v solution is to use the percentage strength of a w/v solution formula: dividing the known grams of solute by the known milliliters of solution and multiplying the resulting quotient by 100.

$$\text{Percentage strength of a weight-in-volume (w/v) solution} = \frac{x \text{ g of solute}}{y \text{ mL of solution}} \times 100$$

Consider the same w/v solution containing 2 g of solute and 4 mL of solution. To determine the percentage strength, you would divide the known grams of solute (2 g) by the known amount of milliliters of solution (4 mL) and multiply by 100.

$$\frac{2 \text{ g}}{4 \text{ mL}} \times 100 = 50\%$$

The strength of the solution is 50%. While the method to calculate percentage strength was different, both methods resulted in the same answer.

The following examples calculate the percentage strength of w/v solutions.

Example 9.1.5

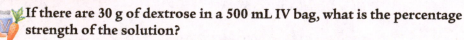 **If there are 30 g of dextrose in a 500 mL IV bag, what is the percentage strength of the solution?**

This problem can be solved by using the formula for percentage strength of a w/v solution or by using the ratio-proportion method.

Percentage Strength of a w/v Solution Formula

To begin, recall the formula for percentage strength of a w/v solution.

$$\text{percentage strength of a w/v solution} = \frac{x \text{ g of solute}}{y \text{ mL of solution}} \times 100$$

Then insert the known values into this equation.

$$\text{percentage strength of a w/v solution} = \frac{30 \text{ g}}{500 \text{ mL}} \times 100 = 6\%$$

Ratio-Proportion Method

To begin, set up a proportion by placing the unknown amount (x g) over 100 mL on the left side and the known amount (30 g/500 mL) on the right side of the proportion. Be sure that the units in the numerators and in the denominators match. Then cross multiply, cancel similar units (like terms), and divide to solve for x.

$$\frac{x\text{ g}}{100\text{ mL}} = \frac{30\text{ g}}{500\text{ mL}}$$

$$x\text{ g (500 mL)} = 30\text{ g (100 mL)}$$

$$x = 6\text{ g}$$

$$\frac{6\text{ g}}{100\text{ mL}} = 6\%$$

Answer: The percentage strength of the solution is 6%.

Example 9.1.6

 If there are 5 g of fat in a 250 mL IV fat emulsion, what is the percentage strength of the solution?

This problem can be solved by using either the formula for percentage strength of a w/v solution or by using the ratio-proportion method.

Percentage Strength of a w/v Solution Formula

To begin, recall the formula for percentage strength of a w/v solution.

$$\text{percentage strength of a w/v solution} = \frac{x\text{ g of solute}}{y\text{ mL of solution}} \times 100$$

Then insert the known values into this equation.

$$\text{percentage strength of a w/v solution} = \frac{5\text{ g}}{250\text{ mL}} \times 100 = 2\%$$

Ratio-Proportion Method

To begin, set up a proportion by placing the unknown amount (x g) over 100 mL on the left side and the known amount (5 g/250 mL) on the right side of the proportion. Be sure that the units in the numerators and in the denominators match. Then cross multiply, cancel similar units (like terms), and divide to solve for x.

$$\frac{x\text{ g}}{100\text{ mL}} = \frac{5\text{ g}}{250\text{ mL}}$$

$$x\text{ g (250 mL)} = 5\text{ g (100 mL)}$$

$$x = 2\text{ g}$$

$$\frac{2\text{ g}}{100\text{ mL}} = 2\%$$

Answer: The percentage strength of the solution is 2%.

WORKPLACE WISDOM

There are several concentrations of sodium chloride available for IV use, including 0.45%, 0.9%, 3%, 14.6%, and 23.4%. It is also common for IV solutions to contain dextrose (a sugar) in addition to sodium chloride. Lactated Ringer's (LR) is another commonly used IV fluid that contains several electrolytes. Unlike sodium chloride, the label for LR is not written using a percentage strength. When preparing a solution, you must read labels carefully to ensure that the correct product and concentration are used. Patients can be harmed if their IV fluids are prepared incorrectly.

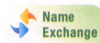
Name Exchange

The generic medication furosemide is commonly known among pharmacy personnel by the brand name Lasix.

Example 9.1.7

Use the label provided to determine the percentage strength of the solution.

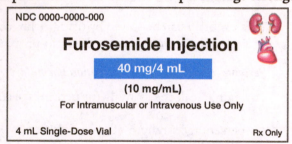

NDC 0000-0000-000

Furosemide Injection

40 mg/4 mL

(10 mg/mL)

For Intramuscular or Intravenous Use Only

4 mL Single-Dose Vial   Rx Only

This problem can be solved by using the formula for percentage strength of a w/v solution or by using the ratio-proportion method.

Percentage Strength of a w/v Solution Formula

To begin, convert 40 mg to grams: 40 mg equals 0.04 g. Then recall the formula for percentage strength of a w/v solution.

$$\text{percentage strength of a w/v solution} = \frac{x \text{ g of solute}}{y \text{ mL of solution}} \times 100$$

Then insert the known values into this equation.

$$\text{percentage strength of a w/v solution} = \frac{0.04 \text{ g}}{4 \text{ mL}} \times 100 = 1\%$$

Ratio-Proportion Method

To begin, convert 40 mg to grams. Set up a proportion by placing the unknown amount (x g) over 40 mg on the left side and the known conversion (1 g/1,000 mg) on the right side of the proportion. Be sure that the units in the numerators and in the denominators match. Then cross multiply, cancel similar units (like terms), and divide to solve for x.

$$\frac{x \text{ g}}{40 \text{ mg}} = \frac{1 \text{ g}}{1,000 \text{ mg}}$$

$$x \text{ g } (1,000 \text{ mg}) = 1 \text{ g } (40 \text{ mg})$$

$$x = 0.04 \text{ g}$$

Now, set up a proportion by placing the unknown amount (x g) over 100 mL on the left side and the known amount (0.04 g/4 mL) on the right side of the proportion. Be sure that the units in the numerators and in the denominators match. Then cross multiply, cancel similar units (like terms), and divide to solve for x.

$$\frac{x \text{ g}}{100 \text{ mL}} = \frac{0.04 \text{ g}}{4 \text{ mL}}$$

$$x \text{ g (4 mL)} = 0.04 \text{ g (100 mL)}$$

$$x = 1 \text{ g}$$

$$\frac{1 \text{ g}}{100 \text{ mL}} = 1\%$$

Answer: The percentage strength of the solution is 1%.

9.1 Problem Set

Express the following items as weight-in-volume (w/v) solutions.

1. the components of dextrose 10% as a w/v solution

2. the components of NaCl 0.45% as a w/v solution

Perform calculations to answer questions 3–5.

3. A patient receives an IV solution containing 500 mL of a 10% IV fat emulsion. How many grams of fat did the patient receive?

4. A patient receives an injection of 1.3 mL of lidocaine 2%. Use the medication label below to determine how many milligrams of lidocaine are in this injection.

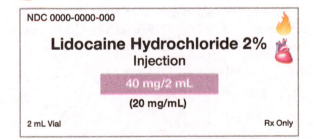

NDC 0000-0000-000

Lidocaine Hydrochloride 2%
Injection

40 mg/2 mL

(20 mg/mL)

2 mL Vial   Rx Only

5. A patient receives NaCl 20 g in a 500 mL solution. What is the percentage strength of the solution?

Based on the labels provided, determine the percentage strength of each medication.

6.

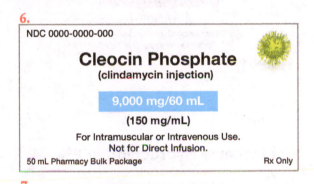

NDC 0000-0000-000

Cleocin Phosphate
(clindamycin injection)

9,000 mg/60 mL

(150 mg/mL)

For Intramuscular or Intravenous Use.
Not for Direct Infusion.

50 mL Pharmacy Bulk Package   Rx Only

7.

NDC 0000-0000-000

Ketorolac Tromethamine
Injection

60 mg/2 mL

(30 mg/mL)

For Intramuscular Use Only

2 mL Single-Dose Vial   Rx Only

8.

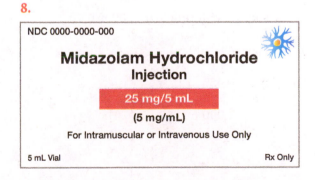

NDC 0000-0000-000

Midazolam Hydrochloride
Injection

25 mg/5 mL

(5 mg/mL)

For Intramuscular or Intravenous Use Only

5 mL Vial   Rx Only

9.

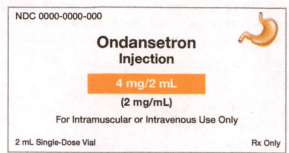

NDC 0000-0000-000

Ondansetron
Injection

4 mg/2 mL

(2 mg/mL)

For Intramuscular or Intravenous Use Only

2 mL Single-Dose Vial   Rx Only

10.

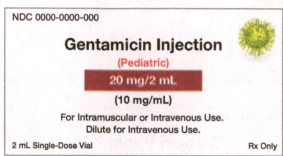

NDC 0000-0000-000

Gentamicin Injection
(Pediatric)

20 mg/2 mL

(10 mg/mL)

For Intramuscular or Intravenous Use.
Dilute for Intravenous Use.

2 mL Single-Dose Vial   Rx Only

11.

NDC 0000-0000-000

Lidocaine Hydrochloride 2%
Injection

40 mg/2 mL

(20 mg/mL)

2 mL Vial   Rx Only

Calculate the amount of solute (in grams) for each of the following solutions.

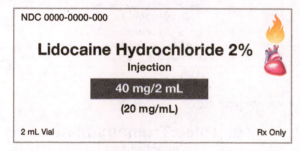

12.   amino acid 3.5%, 2.5 L

13.   dextrose 10%, 1,000 mL

14.   sodium chloride 0.9%, 100 mL

15.   NaCl 4%, 500 mL

16.   NaCl 0.45%, 1 L

17. D_5W, 1,000 mL

18.   aminophylline 0.4%, 500 mL

19.   lidocaine 4%, 0.5 L

20.   dopamine 2%, 250 mL

Calculate the amount of solute (in milligrams) in the following solutions.

21.   5 mL of a dextrose 7.5% solution

22.   50 mL of a 0.5% solution

23.   0.5 mL of a 1% solution

24.   1 mL of a 0.1% solution

25.   5 mL of a 0.2% solution

Use the label provided below to determine how many grams of NaCl are in the following volumes of NS (0.9% NaCl). Round your answer to the nearest hundredth.

NDC 0000-0000-000

0.9% Sodium Chloride
Injection

Each 100 mL contains 0.9 g of sodium chloride

1,000 mL   Rx Only

26.   250 mL

27.   500 mL

28.   1,000 mL

29.   2,225 mL

Determine how many grams of NaCl are in the following volumes of ½ NS (0.45% NaCl). Round your answer to the nearest hundredth.

30.   125 mL

31.   250 mL

32.   750 mL

33.   1,800 mL

34.   2,600 mL

Use the label provided below to determine how many grams of dextrose are in the following volumes of D_5W.

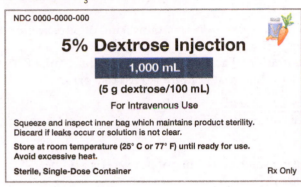

NDC 0000-0000-000

5% Dextrose Injection

1,000 mL

(5 g dextrose/100 mL)

For Intravenous Use

Squeeze and inspect inner bag which maintains product sterility.
Discard if leaks occur or solution is not clear.

Store at room temperature (25° C or 77° F) until ready for use.
Avoid excessive heat.

Sterile, Single-Dose Container   Rx Only

35.   75 mL

36.   385 mL

37.   525 mL

38.   1,350 mL

Determine how many grams of dextrose are in the following volumes of dextrose 10% in water ($D_{10}W$).

39.   100 mL

40.   325 mL

41.   450 mL

42.   875 mL

Self-check your work in Appendix A.

9.2 Volume-in-Volume Calculations

For a **liquid-in-liquid solution**, both the solute and solvent are liquid. Because both the solute and solvent are measured as volumes, a liquid-in-liquid solution is also referred to as a ***volume-in-volume (v/v) solution***. When both solute and solvent are liquid, usually the component representing the greater volume is the solvent. Likewise, the component representing the smaller volume is the solute.

Expressing Volume-in-Volume Solutions

Recall that the concentration of one substance dissolved in another substance may be expressed as a percentage strength or as a ratio strength. The ratio strength of a v/v solution refers to the number of milliliters of solute per 100 mL of solution.

$$\text{ratio strength of a volume-in-volume (v/v) solution} = \frac{x \text{ g of solute}}{100 \text{ mL of solution}}$$

The percentage strength of a v/v solution is expressed as the number of milliliters of solute per 100 mL of solution multiplied by 100.

$$\text{percentage strength of a volume-in-volume (v/v) solution} = \frac{x \text{ g of solute}}{100 \text{ mL of solution}} \times 100$$

Example 9.2.1

Your pharmacy stocks a 12% liquid in a liquid solution. Express this percentage strength as a ratio strength.

A volume-in-volume solution, by definition, is expressed in milliliters of solute per 100 mL of solution.

Answer: A 12% liquid in a liquid solution is 12 mL of solute per 100 mL of solution.

Example 9.2.2

Express the components of an acetic acid 3% irrigation solution in the form of a v/v solution.

By definition, an acetic acid 3% irrigation solution contains 3 mL of pure acetic acid in each 100 mL of fluid. Another way to express this strength is that an irrigation solution with a concentration of acetic acid 3% will provide 3 mL of pure acetic acid for every 100 mL of fluid that is administered to a patient.

$$\frac{3 \text{ mL of pure acetic acid}}{100 \text{ mL of solution}} \text{ or } \frac{3 \text{ mL}}{100 \text{ mL}}$$

Answer: An acetic acid 3% irrigation solution is 3 mL of pure acetic acid per 100 mL of solution, or 3 mL/100 mL.

Calculating Volumes Based on Percentage Strength

The volume of medication in a v/v solution is not always explicitly given. For instance, topical alcohol solutions are labeled as a percentage strength, such as isopropyl alcohol 70%, isopropyl alcohol 91%, or isopropyl alcohol 99%. These examples list percentage strength instead of volume of solute per volume of solution. However, the volume of solute can be calculated from percentage strength, as shown in the following example.

Example 9.2.3

The label from a container of stock isopropyl alcohol 70% is shown below. How many milliliters of pure isopropyl alcohol are contained in 1 qt (946 mL) of isopropyl alcohol 70% solution?

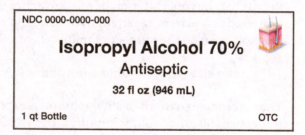

NDC 0000-0000-000

Isopropyl Alcohol 70%
Antiseptic
32 fl oz (946 mL)

1 qt Bottle   OTC

You can solve this problem by using the ratio-proportion method or by using the dimensional analysis method.

Ratio-Proportion Method

To begin, set up a proportion by placing the unknown amount (*x* mL) over 946 mL on the left side of the equation and the strength (70 mL/100 mL) on the right side of the equation. Be sure that the units in the numerators and in the denominators match. Then cross multiply, cancel similar units (like terms), and divide to solve for *x*.

$$\frac{x \text{ mL pure isopropyl alcohol}}{946 \text{ mL of solution}} = \frac{70 \text{ mL pure isopropyl alcohol}}{100 \text{ mL of solution}}$$

x mL pure isopropyl alcohol (100 mL solution) = 70 mL pure isopropyl alcohol
(946 mL solution)

$$x = 662.2 \text{ mL pure isopropyl alcohol}$$

Dimensional Analysis Method

$$\frac{946 \text{ mL solution}}{1} \times \frac{70 \text{ mL pure isopropyl alcohol}}{100 \text{ mL of solution}} = 662.2 \text{ mL pure isopropyl alcohol}$$

Answer: There are 662.2 mL of pure isopropyl alcohol in 1 qt (946 mL) of isopropyl alcohol 70% solution.

Calculating Percentage Strength

When the amount of solute and the total volume of the final solution are known for a v/v solution, you can calculate the percentage strength in several different ways. As previously discussed, percentage strength of a v/v solution is milliliters of solute per 100 mL of solution multiplied by 100. As we saw in the discussion of w/v solutions, you can also determine percentage strength of a v/v solution by dividing the milliliters of solute by the milliliters of solution and multiplying the resulting quotient by 100.

$$\text{percentage strength of a volume-in-volume (v/v) solution} = \frac{x \text{ mL of solute}}{y \text{ mL of solution}} \times 100$$

The following example calculates percentage strength of a v/v solution.

Example 9.2.4

If there are 25 mL of medication in a 1,000 mL IV bag, what is the percentage strength of the solution?

This problem can be solved by using the formula for percentage strength of a v/v solution or by using the ratio-proportion method.

Percentage Strength of a v/v Solution Formula

To begin, recall the formula for percentage strength of a v/v solution.

$$\text{percentage strength of a v/v solution} = \frac{x \text{ mL of solute}}{y \text{ mL of solution}} \times 100$$

Then insert the known values into this equation.

$$\text{percentage strength of v/v solution} = \frac{25 \text{ mL}}{1,000 \text{ mL}} \times 100 = 2.5\%$$

Ratio-Proportion Method

To begin, set up a proportion by placing the unknown amount (x mL) over 100 mL on the left side of the equation and the known amount (25 mL/1,000 mL) on the right side of the equation. Be sure that the units in the numerators and in the denominators match. Then cross multiply, cancel similar units (like terms), and divide to solve for x.

$$\frac{x \text{ mL solute}}{100 \text{ mL of solution}} = \frac{25 \text{ mL solvent}}{1,000 \text{ mL of solution}}$$

$$x \text{ mL solute} (1,000 \text{ mL solution}) = 25 \text{ mL solute} (100 \text{ mL solution})$$

$$x = 2.5 \text{ mL solute}$$

$$\frac{2.5 \text{ mL solute}}{100 \text{ mL of solution}} = 2.5\%$$

Answer: The percentage strength of the solution is 2.5%.

9.2 Problem Set

For items 1–4, express the ratio strength of the following components as a v/v solution.

1. acetic acid 0.25%

2. acetic acid 2%

3. isopropyl alcohol 70%

4. isopropyl alcohol 99%

For items 5–8, calculate the volume based on percentage strength.

5. If a patient receives 2 L of an IV solution containing 10% of a liquid solute, how many milliliters of solute did the patient receive?

6. If a patient receives 500 mL of an IV solution containing 2% of a liquid solute, how many milliliters of solute did the patient receive?

7. If a patient receives 50 mL of an IV solution containing 7.5% of a liquid solute, how many milliliters of solute did the patient receive?

8. If a patient receives 1.5 L of an IV solution containing 0.25% of a liquid solute, how many milliliters of solute did the patient receive?

Use the following label to answer questions 9–12.

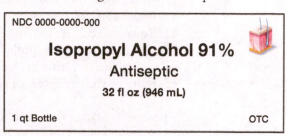

NDC 0000-0000-000

Isopropyl Alcohol 91%
Antiseptic
32 fl oz (946 mL)

1 qt Bottle   OTC

9. How many milliliters of pure isopropyl alcohol are contained in 1 qt (946 mL) of isopropyl alcohol 91% solution?

10. How many milliliters of pure isopropyl alcohol are contained in 750 mL of isopropyl alcohol 91% solution?

11. How many milliliters of pure isopropyl alcohol are contained in 100 mL of isopropyl alcohol 91% solution?

12. How many milliliters of pure isopropyl alcohol are contained in 75 mL of isopropyl alcohol 91% solution?

Calculate the amount of solute (in milliliters) for each of the following solutions. Round your answer to the nearest hundredth of a milliliter.

13. acetic acid 0.25%, 1,000 mL

14. acetic acid 0.25%, 375 mL

15. acetic acid 0.5%, 500 mL

16. acetic acid 0.5%, 750 mL

Calculate the percentage strength for each of the following solutions. Round your answer to the nearest hundredth of a percent.

17. If there are 75 mL of medication in a 1,000 mL IV bag, what is the percentage strength of the solution?

18. If there are 75 mL of medication in a 500 mL IV bag, what is the percentage strength of the solution?

19. If there are 90 mL of medication in a 500 mL IV bag, what is the percentage strength of the solution?

20. If there are 90 mL of medication in a 1,500 mL IV bag, what is the percentage strength of the solution?

Self-check your work in Appendix A.

9.3 Intravenous Flow Rate Calculations

When a prescriber orders an IV infusion for a patient, the medication order typically includes the type of IV fluid to be administered (called the *base solution*) and any additives (such as medications or electrolytes) that are required. The prescriber also indicates the rate of infusion of the solution. This ordered rate, known as a *flow rate*, refers to the volume of fluid a patient should receive per unit of time. This flow rate is often expressed in milliliters per hour. The nursing staff closely monitors IV fluid administration to ensure that an appropriate volume of fluid—and the corresponding amount or dosage of any additive—is given over the specified period to achieve the intended therapeutic response.

Calculating Flow Rate

Flow rate can be calculated by dividing the volume of fluid a patient should receive by the length of time over which the volume is infused (or infusion time).

$$\text{flow rate (mL/hr)} = \frac{\text{total volume infused (mL)}}{\text{infusion time (hr)}}$$

When using the flow rate formula, be sure that the units used are the same throughout the equation (*milliliters* for volume and *hours* for time). Flow rate can also be calculated by using the ratio-proportion method or by using the dimensional analysis method. When calculating the duration of therapy, always round your answer down to the nearest whole hour.

The following example calculates flow rate utilizing the flow rate equation, the ratio-proportion method, and the dimensional analysis method.

Example 9.3.1

A physician has ordered a 1 liter (L) bag of IV fluid to be infused over 10 hours. What is the IV flow rate in milliliters per hour?

This problem can be solved by using one of three approaches: by using the flow rate formula, the ratio-proportion method, or the dimensional analysis method.

Flow Rate Formula
To begin, recall the flow rate formula.

$$\text{flow rate (mL/hr)} = \frac{\text{total volume infused (mL)}}{\text{infusion time (hr)}}$$

Next, convert 1 L to 1,000 mL.

Then insert the known values into the formula.

$$\text{flow rate (mL/hr)} = \frac{1,000 \text{ mL}}{10 \text{ hr}}$$

$$\frac{1,000 \text{ mL}}{10 \text{ hr}} = \frac{100 \text{ mL}}{\text{hr}}$$

Ratio-Proportion Method
First convert 1 L to 1,000 mL. Now set up a proportion by placing the unknown amount (x mL) over 1 hr on the left side of the equation and the conversion factor over the infusion time (1,000 mL/10 hr) on the right side of the equation. Be sure that the units in the numerators and denominators match. Then cross multiply, cancel similar units (like terms), and divide to solve for x.

$$\frac{x \text{ mL}}{1 \text{ hr}} = \frac{1,000 \text{ mL}}{10 \text{ hr}}$$

$$x \text{ mL (10 hr)} = 1,000 \text{ mL (1 hr)}$$

$$x = \frac{100 \text{ mL}}{\text{hr}}$$

Dimensional Analysis Method:
$$\frac{1 \cancel{\text{L}}}{1} \times \frac{1,000 \text{ mL}}{1 \cancel{\text{L}}} \times \frac{1}{10 \text{ hr}} = \frac{100 \text{ mL}}{\text{hr}}$$

Answer: The IV flow rate for this infusion is 100 mL/hr.

Using the Flow Rate Formula to Solve for Different Variables

The flow rate formula can be rearranged to solve for different parameters. Recognizing this concept is helpful when solving different calculations related to flow rate. For example, you may be told a patient is to receive an IV preparation at a certain flow rate. The pharmacy may stock that IV preparation in specific volumes (such as a 1 L IV bag). Based on this information, you may need to determine the length of time that 1 L IV bag will last. This infusion time can be calculated using a rearranged flow rate formula.

$$\text{infusion time (hr)} = \frac{\text{total volume infused (mL)}}{\text{flow rate (mL/hr)}}$$

The following example shows how to calculate the length of time an IV bag will last.

Example 9.3.2

A 1 L bag of IV fluid is administered at a flow rate of 125 mL/hr. How long will the IV bag last?

This problem can be solved by using one of three approaches: by using the rearranged flow rate formula, the ratio-proportion method, or the dimensional analysis method.

Rearranged Flow Rate Formula

To begin, recall the rearranged flow rate formula.

$$\text{infusion time (hr)} = \frac{\text{total volume infused (mL)}}{\text{flow rate (mL/hr)}}$$

Next, convert 1 L to 1,000 mL.

Then insert the known values into the rearranged formula.

$$\text{infusion time (hr)} = \frac{1,000 \text{ mL}}{125 \text{ mL/hr}}$$

$$\frac{1,000 \text{ mL}}{125 \text{ mL/hr}} = 8 \text{ hr}$$

Ratio-Proportion Method

To begin, convert 1 L to 1,000 mL. Next, set up a proportion by placing the unknown duration of time (*x* hr) over the converted volume (1,000 mL) on the left side of the equation and the flow rate (1 hr/125 mL) on the right side of the equation. Be sure that the units in the numerators and in the denominators match. Then cross multiply, cancel similar units (like terms), and divide to solve for *x*.

$$\frac{x \text{ hr}}{1,000 \text{ mL}} = \frac{1 \text{ hr}}{125 \text{ mL}}$$

$$x \text{ hr (125 mL)} = 1 \text{ hr (1,000 mL)}$$

$$x = 8 \text{ hr}$$

Dimensional Analysis Method

$$\frac{1\,\cancel{L}}{1} \times \frac{1{,}000\,\cancel{mL}}{1\,\cancel{L}} \times \frac{1\,hr}{125\,\cancel{mL}} = 8\,hr$$

Answer: The IV bag will last 8 hr.

Once you determine the length of time an IV bag will last, you can calculate the number of IV bags needed for a 24-hour period. This calculation is useful because institutional pharmacies typically provide patients with a 24-hour supply of medication at a time. To perform this calculation, use the following formula.

$$\text{number of bags needed for a 24-hour period} = \frac{24\,hr}{\text{length of time one bag lasts (hr/bag)}}$$

When determining the number of IV bags needed for a 24-hour supply, pharmacy technicians should round up their calculated answer to the nearest whole bag.

The following example calculates the number of bags needed in a 24-hour period using the rearranged flow rate formula, the ratio-proportion method, and the dimensional analysis method.

Example 9.3.3

The prescriber has ordered a 1 L bag of D$_5$NS to run at 150 mL/hr. How many bags will be needed in a 24-hour period?

This problem can be solved by using one of three approaches: by using the rearranged flow rate formula, the ratio-proportion method, or the dimensional analysis method.

Rearranged Flow Rate Formula

To begin, recall the rearranged flow rate formula.

$$\text{infusion time (hr)} = \frac{\text{total volume infused (mL)}}{\text{flow rate (mL/hr)}}$$

Next, convert 1 L to 1,000 mL.

Then insert the known values into the rearranged formula.

$$\text{infusion time (hr)} = \frac{1{,}000\,mL}{150\,mL/hr}$$

$$\frac{1{,}000\,mL}{150\,mL/hr} = 6.67\,hr$$

Now, determine the number of bags needed for a 24-hour period using the following formula.

$$\text{number of bags needed for a 24-hour period} = \frac{24\,hr}{\text{length of time one bag lasts (hr/bag)}}$$

$$x = \frac{24 \text{ hr}}{6.67 \text{ hr/bag}}$$

$x = 3.6$ bags, rounded to 4 bags (only whole bags are supplied)

Ratio-Proportion Method

To begin, convert 1 L to 1,000 mL. Now, determine how long a single IV bag will last. Set up a proportion by placing the unknown duration of time (x hr) over the converted volume (1,000 mL) on the left side of the equation and the flow rate (1 hr/150 mL) on the right side of the equation. Be sure that the units in the numerators and in the denominators match. Then cross multiply, cancel similar units (like terms), and divide to solve for x.

$$\frac{x \text{ hr}}{1,000 \text{ mL}} = \frac{1 \text{ hr}}{150 \text{ mL}}$$

$$x \text{ hr } (150 \text{ mL}) = 1 \text{ hr } (1,000 \text{ mL})$$

$$x = 6.67 \text{ hr}$$

Now, determine the number of bags needed for a 24-hour period using the following formula.

$$\text{number of bags needed for a 24-hour period} = \frac{24 \text{ hr}}{\text{length of time one bag lasts (hr/bag)}}$$

$$x = \frac{24 \text{ hr}}{6.67 \text{ hr}} \text{ per bag}$$

$$x = 3.6 \text{ bags, rounded to 4 bags}$$

Dimensional Analysis Method

$$\frac{1 \text{ bag}}{1 \cancel{L}} \times \frac{1 \cancel{L}}{1,000 \cancel{\text{ mL}}} \times \frac{150 \cancel{\text{ mL}}}{1 \cancel{\text{ hr}}} \times \frac{24 \cancel{\text{ hr}}}{\text{day}} = \frac{3.6 \text{ bag}}{\text{day}} \text{ (rounded to 4 bags/day)}$$

Answer: The number of bags needed for a 24-hour period is 4 bags.

Expressing Flow Rate in Different Dosage Units

Although flow rate is typically expressed in volume per unit of time, flow rate may be expressed in other terms depending on the medication. For example, a prescriber may write a medication order that specifies the dosage that is to be infused over a certain period. The dosage of medication is commonly expressed in milligrams per hour (mg/hr). However, variant units such as milliequivalents (mEq) or units may also be used.

The flow rate formula can be altered to account for different dosage units. To determine flow rate calculations based on milligrams, use the following modifications of the flow rate formula.

$$\text{flow rate (mg/hr)} = \frac{\text{total amount of medication infused (mg)}}{\text{infusion time (hr)}}$$

$$\text{infusion time (hr)} = \frac{\text{total amount of medication infused (mg)}}{\text{flow rate (mg/hr)}}$$

To determine flow rate calculations based on milliequivalents, use the following modifications of the flow rate formula.

$$\text{flow rate (mEq/hr)} = \frac{\text{total amount of medication infused (mEq)}}{\text{infusion time (hr)}}$$

$$\text{infusion time (hr)} = \frac{\text{total amount of medication infused (mEq)}}{\text{flow rate (mEq/hr)}}$$

To determine flow rate calculations based on units, use the following modifications of the flow rate formula.

$$\text{flow rate (units/hr)} = \frac{\text{total amount of medication infused (units)}}{\text{infusion time (hr)}}$$

$$\text{infusion time (hr)} = \frac{\text{total amount of medication infused (units)}}{\text{flow rate (units/hr)}}$$

The following examples demonstrate the use of the flow rate formula expressed in amount of medication per unit of time. Note that the ratio-proportion method and dimensional analysis can also be used to perform these calculations.

Example 9.3.4

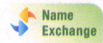

Name Exchange

An IV piggyback is a secondary medication or fluid that is connected to the tubing of a primary medication or fluid. IV piggybacks are abbreviated as IVPBs in some work settings.

 A physician has ordered a 250 mL intravenous piggyback (IVPB) with 500 mg of hydrocortisone to be infused over 4 hours. How many milligrams of medication should be administered per hour?

This problem can be solved by using one of three approaches: by using the modified flow rate formula, the ratio-proportion method, or the dimensional analysis method.

Modified Flow Rate Formula

To begin, recall the rearranged flow rate formula.

$$\text{flow rate (mg/hr)} = \frac{\text{total amount of medication infused (mg)}}{\text{infusion time (hr)}}$$

$$\text{flow rate (mg/hr)} = \frac{500 \text{ mg}}{4 \text{ hr}} = 125 \text{ mg/hr}$$

Ratio-Proportion Method

To begin, set up a proportion by placing the unknown dose (*x* mg) over the time (1 hr) on the left side of the equation and the known flow rate (500 mg/4 hr) on the right side of the equation. Be sure that the units in the numerators and in the denominators match. Then cross multiply, cancel similar units (like terms), and divide to solve for *x*.

$$\frac{x \text{ mg}}{1 \text{ hr}} = \frac{500 \text{ mg}}{4 \text{ hr}}$$

$$x \text{ mg} (4 \text{ hr}) = 500 \text{ mg} (1 \text{ hr})$$

$$x = 125 \text{ mg/hour}$$

Dimensional Analysis Method

$$\frac{500 \text{ mg}}{1 \text{ bag}} \times \frac{1 \text{ bag}}{4 \text{ hr}} = 125 \text{ mg/hr}$$

Answer: This order requires the infusion of 125 mg of medication per hour.

Example 9.3.5

A patient receives 8,100 units of heparin over 6 hours at a constant rate. How many units of heparin does the patient receive each hour?

This problem can be solved by using the modified flow rate formula, by using the ratio-proportion method, or by using dimensional analysis.

Modified Flow Rate Formula

To begin, recall the modified flow rate formula.

$$\text{flow rate (units/hr)} = \frac{\text{total amount of medication infused (units)}}{\text{infusion time (hr)}}$$

$$\text{flow rate (units/hr)} = \frac{8,100 \text{ units}}{6 \text{ hr}} = 1,350 \text{ units/hr}$$

Ratio-Proportion Method

To begin, set up a proportion by placing the unknown dose (x units) over the time (1 hr) on the left side of the equation and the known dosage (8,100 units/ 6 hr) on the right side of the equation. Be sure that the units in the numerators and in the denominators match. Then cross multiply, cancel similar units (like terms), and divide to solve for x.

$$\frac{x \text{ units}}{1 \text{ hr}} = \frac{8,100 \text{ units}}{6 \text{ hr}}$$

$$x \text{ units} (6 \text{ hr}) = 8,100 \text{ units} (1 \text{ hr})$$

$$x = 1,350 \text{ units/hr}$$

Dimensional Analysis Method

$$\frac{8,100 \text{ units}}{\text{bag}} \times \frac{1 \text{ bag}}{6 \text{ hr}} = 1,350 \text{ units/hr}$$

Answer: The patient receives 1,350 units of heparin per hour.

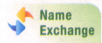

Name Exchange

The anti-infective generic drug cefazolin is also known as the brand name Ancef.

Example 9.3.6

The following medication order is received by the hospital pharmacy.

℞   cefazolin, 1 g

Fluid volume: D$_5$W, 150 mL
Administration rate: over 120 minutes

What volume of fluid is administered per hour? How many milligrams of medication are being given per hour?

This problem can be solved by using one of three approaches: by using the flow rate formula, the ratio-proportion method, or the dimensional analysis method.

Step 1. Determine the volume of fluid administration per hour.

Flow Rate Formula

To begin, convert 120 minutes to hours.

$$120 \text{ minutes} = 2 \text{ hours}$$

Then use the flow rate formula to determine the volume of fluid administered per hour.

$$\text{flow rate (mL/hr)} = \frac{\text{total volume infused (mL)}}{\text{infusion time (hr)}}$$

$$\text{flow rate (mL/hr)} = \frac{150 \text{ mL}}{2 \text{ hr}} = 75 \text{ mL/hr}$$

Ratio-Proportion Method

To begin, convert 120 minutes to hours, as you did for the flow rate formula.

$$120 \text{ minutes} = 2 \text{ hours}$$

Then set up a proportion by placing the unknown dose (x mL) over the time (1 hr) on the left side of the equation and the known dosage (150 mL/2 hr) on the right side of the equation. Be sure that the units in the numerators and in the denominators match. Then cross multiply, cancel similar units (like terms), and divide to solve for x.

$$\frac{x \text{ mL}}{1 \text{ hr}} = \frac{150 \text{ mL}}{2 \text{ hr}}$$

$$x \text{ mL} (2 \text{ hr}) = 150 \text{ mL} (1 \text{ hr})$$

$$x = 75 \text{ mL/hour}$$

Dimensional Analysis Method

$$\frac{150 \text{ mL}}{120 \text{ min}} \times \frac{60 \text{ min}}{\text{hr}} = 75 \text{ mL/hr}$$

Step 2. Now calculate the amount of medication given per hour (in milligrams per hour). This part of the problem can be solved by using one of three approaches: by using the flow rate formula, the ratio-proportion method, or the dimensional analysis method.

Flow Rate Formula

To begin, convert the medication dose from grams to milligrams.

$$1 \text{ g} = 1{,}000 \text{ mg}$$

Then use the flow rate formula to determine the amount of medication administered per hour.

$$\text{flow rate (mg/hr)} = \frac{\text{total amount of medication infused (mg)}}{\text{infusion time (hr)}}$$

$$\text{flow rate (mg/hr)} = \frac{1{,}000 \text{ mg}}{2 \text{ hr}} = 500 \text{ mg/hr}$$

Ratio-Proportion Method

To begin, convert 120 minutes to hours and 1 g to milligrams.

$$120 \text{ minutes} = 2 \text{ hours}$$

$$1 \text{ g} = 1{,}000 \text{ mg}$$

Then set up a proportion by placing the unknown dose (*x* mg) over the time (1 hr) on the left side of the equation and the known dosage (1,000 mg/2 hr) on the right side of the equation. Be sure that the units in the numerators and in the denominators match. Then cross multiply, cancel similar units (like terms), and divide to solve for *x*.

$$\frac{x \text{ mg}}{1 \text{ hr}} = \frac{1{,}000 \text{ mg}}{2 \text{ hr}}$$

$$x \text{ mg} (2 \text{ hr}) = 1{,}000 \text{ mg} (1 \text{ hr})$$

$$x = 500 \text{ mg/hour}$$

Dimensional Analysis Method

$$\frac{1 \cancel{\text{g}}}{120 \cancel{\text{min}}} \times \frac{1{,}000 \text{ mg}}{1 \cancel{\text{g}}} \times \frac{60 \cancel{\text{min}}}{\text{hr}} = 500 \text{ mg/hr}$$

Answer: The volume of fluid administered per hour is 75 mL. The amount of medication being given per hour is 500 mg.

9.3 Problem Set

Perform calculations to answer questions 1–5.

1. A 1 L bag of IV fluid is running at 50 mL/hour. How long will the fluid last?

2. A 1 L bag of IV fluid is hung at 1900 and has a flow rate of 100 mL/hr. What time will the next bag be needed?

3. A 500 mL bag of IV fluid has a flow rate of 30 mL/hr. How long will the fluid last?

4. If a patient is given 60 mg of medication in 75 mL over 45 minutes, what is the flow rate in milliliters per hour?

5. A patient receives 20,000 units of heparin in an IV of 100 mL over 45 minutes. What is the flow rate in milliliters per hour?

Use the IVPB label below to answer questions 6 and 7.

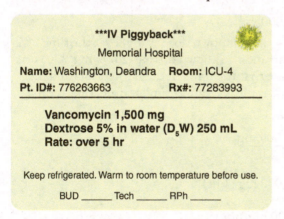

> *****IV Piggyback*****
> Memorial Hospital
> **Name:** Washington, Deandra   **Room:** ICU-4
> **Pt. ID#:** 776263663   **Rx#:** 77283993
>
> **Vancomycin 1,500 mg**
> **Dextrose 5% in water (D₅W) 250 mL**
> **Rate: over 5 hr**
>
> Keep refrigerated. Warm to room temperature before use.
>
> BUD _____ Tech _____ RPh _____

6. What is the flow rate in milliliters per hour?

7. What is the vancomycin dosage in milligrams per hour?

Use the IVPB label below to answer questions 8 and 9.

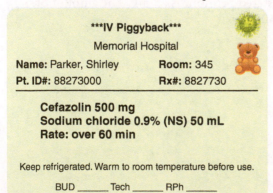

> *****IV Piggyback*****
> Memorial Hospital
> **Name:** Parker, Shirley   **Room:** 345
> **Pt. ID#:** 88273000   **Rx#:** 8827730
>
> **Cefazolin 500 mg**
> **Sodium chloride 0.9% (NS) 50 mL**
> **Rate: over 60 min**
>
> Keep refrigerated. Warm to room temperature before use.
>
> BUD _____ Tech _____ RPh _____

8. What is the flow rate in milliliters per hour?

9. What is the cefazolin dosage in milligrams per hour?

Use the IV label below to answer questions 10–15.

> *****Large-Volume Parenteral*****
> Memorial Hospital
> **Name:** Le, Thu   **Room:** OB-14
> **Pt. ID#:** 449009288   **Rx#:** 7200182
>
> **Potassium chloride 20 mEq**
> **D₅NS 1,000 mL**
> **Rate: 100 mL/hr**
>
> Keep refrigerated. Warm to room temperature before use.
>
> BUD _____ Tech _____ RPh _____

10. What is the flow rate in milliliters per hour?

11. How many hours will this IV bag last?

12. How many IV bags will be needed in a 24-hour period? (Round up your answer to the nearest 1 L bag.)

13. What is the potassium chloride dosage in milliequivalents per hour?

For each flow rate in questions 14–23, determine the quantity of 1 L bags needed for 24 hours. (Round up your answer to the nearest 1 L bag.)

14. 50 mL/hr _____

15. 75 mL/hr _____

16. 100 mL/hr _____

17. 120 mL/hr _____

18. 125 mL/hr _____

19. 130 mL/hr _____

20. 150 mL/hr _____

21. 175 mL/hr _____

22. 200 mL/hr _____

23. 225 mL/hr _____

Using what you have learned, interpret the prescriptions and perform the necessary calculations to answer questions 24–28.

24.
R̸ **Hydrocortisone 250 mg**
Fluid volume: 250 mL
Time of infusion: 4 hr

a. What is the flow rate in milliliters per hour?

b. How many milligrams will be administered per hour?

25.
R̸ **Penicillin G**
12 million units
Fluid volume: 500 mL
Time of infusion: 12 hr

a. What is the flow rate in milliliters per hour?

b. How many units will be administered per hour?

26.
R̸ **Lidocaine 4%**
Fluid volume: 500 mL
Flow rate: 800 mg/hr

a. What is the flow rate in milliliters per hour?

b. How many hours will it take until the entire IV bag has been administered?

27.
R̸ **Methylprednisolone 250 mg**
Fluid volume: 500 mL
Flow rate: 20 mg/hr

a. What is the flow rate in milliliters per hour?

b. How many hours will it take until the entire dose has been administered?

28.
R̸ **Dopamine 1,600 mcg in D_5W**
Fluid volume: 500 mL
Dosage: 4 mcg/min

a. What is the flow rate in milliliters per hour?

b. How many micrograms will be administered per hour?

29. A physician has ordered an IV infusion of dopamine hydrochloride 800 mg in 250 mL of D_5W to run at 5 mg/hr. Dopamine is available in a 20 mL vial at a concentration of 200 mg/5 mL.

a. How many milliliters of dopamine must be drawn up to prepare this dose?

b. What is the IV flow rate in milliliters per hour?

30. A physician has ordered an IVPB of gentamicin 2 mg/kg q8h for a patient who weighs 176 lb. The IVPB will be prepared in a base solution of D_5W 100 mL and will be administered over 60 min. Gentamicin is available in a 20 mL vial at a concentration of 40 mg/mL.

a. How many milliliters of gentamicin must be drawn up to prepare a single dose?

b. What is the administration rate in milliliters per hour?

Self-check your work in Appendix A.

9.4 Drop Factor Calculations

Nursing staff—and, occasionally, pharmacy staff—are required to calculate the rate of administration for an IV fluid in drops per minute (gtts/min). Most institutions now use electronic infusion pumps to regulate both the volume and the rate of a patient's IV medication. Nursing personnel program the prescribed rate into the electronic infusion pump at the patient's bedside to administer the prescribed number of drops per minute. The rate can be digitally adjusted, which causes the pump's internal clamp to slow or quicken the rate at which the fluid flows through tubing routed through a chamber in the pump. Pumps can be set to administer IV fluids in milliliters per hour or drops per minute.

Occasionally, nursing staff must manually adjust the IV flow rate using the tubing's roll clamp, which controls the rate of the fluid volume being administered to the patient. The rate in drops per minute can be calculated manually by counting the number of drops of fluid that fall into the drip chamber in one minute. The nurse can then manually adjust the rate up or down by using the roll clamp.

Calculating Flow Rate in Drops per Minute

Calculating the flow rate in drops per minute is complicated by the variety of IV tubing sets, commonly referred to as *IV sets*, that are available. Manufacturers produce calibrated IV sets that result in different-sized drops. An IV set is identified by the number of drops it takes to produce 1 mL. This calibration may be referred to as a *drop set* or a *drip set* but is most commonly called the IV set's ***drop factor***.

IV sets typically come in two types: macrodrip sets and microdrip (minidrip) sets. A **macrodrip set** with a drop factor of 10 gtts/mL, 15 gtts/mL, or 20 gtts/mL produces large drops in the IV set's drip chamber. A **microdrip (minidrip) set** with a drop factor of 60 gtts/mL produces small drops in the IV set's drip chamber. Figure 9.1 illustrates these two types of IV sets.

The drop factor for an IV set is prominently displayed on the outside of the IV tubing package. The 10-drop and 15-drop sets are commonly used for adult patients, whereas the 60-drop set is used for pediatric patients or patients who are critically ill and are being given **narrow therapeutic index drugs**, or drugs that have a small difference between toxic and therapeutic doses (see Table 9.1).

TABLE 9.1 Common Drop Factors

Drop Factor	Drops per Milliliter
Macrodrops	
10	10 gtts/mL
15	15 gtts/mL
20	20 gtts/mL
Microdrops	
60	60 gtts/mL

To determine the IV flow rate in drops per minute when the total volume and infusion time are known, use the following formula.

$$\text{IV flow rate or IVFR in Drops per Minute (gtts/min)} = \frac{\text{total volume or TV (mL)}}{\text{infusion time or IT (min)}} \times \text{drop factor or DF (gtts/mL)}$$

or

$$\text{IVFR in gtts/min} = \frac{\text{TV}}{\text{IT}} \times \text{DF}$$

FIGURE 9.1
IV Drop Sets

IV fluids are
administered
using IV sets,
which have
different-sized
drops.

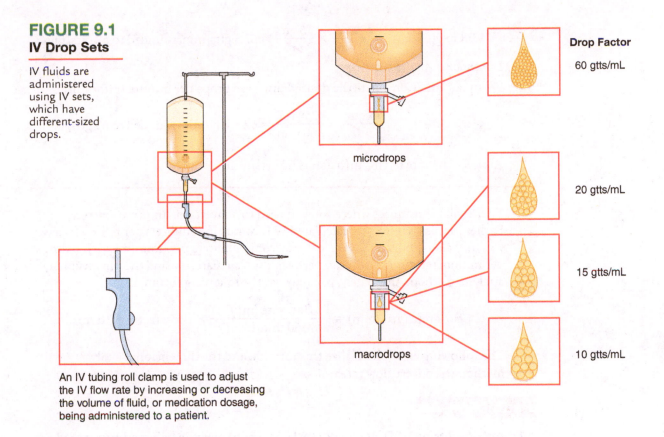

Drop Factor

60 gtts/mL

microdrops

20 gtts/mL

15 gtts/mL

macrodrops

10 gtts/mL

An IV tubing roll clamp is used to adjust
the IV flow rate by increasing or decreasing
the volume of fluid, or medication dosage,
being administered to a patient.

**Quick
Study**

If remembering the
IV flow rate formula
is difficult, dimen-
sional analysis may
be used instead. To
use the dimensional
analysis method,
set up an equation
to solve for the
desired units of
drops per minute.

**Math
Morsel**

When a drop per
minute calculation
results in a partial
drop, pharmacy
technicians should
round down to the
nearest whole drop.

To better understand this flow rate formula, consider the units that may be used.

$$\frac{mL}{min} \times \frac{drops}{mL} = drops/min$$

Dimensional analysis may also be used to solve this type of equation. Be aware
that in the event your calculation results in a partial drop per minute you should
round down your answer to the nearest whole drop. For example, 20.6 gtts/min would
be rounded down to 20 gtts/min. The following examples demonstrate how to use the
flow rate formula in various scenarios.

Example 9.4.1

**An IV solution has a total volume of 250 mL and is being administered over
60 minutes using macrodrip tubing with a drop factor of 15 gtts/mL. What
is the rate in drops per minute?**

This problem can be solved by using the IV flow rate formula or by using the
dimensional analysis method.

IV Flow Rate Formula

Recall the drop factor formula.

$$IVFR \text{ in gtts/min} = \frac{TV}{IT} \times DF$$

$$\text{IVFR in gtts/min} = \frac{250 \ \cancel{mL}}{60 \ \text{min}} \times \frac{15 \ \text{gtts}}{\cancel{mL}} = 62.5 \ \text{gtts/min, rounded to 62 gtts/min}$$

Dimensional Analysis Method

Set up an equation where the desired units are drops per minute (gtts/min).

$$\frac{15 \ \text{gtts}}{\cancel{mL}} \times \frac{250 \ \cancel{mL}}{60 \ \text{min}} = 62.5 \ \text{gtts/min, rounded to 62 gtts/min}$$

Answer: The rate of this infusion is 62 gtts/min.

There will be instances where you will need to convert the units of flow rate. Earlier in this chapter, you calculated IV flow rate in milliliters per hour. However, you may also need to convert flow rate from milliliters per hour (mL/hr) to drops per minute (gtts/min). You can perform this calculation using the dimensional analysis method. Alternately, you may use the following formula.

$$\text{IV flow rate (gtts/min)} = \frac{\text{IV flow rate (mL/hr)}}{60 \ \text{min/hr}} \times \text{drop factor (gtts/mL)}$$

The following examples utilize this formula and the dimensional analysis method to convert flow rate units.

Example 9.4.2

 An IV solution of D$_5$W with 20,000 units of heparin is being administered at a rate of 40 mL/hr using macrodrip tubing with a drop factor of 20 gtts/mL. How many drops per minute are being administered?

This problem can be solved by using the IV flow rate conversion formula or by using the dimensional analysis method.

IV Flow Rate Conversion Formula

To begin, recall the IV flow rate conversion formula.

$$\text{IV flow rate (gtts/min)} = \frac{\text{IV flow rate (mL/hr)}}{60 \ \text{min/hr}} \times \text{drop factor (gtts/mL)}$$

Then insert the values from the word problem into the formula and cancel like units.

$$\text{IV flow rate (gtts/min)} = \frac{40 \ \text{mL/hr}}{60 \ \text{min/hr}} \times 20 \ \text{gtts/mL}$$

$$\frac{40 \ \cancel{mL/hr}}{60 \ \cancel{min/hr}} \times \frac{20 \ \text{gtts}}{\cancel{mL}} = 13.33 \ \text{gtts/min, rounded to 13 gtts/min}$$

Dimensional Analysis Method

$$\frac{40 \ \cancel{mL}}{1 \ \cancel{hr}} \times \frac{20 \ \text{gtts}}{\cancel{mL}} \times \frac{1 \ \cancel{hr}}{60 \ \text{min}} = 13.33 \ \text{gtts/min, rounded to 13 gtts/min}$$

Answer: The flow rate of this infusion is 13 gtts/min.

Expressing Flow Rate in Milligrams per Drop

Occasionally, pharmacy personnel use drop factor calculations to determine the milligrams of medication that will be infused per drop. These calculations can be solved by first determining the solution concentration in milligrams per milliliter (mg/mL). Then this concentration in milligrams per milliliter must be converted to milligrams per drop (mg/gtt). This calculation requires you to divide the concentration (mg/mL) by the drop factor (gtts/mL). The following formula is used in these calculations.

$$\text{concentration (mg/gtt)} = \frac{\text{concentration (mg/mL)}}{\text{drop factor (gtts/mL)}}$$

The following examples demonstrate both the use of this formula and the use of the dimensional analysis method to solve this type of calculation.

Example 9.4.3

 A prescriber has ordered a dopamine drip of 800 mg in 250 mL of D$_5$W. The IV solution will be administered at 10 mL/hr through tubing that has a drop factor of 10 gtts/mL. How many milligrams of dopamine are in each drop?

This problem can be solved by using the concentration in milligrams per drop formula or by using the dimensional analysis method.

Concentration in Milligrams per Drop (mg/gtt) Formula

To begin, determine the concentration (in milligrams per milliliter) of dopamine in D$_5$W.

$$\frac{800 \text{ mg}}{250 \text{ mL}} = 3.2 \text{ mg/mL}$$

Then use the concentration in milligrams per drop (mg/gtt) formula to solve the problem. To do so, insert the milligrams per milliliter value you just calculated (3.2 mg/mL) above into the formula and divide by the drop factor given in the problem (10 gtts/mL).

$$\text{concentration (mg/gtt)} = \frac{\text{concentration (mg/mL)}}{\text{drop factor (gtts/mL)}}$$

$$\text{concentration (mg/gtt)} = \frac{3.2 \text{ mg/mL}}{10 \text{ gtts/mL}}$$

$$\text{concentration (mg/gtt)} = 0.32 \text{ mg/gtt}$$

Dimensional Analysis Method

$$\frac{800 \text{ mg}}{250 \text{ mL}} \times \frac{1 \text{ mL}}{10 \text{ gtts}} = 0.32 \text{ mg/gtt}$$

Answer: There are 0.32 mg of dopamine in each drop.

Example 9.4.4

A physician has ordered vancomycin 250 mg in 100 mL of NS every six hours for a pediatric patient. The IV solution will be administered at 50 mL/hr through 20 gtts/mL macrodrip tubing. How many milligrams of vancomycin are in each drop?

This problem can be solved by using the concentration in milligrams per drop formula or by using the dimensional analysis method.

Concentration in Milligrams per Drop (mg/gtt) Formula

To begin, determine the concentration (in milligrams per milliliter) of vancomycin in NS.

$$\frac{250 \text{ mg/mL}}{100 \text{ mL}} = 2.5 \text{ mg/mL}$$

Then use the concentration in milligrams per drop (mg/gtt) formula to solve the problem. To do so, insert the milligrams per milliliter value you just calculated above (2.5 mg/mL) into the formula and divide by the drop factor in the problem (20 gtts/mL).

$$\text{concentration (mg/gtt)} = \frac{\text{concentration (mg/mL)}}{\text{drop factor (gtts/mL)}}$$

$$\text{concentration (mg/gtt)} = \frac{2.5 \text{ mg/mL}}{20 \text{ gtts/mL}}$$

$$\text{concentration (mg/gtt)} = 0.125 \text{ mg/gtt}$$

Dimensional Analysis Method

$$\frac{250 \text{ mg}}{100 \text{ mL}} \times \frac{1 \text{ mL}}{20 \text{ gtts}} = 0.125 \text{ mg/gtt}$$

Answer: There are 0.125 mg of vancomycin in each drop.

9.4 Problem Set

Perform calculations to answer the following questions. Round down your answers to the nearest drop.

1. An IV rate is 10 mL/hr. Using an IV set with a drop factor of 10 gtts/mL, what is the rate in drops per minute?

2. What is the IV flow rate in drops per minute for an IV solution that is administered at 35 mL/hr using a 60-drop set?

3. A patient is to receive 1 g of cefazolin in 100 mL of ½ NS over one hour using a 10-drop set. What is the rate in drops per minute?

4. A nurse will be administering 500 mg of medication in 50 mL over 30 minutes using microdrip tubing. What is the flow rate in drops per minute?

5. A physician orders 20,000 units of heparin in an IV solution of D_5NS 500 mL to be administered continuously over 24 hours. Using a 15-drop set, what is the rate in drops per minute?

6. A physician orders 750 mg of vancomycin in a 250 mL IVPB over one hour using a 15-drop set. How many drops per minute will be administered?

7. A patient is to be given 1,000 mL of Lactated Ringer's (LR) solution at 50 mL/hr. If tubing with a drop factor of 15 is used, what is the rate in drops per minute?

8. A patient is to be given an infusion at 95 mL/hr. What will the drip rate (gtts/min) be if a 20-drop set is used?

9. A physician orders 40 mEq of potassium chloride in 100 mL of D_5W to be administered over 4 hours. If a 10-drop set is used, how many milliequivalents of potassium will be in each drop?

10. A patient is to receive 20,000 units of heparin in 500 mL of D_5 ½ NS at a flow rate of 25 mL/hr. If tubing with a drop factor of 15 is used, what will be the rate in drops per minute?

11. A pharmacy receives the medication order below. What is the rate in drops per minute if microdrip tubing is used?

ID#: Y7HH7992			Memorial Hospital
Name: Baldwin, Flora			
DOB: 11/22/90			
Room: 514			Physician's
Dr: Ahmed Vincelette, MD			Medication Order
ALLERGY OR SENSITIVITY		DIAGNOSIS	
aspirin, latex		pancreatitis	
DATE	TIME	ORDERS	PHYSICIAN'S SIG.
10/28/2024	2316	IV fluid — D5NS 1L w/20	
		mEq potassium chloride,	
		1 mg folic acid, and	
		1 ampule of multivitamins	
		@ 50 mL/hr	
			Ahmed Vincelette, M.D.

12. A pharmacy receives the medication order below. What is the rate in drops per minute if tubing with a drop factor of 20 is used?

ID#: MBYUU97II			Memorial Hospital
Name: Mosier, Bud			
DOB: 02/22/59			
Room: 716			Physician's
Dr: Jeremiah King, M.D.			Medication Order
ALLERGY OR SENSITIVITY		DIAGNOSIS	
penicillin, sulfa, shellfish, tape		asthmatic bronchitis	
DATE	TIME	ORDERS	PHYSICIAN'S SIG.
5/15/2024	1527	Aminophylline 1 g in	
		250 mL D5W	
		@ 10 mL/hr	
			Jeremiah King, M.D.

13. A pharmacy receives the medication order below. If microdrip tubing is used, how many milligrams of amiodarone will be in each drop?

ID#: 9927739992			Memorial Hospital
Name: Brzyznski, Martha			
DOB: 01/09/48			
Room: ICU-24			Physician's
Dr: Amarite Gaya, M.D.			Medication Order
ALLERGY OR SENSITIVITY		DIAGNOSIS	
no known drug allergies		myocardial infarction	
DATE	TIME	ORDERS	PHYSICIAN'S SIG.
5/15/2024	0624	Administer amiodarone	
		drip	
		450 mg in 250 mL NS	
		at 8 mL/hr	
			Amarite Gaya, M.D.

14. A pharmacy receives the medication order below. Using tubing with a drop factor of 10, how many milligrams per drop will be administered?

ID#: UHy08llieX			Memorial Hospital
Name: Lazaar, Howard			
DOB: 07/20/50			R_x
Room: CCU -03			Physician's
Dr: Thu Singh, M.D.			Medication Order

ALLERGY OR SENSITIVITY			DIAGNOSIS	
aspirin, sulfa, penicillin, milk			heart failure	
DATE	TIME	ORDERS		PHYSICIAN'S SIG.
10/30/2024	0740	Norepinephrine		
		8 mg/250 mL		
		D5W over 24 hours		
				Thu Singh, M.D.

15. The label below is received in the inpatient pharmacy. If the nurse administers this IVPB using tubing with a drop factor of 10, how many drops per minute will be administered?

> ***IV Piggyback***
> Memorial Hospital
>
> Name: Geist, Polly   Room: PICU
> Pt. ID#: KKU882799   Rx#: 66729937
> _____
>
> **Tobramycin 40 mg**
> **Dextrose 5% in water (D$_5$W) 25 mL**
> **Rate: over 60 min**
>
> Keep refrigerated. Warm to room temperature.
>
> BUD _____ Tech _____ RPh _____

16. The following label is received in the IV room. If the nurse administers it using microdrip tubing, how many milliequivalents will be administered with each drop?

> ***Large-Volume Parenteral***
> Memorial Hospital
>
> Name: Briggs, Jennifer   Room: NICU
> Pt. ID#: H68YY7   Rx#: 6638927
> _____
>
> **D$_{10}$W 500 mL**
> **Potassium acetate 10 mEq**
> **Rate: 5 mL/hr**
>
> Keep refrigerated. Warm to room temperature.
>
> BUD _____ Tech _____ RPh _____

Self-check your work in Appendix A.

9.5 Special Dilution and Parenteral Nutrition Calculations

Safety Alert

Pharmacy technicians should always exercise special caution when performing pediatric dosing calculations. Calculations should always be double checked or triple checked by pharmacists.

As you learned in Chapter 7, physicians may prescribe IV preparations in concentrations of medications that are not commercially available. When a desired concentration or dose is not commercially available, you can use the alligation method to combine two *similar*, commercially available products (one with a high concentration and one with a low concentration) to make a desired concentration. However, there are other instances in which the high concentrations of commercially available medications make dilutions to smaller doses difficult or impractical. In these situations, the desired doses are such small volumes that they are too difficult to draw up accurately in a syringe or to administer. Consequently, you may need to dilute commercially available formulations with a diluent (such as sterile water for injection [SWFI], normal saline, or D_5W). This customized, diluted formulation, known as a *special dilution*, may be ordered for a pediatric patient.

Calculating Special Dilutions

There are three basic steps to calculating special dilutions. The first step is to determine the total amount of drug needed for the special dilution. The second step is to determine the volume of concentrated medication required to prepare the special dilution. Both these steps can be done by using the ratio-proportion method or by using the dimensional analysis method. The third step is to determine the volume of diluent needed for dilution of the concentrated medication. This step is achieved by calculating the difference between the total volume of the special dilution and the volume of drug required, as shown in the following formula:

$$\text{diluent volume} = \text{total volume (TV)} - \text{drug volume (DV)}$$

The following example takes you through the steps required to calculate a special dilution.

Example 9.5.1

Prepare a special dilution of gentamicin with a total volume of 4 mL and a concentration of 5 mg/mL. Use a stock solution of gentamicin 10 mg/mL and SWFI to prepare this special dilution.

You can solve this problem by using the ratio-proportion method or by using the dimensional analysis method. The ratio-proportion method will be demonstrated in this example.

Step 1. Determine the total amount of medication needed for the special dilution.

desired final product = 5 mg/mL
total volume (TV) = 4 mL

Use the ratio-proportion method to determine the number of milligrams of medication needed for the special dilution. Set up a proportion by placing the unknown amount (*x* mg) over the total volume

(4 mL) on the left side of the equation and the known concentration (5 mg/1 mL) on the right side of the equation. Be sure that the units in the numerators and in the denominators match. Then cross multiply, cancel similar units (like terms), and divide to solve for x.

$$\frac{x \text{ mg}}{4 \text{ mL}} = \frac{5 \text{ mg}}{1 \text{ mL}}$$

$$x \text{ mg} (1 \text{ mL}) = 5 \text{ mg} (4 \text{ mL})$$

$$x = 20 \text{ mg}$$

The total number of milligrams of gentamicin needed for the special dilution is 20 mg.

Note: Dimensional analysis could also be used to determine this step.

Step 2. Determine the volume of concentrated medication (in this case, the 10 mg/mL stock solution) needed to prepare the special dilution. Set up a proportion by placing the unknown volume (x mL) over the number of milligrams calculated in Step 1 (20 mg) on the left side of the equation and the known stock solution concentration (1 mL/10 mg) on the right side of the equation. Be sure that the units in the numerators and in the denominators match. Then cross multiply, cancel similar units (like terms), and divide to solve for x.

$$\frac{x \text{ mL}}{20 \text{ mg}} = \frac{1 \text{ mL}}{10 \text{ mg}}$$

$$x \text{ mL} (10 \text{ mg}) = 1 \text{ mL} (20 \text{ mg})$$

$$x = 2 \text{ mL}$$

The total number of milliliters of gentamicin stock solution (10 mg/mL) needed to prepare the special dilution is 2 mL.

Note: Dimensional analysis could also be used to determine this step.

Step 3. Determine the volume of diluent (SWFI) needed to prepare the special dilution by using the following formula.

$$\text{diluent volume} = \text{total volume (TV)} - \text{drug volume (DV)}$$

Identify the variables:

TV = 4 mL (stated in problem)
DV = 2 mL (determined in Step 2)

Then insert the known variables into the formula.

$$\text{diluent volume} = 4 \text{ mL} - 2 \text{ mL} = 2 \text{ mL}$$
$$\text{diluent volume} = 2 \text{ mL}$$

Answer: You must draw up 2 mL of the gentamicin 10 mg/mL stock solution into a syringe and 2 mL of the SWFI diluent into a syringe. Both syringes will be injected into a sterile, empty vial, and the resulting 4 mL special dilution is a gentamicin solution with a concentration of 5 mg/mL.

Other special dilutions you may need to compound are IV solutions that have percentage strengths not commercially available, such as IV dextrose solutions. In some instances, you can combine a higher-strength concentration of a dextrose solution with a lower-strength concentration of a dextrose solution to formulate the ordered percentage-strength solution. If you recall from Chapter 7, you used an alligation grid to help you set up the calculations to formulate this customized percentage-strength solution. However, in other instances, a prescriber may order a special dilution of a concentrated dextrose solution mixed with SWFI to achieve a specific percentage-strength solution. To compound this type of special dilution, you will follow a process of three calculations, as outlined below.

The first calculation in this process determines the volume of dextrose solution needed. To perform these calculations, you can use either the ratio-proportion method or the dimensional analysis method. You can also use the following formula to calculate the volume of concentrated solution needed.

$$\text{volume of concentrated solution needed for special dilution (mL)} = \frac{\text{total volume or TV (mL)}}{\text{concentrated solution percent (\%)}} \times \text{desired percent (\%)}$$

The second calculation in this process determines the volume of diluent needed. To perform this process, you will use the following formula.

$$\text{diluent volume} = \text{total volume (TV)} - \text{concentrated solution volume}$$

The third calculation in this process verifies the accuracy of your calculated volumes. The sum of the volumes determined in the first two calculation processes should equal the total volume of the special dilution. The following example demonstrates these three processes for compounding this type of special dilution.

Example 9.5.2

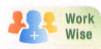

Work Wise

Pharmacy personnel often use technical jargon to relay information to one another. For example, a dextrose 10% in water solution is often spoken using its abbreviation: "D10" or "$D_{10}W$."

A medication order for 1,000 mL of dextrose 10% in water ($D_{10}W$) for IV use is received by a pharmacy. Currently, the pharmacy has stock solutions of $D_{70}W$ and SWFI for injection. How much $D_{70}W$ and how much SWFI are needed to prepare the ordered IV solution?

Step 1. Calculate the volume of concentrated dextrose solution needed. Use the following formula to determine this volume.

$$\text{volume of concentrated solution needed for special dilution (mL)} = \frac{\text{total volume or TV (mL)}}{\text{concentrated solution percent (\%)}} \times \text{desired percent (\%)}$$

Identify the variables:
TV = 1,000 mL
concentrated solution % = 70
desired solution % = 10

Then insert the known variables into the formula.

$$\text{volume of concentrated solution needed for special dilution (mL)} = \left(\frac{1{,}000\ \text{mL}}{70\%}\right) \times 10\% = 142.86\ \text{mL, rounded to } 142.9\ \text{mL}$$

The amount of $D_{70}W$ needed is 142.9 mL.

Step 2. Calculate the volume of diluent (SWFI) needed.

$$1{,}000\ \text{mL} - 142.9\ \text{mL} = 857.1\ \text{mL}$$

The amount of diluent (sterile water) needed is 857.1 mL.

Step 3. Verify the accuracy of your calculations by adding the volumes that you determined in Steps 1 and 2. If you have performed each of the calculations correctly, the sum should equal the total volume ordered by the physician—in this case, 1,000 mL.

$$142.9\ \text{mL} + 857.1\ \text{mL} = 1{,}000\ \text{mL}$$

Answer: You will need 142.9 mL of $D_{70}W$ and 857.1 mL of SWFI to prepare the ordered solution.

Calculating Parenteral Nutrition

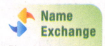
Name Exchange

Pharmacy technicians may hear parenteral nutrition referred to by its abbreviation *PN.* You may also hear it referred to as as *hyperalimentation* in your practice setting.

Parenteral nutrition (PN) is a means of supplying needed nourishment to patients who cannot or will not take in sufficient (or any) food or water through their mouths or a port in the gastrointestinal (GI) system. Parenteral nutrition can be peripheral parenteral nutrition (PPN) or **total parenteral nutrition (TPN)**. PPN provides partial nutritional support for patients who have short-term hospital stays. TPN provides complete and sustaining nutritional support for patients who cannot receive food, water, or medication by mouth. This inability to take nutrition by mouth can be the result of surgery, infection, or inflammation in the GI tract. TPN administration is generally for extended stays in the hospital (or sometimes even at home with home health care). The focus of this discussion is TPN.

WORKPLACE WISDOM

Sterile water for injection (SWFI) may be used to prepare IV solutions. Although the term "sterile water" might sound harmless, this diluent can be dangerous if used improperly. Sterile water is a hypotonic solution, meaning it has a lower osmotic pressure than plasma. When too much of a hypotonic solution is administered intravenously to a patient, the water that lies outside of a patient's cells moves to the inside of the cells. This movement results in cell swelling and, in some cases, cell rupture, or *hemolysis*. Hemolysis can have negative health consequences and can even result in death. For that reason, be sure to always double check your calculations and measurements when using SWFI.

TPN is typically a large-volume IV solution compounded from multiple solutions, such as dextrose, amino acids, sterile water, fat emulsion, electrolytes, multivitamins (MVIs), and minerals. The major component and volumetric source of a TPN solution is called the **TPN base solution**, which comprises dextrose, amino acids, SWFI, and, in some cases, fat emulsion. The electrolytes, minerals, and MVIs are considered **TPN additives**.

TPN calculations require special pharmacy calculations that involve multiple steps. The first step requires calculation of the components of the base solution, with the exception of sterile water (which is calculated in Step 4). In this step, the volumes of dextrose, amino acids, and, in some cases, fat emulsions are calculated using the following formula.

$$\text{volume of base solution (mL)} = \frac{\text{total volume or TV (mL)}}{\text{stock solution percent (\%)}} \times \text{desired percent (\%)}$$

Note that this formula is similar to the one used to calculate special dilutions.

The second step in TPN calculations is to determine the volume of the additives (electrolytes, minerals, and MVIs). To complete this calculation, you can use one of three approaches: the ratio-proportion method, the dimensional analysis method, or the following formula.

$$\text{volume of additive needed (mL)} = \frac{\text{desired dose or D}}{\text{concentration on hand or H (per mL)}}$$

Keep in mind that additives may be ordered in a specific dose (such as mEq) or in doses per volume of TPN (such as mEq/L). If the TPN is ordered in doses per volume of TPN (such as mEq/L), you must determine the desired dose (D) by multiplying the dose per volume by the total TPN volume.

The third step is to add the volumes of the base solutions calculated in Step 1 and the additives calculated in Step 2.

The fourth step is determining the amount of SWFI needed to make the TPN the appropriate total volume. This step is done by finding the difference between the total TPN volume and the volume of the base solutions and additives (determined in Step 3).

The fifth step verifies the accuracy of volume calculations. This step involves finding the sum of all the base solutions (dextrose, amino acids, fat emulsions, and SWFI) and the additives (electrolytes, minerals, and MVIs). The sum should equal the total ordered volume of the TPN.

The following example demonstrates the five-part procedure for solving typical TPN problems.

Put Down Roots

The word *parenteral* comes from the Greek roots *para*, meaning "beside," and *enteron*, meaning "intestine." Therefore, a parenteral preparation refers to a product that bypasses—or goes "beside" rather than through—the GI tract.

Example 9.5.3

A physician has ordered a 2,000 mL TPN with the base solution and additives shown below. What is the volume of each base solution and additive needed to make the TPN? The stock solutions available in the pharmacy are listed.

Base Solution

Dextrose 15%

Aminosyn (amino acid solution) 3.5%

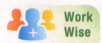

Work Wise

Neonatal and pediatric TPN solutions involve complex calculations that require additional steps. These types of pharmacy calculations are performed by pharmacy technicians as they gain practical experience in advanced pharmacy settings.

Liposyn (fat emulsion) 5%

SWFI QSAD to 2,000 mL

Additives

Sodium chloride 40 mEq

Potassium chloride 10 mEq

Potassium phosphate 6 mM

MVIs 10 mL/day

Prepared Using the Following Pharmacy Stock Solutions (i.e., concentrations kept on hand in the pharmacy)

Dextrose 70%

Aminosyn 10%

Liposyn 20%

Sodium chloride 4 mEq/mL

Potassium chloride 2 mEq/mL

Potassium phosphate 3 mM/mL

MVIs 10 mL/day

KEY

TV = total volume of TPN ordered by prescriber

stock % = percentage strength of the solution that is stocked in the pharmacy

desired % = percentage strength of the solution ordered by the prescriber

mL = number of milliliters of stock solution needed to prepare the TPN solution

Step 1. Calculate the volume of the TPN base components—dextrose, Aminosyn, and Liposyn. (*Note:* The SWFI volume will be calculated in Step 4.) Use the following formula for each base component calculation.

$$\text{volume of base solution (mL)} = \left(\frac{\text{total volume or TV [mL]}}{\text{stock solution percent [\%]}} \right) \times \text{desired percent (\%)}$$

A. To begin, determine the amount of dextrose needed. Identify the variables:

TV = 2,000 mL
stock % = 70
desired % = 15

Then insert the variables into the following formula.

$$\text{volume of base solution (mL)} = \left(\frac{\text{total volume or TV [mL]}}{\text{stock solution percent [\%]}} \right) \times \text{desired percent (\%)}$$

$$\text{volume of base solution (mL)} = \left(\frac{2,000 \text{ mL}}{70\%} \right) \times 15\%$$

Then cancel similar units (like terms) and solve.

$$\left(\frac{2{,}000 \text{ mL}}{70\%}\right) \times 15\% = 428.57, \text{ rounded to } 429$$

The amount of dextrose needed is 429 mL.

B. Next, determine the amount of Aminosyn needed.

Identify the variables:
TV = 2,000 mL
stock % = 10
desired % = 3.5

Then insert the variables into the following formula.

$$\text{volume of base solution (mL)} = \left(\frac{\text{total volume or TV [mL]}}{\text{stock solution percent [\%]}}\right) \times \text{desired percent (\%)}$$

$$\text{volume of base solution (mL)} = \left(\frac{2{,}000 \text{ mL}}{10\%}\right) \times 3.5\%$$

Then cancel similar units (like terms) and solve.

$$\left(\frac{2{,}000 \text{ mL}}{10\%}\right) \times 3.5\% = 700 \text{ mL}$$

The amount of Aminosyn needed is 700 mL.

C. Now, determine the amount of Liposyn needed.

Identify the variables:
TV = 2,000 mL
stock % = 20
desired % = 5

Then insert the variables into the following formula.

$$\text{volume of base solution (mL)} = \left(\frac{\text{total volume or TV [mL]}}{\text{stock solution percent [\%]}}\right) \times \text{desired percent (\%)}$$

$$\text{volume of base solution (mL)} = \left(\frac{2{,}000 \text{ mL}}{20\%}\right) \times 5\%$$

Then cancel similar units (like terms) and solve.

$$\left(\frac{2{,}000 \text{ mL}}{20\%}\right) \times 5\% = 500 \text{ mL}$$

The amount of Liposyn needed is 500 mL.

Step 2. This TPN orders additives in specific doses. Because it is given in the order, you do not need to calculate the desired dose. Calculate the volume of each additive based on the following formula:

$$\text{volume of additive needed (mL)} = \frac{\text{desired dose or D}}{\text{concentration on hand or H (per mL)}}$$

A. To begin, determine the amount of sodium chloride needed.

Identify the variables:
D = 40 mEq
H = 4 mEq/mL

Then insert the variables into the formula.

$$\text{volume of additive needed (mL)} = \frac{40 \text{ mEq}}{4 \text{ mEq/mL}}$$

Cancel similar units (like terms) and solve.

$$\frac{40 \text{ mEq}}{4 \text{ mEq/mL}} = 10 \text{ mL}$$

The amount of sodium chloride needed is 10 mL.

B. Next, determine the amount of potassium chloride needed.

Identify the variables:
D = 10 mEq
H = 2 mEq/mL

Then insert the variables into the formula.

$$\text{volume of additive needed (mL)} = \frac{10 \text{ mEq}}{2 \text{ mEq/mL}}$$

Cancel like units and solve.

$$\frac{10 \text{ mEq}}{2 \text{ mEq/mL}} = 5 \text{ mL}$$

The amount of potassium chloride needed is 5 mL.

C. Now, determine the amount of potassium phosphate needed.

Identify the variables:
D = 6 mM
H = 3 mM/mL

Then insert the variables into the formula.

$$\text{volume of additive needed (mL)} = \frac{6 \text{ mM}}{3 \text{ mM/mL}}$$

Cancel similar units (like terms) and solve.

$$\frac{6 \text{ mM}}{3 \text{ mM/mL}} = 2 \text{ mL}$$

The amount of potassium phosphate needed is 2 mL.

D. Finally, determine the amount of MVIs needed. (*Note:* Because the prescriber has ordered a specific volume of MVIs for the entire order, you will simply draw up the ordered volume.)

The amount of MVIs needed is 10 mL.

Step 3. Add the volumes of the base solutions calculated in Step 1 and the additives calculated in Step 2.

$$
\begin{array}{r}
429 \text{ mL} \\
700 \text{ mL} \\
500 \text{ mL} \\
10 \text{ mL} \\
5 \text{ mL} \\
2 \text{ mL} \\
+ 10 \text{ mL} \\
\hline
1{,}656 \text{ mL}
\end{array}
$$

Step 4. Determine the amount of SWFI needed to make the total volume of the TPN 2,000 mL. Subtract the total determined in Step 3 (the volume of base solution and additives) from the total volume of the TPN solution.

$$
\begin{array}{r}
2{,}000 \text{ mL} \\
-1{,}656 \text{ mL} \\
\hline
344 \text{ mL}
\end{array}
$$

The amount of sterile water needed is 344 mL.

Step 5. Verify the accuracy of your calculations by adding together all of the volumes. If you have performed each of the calculations correctly, they should equal the total volume ordered by the physician—in this case, 2,000 mL.

$$
\begin{array}{r}
429 \text{ mL} \\
700 \text{ mL} \\
500 \text{ mL} \\
10 \text{ mL} \\
5 \text{ mL} \\
2 \text{ mL} \\
10 \text{ mL} \\
+ 344 \text{ mL} \\
\hline
2{,}000 \text{ mL}
\end{array}
$$

Answer: The TPN requires 429 mL of $D_{70}W$, 700 mL of Aminosyn 10%, 500 mL of Liposyn 20%, 10 mL of sodium chloride, 5 mL of potassium chloride, 2 mL of potassium phosphate, 10 mL of MVIs, and 344 mL of SWFI.

9.5 Problem Set

1. Prepare a special dilution of acyclovir with a total volume of 10 mL and a concentration of 10 mg/mL. To create this special dilution, use a stock solution of acyclovir with a concentration of 100 mg/mL and sterile water. Round your answers to the nearest whole milliliter.

   a. How many milligrams of acyclovir do you need for this special dilution?

   b. How many milliliters of the acyclovir stock solution do you need to draw up for this special dilution?

   c. How many milliliters of SWFI do you need to draw up for this special dilution?

2. Prepare a special dilution of tobramycin with a total volume of 5 mL and a concentration of 10 mg/mL. To create this special dilution, use a stock solution of tobramycin with a concentration of 40 mg/mL and SWFI. Round your answers to the nearest whole milligram or hundredth of a milliliter.

   a. How many milligrams of tobramycin do you need for this special dilution?

   b. How many milliliters of the tobramycin stock solution do you need to draw up for this special dilution?

   c. How many milliliters of sterile water do you need to draw up for this special dilution?

3. Prepare a special dilution of vancomycin with a total volume of 10 mL and a concentration of 10 mg/mL. To create this special dilution, use a stock solution of vancomycin with a concentration of 500 mg/5 mL and SWFI. Round your answers to the nearest whole milligram or milliliter.

   a. How many milligrams of vancomycin do you need for this special dilution?

   b. How many milliliters of the vancomycin stock solution do you need to draw up for this special dilution?

   c. How many milliliters of SWFI do you need to draw up for this special dilution?

4. Prepare a special dilution of dexamethasone with a total volume of 5 mL and a concentration of 1 mg/mL. To create this special dilution, use a stock solution of dexamethasone with a concentration of 4 mg/mL and SWFI. Round your answers to the nearest whole milligram or hundredth of a milliliter.

   a. How many milligrams of dexamethasone do you need for this special dilution?

   b. How many milliliters of the dexamethasone stock solution do you need to draw up for this special dilution?

   c. How many milliliters of SWFI do you need to draw up for this special dilution?

5. Prepare a special dilution of gentamicin with a total volume of 10 mL and a concentration of 1 mg/mL. To create this special dilution, use SWFI and the following gentamicin stock solution. Round your answers to the nearest whole milligram or milliliter.

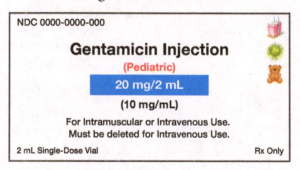

   a. How many milligrams of gentamicin do you need for this special dilution?

   b. How many milliliters of the gentamicin stock solution shown above do you need to draw up for this special dilution?

   c. How many milliliters of SWFI do you need to draw up for this special dilution?

For questions 6–10, determine how much dextrose solution and how much SWFI are needed to make each dilution. Round your answers to the nearest whole milliliter.

6. Prepare 500 mL of $D_{15}W$ using dextrose 70% and SWFI.

7. Prepare 2,000 mL of $D_{10}W$ using dextrose 50% and SWFI.

8. Prepare 1,000 mL of $D_{10}W$ using $D_{50}W$ and SWFI.

9. Prepare 750 mL of D_8W using $D_{50}W$ and SWFI.

10. Prepare 250 mL of $D_{7.5}W$ using $D_{70}W$ and SWFI.

11. Your pharmacy receives the TPN order shown below. Use the TPN order, along with the various pharmacy stock solutions carried by your pharmacy, to determine the volume of each base solution and additive. Round your answers to the nearest hundredth of a milliliter.

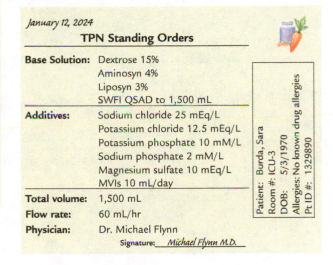

November 9, 2024

TPN Standing Orders

Base Solution: Dextrose 17%
Aminosyn 3%
Liposyn 2.5%
SWFI QSAD to 1,500 mL

Additives: Sodium chloride 20 mEq/L
Potassium chloride 15 mEq/L
Potassium phosphate 10 mM/L
Sodium phosphate 3 mM/L
Magnesium sulfate 10 mEq/L
MVIs 10 mL/day

Patient: McGraw, Tilly
Room #: ICU-15
DOB: 3/26/41
Allergies: Penicillin
Pt. ID #: WWIKKD6773

Total volume: 1,500 mL
Flow rate: 60 mL/hr
Physician: Dr. Serena Martinez
Signature: *Serena Martinez, M.D.*

Your pharmacy carries the following stock solutions:

Dextrose 70%
Aminosyn 10%
Liposyn 20%
Sodium chloride 4 mEq/mL
Potassium chloride 2 mEq/mL
Potassium phosphate 3 mM/mL
Sodium phosphate 3 mM/mL
Magnesium sulfate 4.06 mEq/mL
MVIs10 mL/day

Determine the volume of each of the following components:

a. Dextrose = _____ mL

b. Aminosyn = _____ mL

c. Liposyn = _____ mL

d. Sodium chloride = _____ mL

e. Potassium chloride = _____ mL

f. Potassium phosphate = _____ mL

g. Sodium phosphate = _____ mL

h. Magnesium sulfate = _____ mL

i. MVIs = _____ mL

j. SWFI = _____ mL

k. Total volume = _____ mL

12. Your pharmacy receives the TPN order shown below. Use the TPN order, along with the various pharmacy stock solutions carried by your pharmacy, to determine the volume of each base solution and additive. Round your answers to the nearest hundredth of a milliliter.

January 12, 2024

TPN Standing Orders

Base Solution: Dextrose 15%
Aminosyn 4%
Liposyn 3%
SWFI QSAD to 1,500 mL

Additives: Sodium chloride 25 mEq/L
Potassium chloride 12.5 mEq/L
Potassium phosphate 10 mM/L
Sodium phosphate 2 mM/L
Magnesium sulfate 10 mEq/L
MVIs 10 mL/day

Patient: Burda, Sara
Room #: ICU-3
DOB: 5/3/1970
Allergies: No known drug allergies
Pt ID #: 1329890

Total volume: 1,500 mL
Flow rate: 60 mL/hr
Physician: Dr. Michael Flynn
Signature: *Michael Flynn M.D.*

Your pharmacy carries the following stock solutions:

Dextrose 70%
Aminosyn 10%
Liposyn 20%
Sodium chloride 4 mEq/mL
Potassium chloride 2 mEq/mL
Potassium phosphate 3 mM/mL
Sodium phosphate 3 mM/mL
Magnesium sulfate 4.06 mEq/mL
MVIs 10 mL/day

Determine the volume of each of the following components:

a. Dextrose = _____ mL

b. Aminosyn = _____ mL

c. Liposyn = _____ mL

d. Sodium chloride = _____ mL

e. Potassium chloride = _____ mL

f. Potassium phosphate = _____ mL

g. Sodium phosphate = _____ mL

h. Magnesium sulfate = _____ mL

i. MVIs = _____ mL

j. SWFI = _____ mL

k. Total volume = _____ mL

Self-check your work in Appendix A.

Review and Assessment

CHAPTER SUMMARY

- Solutions are a mixture of solute and solvent.

- Pharmacy practice commonly involves the use of solid-in-liquid (weight-in-volume) solutions and liquid-in-liquid (volume-in-volume) solutions.

- The concentration of a solution can be expressed as a ratio strength or as a percentage strength.

- The concentration of a weight-in-volume solution is expressed in grams of solute per 100 mL of solution.

- The concentration of a volume-in-volume solution is expressed in milliliters of solute per 100 mL of solution.

- In volume-in-volume solutions, the component representing the greater volume is referred to as the *solvent*, and the component representing the smaller volume is referred to as the *solute*.

- IV solutions are administered at a certain rate, which is known as the *flow rate*.

- Flow rate is typically expressed as a volume per hour.

- Flow rate may also be expressed as an amount or dosage of medication per hour, such as milligrams per hour, milliequivalents per hour, or units per hour.

- Special dilutions are used when desired concentrations of a product are not available commercially.

- Special dilutions are made by diluting higher concentrations of commercially available products to a desired lower concentration.

- TPN is compounded from base solutions and additives.

- TPN calculations require multiple steps.

FORMULAS FOR SUCCESS

Ratio Strength of a Weight-in-Volume (w/v) Solution (Section 9.1)

$$\text{ratio strength of a weight-in-volume (w/v) solution} = \frac{x \text{ g of solute}}{100 \text{ mL of solution}}$$

Percentage Strength of a Weight-in-Volume (w/v) Solution (Section 9.1)

$$\text{percentage strength of a weight-in-volume (w/v) solution} = \frac{x \text{ g of solute}}{100 \text{ mL of solution}} \times 100$$

Alternate Percentage Strength of a Weight-in-Volume (w/v) Solution (Section 9.1)

$$\text{percentage strength of a weight-in-volume (w/v) solution} = \frac{x \text{ g of solute}}{y \text{ mL of solution}} \times 100$$

Ratio Strength of a Volume-in-Volume (v/v) Solution (Section 9.2)

$$\text{ratio strength of a volume-in-volume (v/v) solution} = \frac{x \text{ mL of solute}}{100 \text{ mL of solution}} \times 100$$

Percentage Strength of a Volume-in-Volume (v/v) Solution (Section 9.2)

$$\text{percentage strength of a volume-in-volume (v/v) solution} = \frac{x \text{ mL of solute}}{100 \text{ mL of solution}} \times 100$$

Alternate Percentage Strength of a Volume-in-Volume (w/v) Solution (Section 9.1)

$$\text{percentage strength of a volume-in-volume (w/v) solution} = \frac{x \text{ mL of solute}}{y \text{ mL of solution}} \times 100$$

IV Flow Rate and Its Modifications (Section 9.3)

$$\text{flow rate (mL/hr)} = \frac{\text{total volume infused (mL)}}{\text{infusion time (hr)}}$$

$$\text{number of bags needed for a 24-hour period} = \frac{24 \text{ hr}}{\text{length of time one bag lasts (hr/bag)}}$$

$$\text{flow rate (mg/hr)} = \frac{\text{total amount of medication infused (mg)}}{\text{infusion time (hr)}}$$

$$\text{infusion time (hr)} = \frac{\text{total amount of medication infused (mg)}}{\text{flow rate (mg/hr)}}$$

$$\text{flow rate (mEq/hr)} = \frac{\text{total amount of medication infused (mEq)}}{\text{infusion time (hr)}}$$

$$\text{infusion time (hr)} = \frac{\text{total amount of medication infused (mEq)}}{\text{flow rate (mEq/hr)}}$$

$$\text{flow rate (units/hr)} = \frac{\text{total amount of medication infused (units)}}{\text{infusion time (hr)}}$$

$$\text{infusion time (hr)} = \frac{\text{total amount of medication infused (units)}}{\text{flow rate (units/hr)}}$$

IV Flow Rate in Drops per Minute (Section 9.4)

$$\text{IV flow rate or IVFR in Drops per Minute (gtts/min)} = \frac{\text{total volume or TV (mL)}}{\text{infusion time or IT (min)}} \times \text{drop factor or DF (gtts/mL)}$$

Concentration for Milligrams per Drop (Section 9.4)

$$\text{concentration (mg/gtt)} = \frac{\text{concentration (mg/mL)}}{\text{drop factor (gtts/mL)}}$$

Diluent Volume in Special Dilutions (Section 9.5)

$$\text{diluent volume} = \text{total volume (TV)} - \text{drug volume (DV)}$$

Concentrated Solution Volume in Special Dilutions (Section 9.5)

$$\begin{array}{l}\text{volume of concentrated solution needed} \\ \text{for special dilution (mL)}\end{array} = \left(\frac{\text{total volume or TV [mL]}}{\text{concentrated solution percent [\%]}}\right) \times \text{desired percent (\%)}$$

Diluent Volume in Special Dilutions (Section 9.5)

$$\text{diluent volume} = \text{total volume (TV)} - \text{concentrated solution volume}$$

Base Solution Volume in PN Solutions (Section 9.5)

$$\text{volume of base solution (mL)} = \left(\frac{\text{total volume or TV [mL]}}{\text{stock solution percent [\%]}}\right) \times \text{desired percent (\%)}$$

Additives Volume in PN Solutions (Section 9.5)

$$\text{volume of additive needed (mL)} = \frac{\text{desired dose or D}}{\text{concentration on hand or H (per mL)}}$$

CHECK YOUR UNDERSTANDING

Take a moment to review what you have learned in this chapter and answer the following questions.

1. A liquid-in-liquid solution is a solution in which
   a. both the solute and solvent are liquid.
   b. both the solute and solvent are solid.
   c. the solute is liquid and the solvent is solid.
   d. the solute is solid and the solvent is liquid.

2. A pharmacy stocks a 12% weight-in-volume (w/v) solution. Which concentration reflects the components of this solution?
   a. 12 g/100 L
   b. 12 g/100 mL
   c. 12 mL/100 L
   d. 12 mL/100 mL

3. A pharmacy stocks a 0.5% volume-in-volume (v/v) solution. Which concentration reflects the components of this solution?
   a. 0.5 g/100 mL
   b. 0.5 L/100 mL
   c. 0.5 mg/100 mL
   d. 0.5 mL/100 mL

4. How many grams of dextrose are in 1 L of D_5NS?
   a. 5
   b. 50
   c. 0.9
   d. 9

5. What is another term that refers to infusion rate?
   a. concentration rate
   b. dilution rate
   c. flow rate
   d. percentage strength

6. Drop factor related to IV tubing is
   a. the number of drops to produce 1 mL.
   b. the number of drops to produce 100 mL.
   c. the number of milliliters per drop.
   d. the number of milligrams per drop.

7. A prescriber has ordered vancomycin 1 g in 250 mL of 0.45% sodium chloride IVPB. This solution is to be administered over 60 minutes using IV tubing with a drop factor of 10. What is the infusion rate in drops per minute (gtts/min)?
   a. 41 gtts/min
   b. 44 gtts/min
   c. 47 gtts/min
   d. 50 gtts/min

8. Which drop factor is indicative of microdrip tubing?
   a. a drop factor of 10 (10 gtts/mL)
   b. a drop factor of 15 (15 gtts/mL)
   c. a drop factor of 20 (20 gtts/mL)
   d. a drop factor of 60 (60 gtts/mL)

9. Determine the amount of dextrose and sterile water for injection (SWFI) needed to make the following solution: $D_{12}W$ 500 mL using $D_{70}W$ and SWFI.
   a. $D_{70}W$ 85.7 mL; SWFI 414.3 mL
   b. $D_{70}W$ 41.7 mL; SWFI 458.3 mL
   c. $D_{70}W$ 7.1 mL; SWFI 492.9 mL
   d. $D_{70}W$ 1.7 mL; SWFI 498.3 mL

10. Determine the amount of dextrose, Aminosyn (AA), and SWFI needed to make the following solution: TPN solution with D18%, AA 3%, and SWFI QSAD to 2 L. The stock solutions in your pharmacy are as follows: $D_{70}W$ and AA 10%.
    a. $D_{70}W$ 514.3 mL; AA 600 mL; SWFI 885.7 mL
    b. $D_{70}W$ 777.7 mL; AA 666.6 mL; SWFI 555.7 mL
    c. $D_{70}W$ 720 mL; AA 120 mL; SWFI 1,160 mL
    d. $D_{70}W$ 514.3 mL; AA 85.7 mL; SWFI 1,400 mL

FIND SOLUTIONS

Take a moment to consider what you have learned in this chapter and respond thoughtfully to the prompts.

 Scenario A: You have just received the following medication order in the pharmacy. Answer the questions below based on this medication order.

ID#: KU88399			Memorial Hospital
Name: Barker, Wally			
DOB: 10/9/45			
Room: 1018			
Dr: Marshall Rutz, M.D.			Physician's Medication Order

ALLERGY OR SENSITIVITY			DIAGNOSIS	
Bactrim, erythromycin			*hypokalemia*	

DATE	TIME	ORDERS	PHYSICIAN'S SIG.
5/22/2024	1551	*Potassium chloride*	
		20 mEq/L D₅NS	
		@ 125 mL/hr	
			Marshall Rutz, M.D.

1. How many milliequivalents of potassium chloride will the patient receive in 24 hours?

2. How many grams of dextrose will the patient receive in 24 hours?

3. How many grams of sodium chloride (through the NS component) will the patient receive in 24 hours?

 Scenario B: The following IV label is received in the hospital pharmacy. Answer the questions below based on this IV label.

Large-Volume Parenteral
Memorial Hospital

Name: Vaughn, Perry	**Room:** TCU
Pt. ID#: YHYTELLL	**Rx#:** 2299388

Aminophylline 1 g
D₅W 500 mL
Rate: 20 mL/hr

Keep refrigerated. Warm to room temperature before use.

BUD _____ Tech _____ RPh _____

4. How many grams of dextrose will the patient receive in 24 hours?

5. How many milligrams of aminophylline will the patient receive in 24 hours?

6. How many milliliters of fluid will the patient receive in 24 hours?

Scenario C: A physician has prescribed the following order. Answer the questions below based on this medication order.

ID#: LK9968811687			Memorial Hospital
Name: Brzyznski, Martha			
DOB: 1/9/48			
Room: 588			Physician's Medication Order
Dr: Amarite Gaya, M.D.			

ALLERGY OR SENSITIVITY			DIAGNOSIS	
penicillins			*cellulitis*	

DATE	TIME	ORDERS	PHYSICIAN'S SIG.
5/20/2024	1551	*Vancomycin 1,500 mg*	
		in 500 mL	
		D₅W IV q12h	
			Amarite Gaya, M.D.

7. A reconstituted vial of vancomycin contains 500 mg/5 mL. How many vials will be needed to prepare the order?

8. What is the percentage strength of vancomycin?

9. The maximum concentration of vancomycin should not exceed 5 mg/mL. Is the ordered concentration appropriate?

10. The recommended infusion time for vancomycin is at least 30 minutes for every 500 mg administered to prevent infusion-related reactions. What is the minimum infusion time for this order?

Scenario D: A physician has prescribed the following order. Answer the questions below based on this medication order. Amiodarone is available in a premixed 450 mg/250 mL solution in the pharmacy.

ID#: SU8447864494			Memorial Hospital
Name: Lazaar, Howard			
DOB: 10/20/50			
Room: 1547			Physician's Medication Order
Dr: Jeremiah King, M.D.			
ALLERGY OR SENSITIVITY		**DIAGNOSIS**	
no known allergies		*atrial fibrillation*	
DATE	TIME	ORDERS	PHYSICIAN'S SIG.
5/22/2024	1531	Amiodarone 0.5 mg/min IV	
		x 18 hr	
			Jeremiah King, M.D.

11. What is the flow rate in milliliters per hour (mL/hr)?

12. If a 15-drop set is being used, what is the flow rate in drops per minute (gtts/min)?

13. How many IV bags will be needed to fulfill the order?

14. If the order was started at 1800, when will the patient need a new IV bag hung?

Scenario E: The following TPN label was received in the inpatient pharmacy. Answer the accompanying questions based on this label. Round your answers to the nearest tenth of a milliliter.

TPN Solution
Memorial Hospital

Name: Burge, April   **Room:** 2284
Pt. ID#: HHUSY0068   **Rx#:** 7728829

Dextrose 15%
Aminosyn 5%
Liposyn 2.5%
SWFI QSAD
Sodium chloride 10 mEq/L
Potassium chloride 10 mEq/L
Magnesium sulfate 2.5 mEq/L
Regular insulin 20 units/L
MVIs 10 mL/day

Flow Rate: 150 mL/hr

Keep refrigerated. Warm to room temperature before use.

BUD _____ Tech _____ RPh _____

Pharmacy Stock Solutions:

$D_{70}W$

Aminosyn 10%

Liposyn 10%

Sodium chloride 4 mEq/mL

Potassium chloride 2 mEq/mL

Magnesium sulfate 4.06 mEq/mL

Regular insulin 100 units/mL

MVIs 10 mL/day

---

15. The TPN flow rate is 150 mL/hr. What is the total volume needed for 24 hours? (*Note:* This volume will be the TPN total volume—the QSAD amount that should be used to determine the SWFI volume.)

16. How much dextrose will you need to make this compound?

17. How much Aminosyn will you need?

18. How much Liposyn will you need?

19. How much sodium chloride will you need?

20. How much potassium chloride will you need?

21. How much magnesium sulfate will you need?

22. How much regular insulin will you need?

23. How much MVIs will you need?

24. How much SWFI will you need?

The online course includes additional review and assessment resources.

Problem Set and Find Solutions Answers

Chapter 1

1.1 Problem Set

1. 10

2. 5

3. 624

   Work:

   $$624 = \frac{\underset{500}{D} + \underset{100}{C} + \underset{10}{X} + \underset{10}{X} + \underset{(5-1)}{IV}}{} = 624$$

4. 2,050

   Work:

   $$2{,}050 = \frac{\underset{1{,}000}{M} + \underset{1{,}000}{M} + \underset{50}{L}}{} = 2{,}050$$

5. 48

   Work:

   $$48 = \frac{\underset{(50-10)}{XL} + \underset{5}{V} + \underset{1}{I} + \underset{1}{I} + \underset{1}{I}}{} = 48$$

6. XVII

   Work:

   $$17 = \frac{10 + 5 + 1 + 1}{X \quad V \quad I \quad I}$$

7. LXVII

   Work:

   $$67 = \frac{50 + 10 + 5 + 1 + 1}{L \quad X \quad V \quad I \quad I}$$

8. MCMXCV

   Work:

   $$1{,}995 = \frac{1{,}000 + (1{,}000 - 100) + (100 - 10) + 5}{M \qquad CM \qquad XC \qquad V}$$

9. XIII

   Work:

   $$13 = \frac{10 + 1 + 1 + 1}{X \quad I \quad I \quad I}$$

10. CCCXXVII

    Work:

    $$327 = \frac{100 + 100 + 100 + 10 + 10 + 5 + 1 + 1}{C \quad C \quad C \quad X \quad X \quad V \quad I \quad I}$$

11. XC

    Work:

    $$90 = 100 - 10 = XC$$

12. LXXV

    Work:

    $$75 = \frac{50 + 10 + 10 + 5}{L \quad X \quad X \quad V}$$

13. 26.5

Work:

$$\frac{\text{VIIss} + \text{XV} + \text{IV}}{7.5 + 15 + 4} = 26.5$$

14. 28

Work:

$$\frac{\text{XLVII} - \text{XIX}}{47 - 19} = 28$$

15. 68

Work:

$$\frac{\text{XVII} \times \text{IV}}{17 \times 4} = 28$$

16. 14

Work:

$$\frac{\text{XLII} \div \text{III}}{42 \div 3} = 14$$

17. 7.5 tablets

Work: VIIss = 5 + 1 + 1 + ½ = 7.5 tablets

18. a. 10 grains

b. 1 tablet daily (10 grains)

c. 100 tablets

19. a. 1 tablet

b. 9 days

Work: XXVII = 10 + 10 + 5 + 1 + 1 = 27 tablets/3 tablets per day = 9 days

20. a. 5 tablets daily

Work: 2 tablets (in am) + 1 tablet (at lunch) + 2 tablets (at dinner)

b. 150 tablets

Work: CL = 100 + 50 = 150

1.2 Problem Set

1. 1

2. 2

3. 5

4. 15

5. 20

6. 3

7. 5

8. 4

9. 12

10. 100

11. ½

12. ⅜

13. $^9/_{10}$

14. $^{15}/_{15}$

15. ⅘

16. $^2/_1$

17. $^2/_6$

18. $^1/_{10}$

19. ¼

20. $^1/_{15}$

21. $^6/_6$, or 1

22. $^8/_{10}$, or ⅘

23. $^{79}/_{100}$

24. 1 $^{14}/_{15}$

Work: *Solution 1.*

Step 1. Create common denominators:

$^5/_6 \times {}^{10}/_{10} = {}^{50}/_{60}$, $^7/_{10} \times {}^6/_6 = {}^{42}/_{60}$, $^2/_6 \times {}^{12}/_{12} = {}^{24}/_{60}$

Step 2. Add the numerators:

$^{50}/_{60} + {}^{42}/_{60} + {}^{24}/_{60} = {}^{116}/_{60}$

Step 3. Simplify:

$^{116}/_{60} = {}^{156}/_{60} = 1\ {}^{14}/_{15}$

Solution 2.

Step 1. Create common denominators:

$^5/_6 \times {}^5/_5 = {}^{25}/_{30}$, $^7/_{10} \times {}^3/_3 = {}^{21}/_{30}$, $^2/_5 \times {}^6/_6 = {}^{12}/_{30}$

Step 2. Add the numerators:

$^{25}/_{30} + {}^{21}/_{30} + {}^{12}/_{30} = {}^{58}/_{30}$

Step 3. Simplify:

$^{58}/_{30} = {}^{29}/_{15} = 1\ {}^{14}/_{15}$

25. $1 \frac{37}{96}$

   Work: Step 1. Create common denominators:

   $\frac{21}{32} \times \frac{3}{3} = \frac{63}{96}$, $\frac{1}{12} \times \frac{8}{8} = \frac{8}{96}$, $\frac{31}{48} \times \frac{2}{2} = \frac{62}{96}$

   Step 2. Add the numerators:

   $\frac{63}{96} + \frac{8}{96} + \frac{62}{96} = \frac{133}{96}$

   Step 3. Simplify:

   $\frac{113}{96} = 1 \frac{37}{96}$

26. $\frac{6}{10}$, reduced to $\frac{3}{5}$

27. $\frac{12}{50}$, reduced to $\frac{6}{25}$

28. $\frac{24}{100}$, reduced to $\frac{6}{25}$

29. $\frac{84}{100}$, reduced to $\frac{21}{25}$

   Work: Step 1. Create common denominators:

   $\frac{9}{10} \times \frac{10}{10} = \frac{90}{100}$

   $\frac{1}{25} \times \frac{4}{4} = \frac{4}{100}$

   $\frac{2}{100}$

   Step 2. Subtract the numerators:

   $\frac{90}{100} - \frac{4}{100} - \frac{2}{100} = \frac{84}{100}$, reduced to $\frac{21}{25}$

30. $\frac{14}{50}$, reduced to $\frac{7}{25}$

   Work: Step 1. Create common denominators:

   $\frac{3}{5} \times \frac{10}{10} = \frac{30}{50}$

   $\frac{2}{50}$

   $\frac{7}{25} \times \frac{2}{2} = \frac{14}{50}$

   Step 2. Subtract the numerators:

   $\frac{30}{50} - \frac{2}{50} - \frac{14}{50} = \frac{14}{50}$, reduced to $\frac{7}{25}$

31. $\frac{1}{4}$

32. $6 \frac{7}{10}$

33. $2 \frac{1}{5}$

34. $\frac{9}{10}$

35. $\frac{2}{5}$

36. $\frac{9}{10}$

37. 3 tablets

   Work Step 1. Create common denominators:

   $\frac{1}{4}$ tablets, $\frac{1}{2}$ tablets $\times \frac{2}{2} = \frac{2}{4}$ tablets, $1 \frac{1}{2}$ tablets $= \frac{3}{2}$ tablets $\times \frac{2}{2} = \frac{6}{4}$ tablets, $\frac{3}{4}$ tablets

   Step 2. Add the numerators:

   $\frac{1}{4}$ tablets $+ \frac{2}{4}$ tablets $+ \frac{6}{4}$ tablets $+ \frac{3}{4}$ tablets $= \frac{12}{4}$ tablets

   Step 3. Simplify:

   $\frac{12}{4}$ tablets = 3 tablets

38. 2 tablets containing $\frac{1}{100}$ grain in each tablet

   Work: $2 \times \frac{1}{100}$ grain $= \frac{2}{100}$ grain $= \frac{1}{50}$ grain

   Because the denominator is smaller, $\frac{1}{50}$ grain $> \frac{1}{150}$ grain

39. 1,500 containers

   Work: 375 grains $\times$ 1 unit dose/1⁄4 grain $= 375 \times 4 = 1,500$ containers

40. 17 bags

   Work: Step 1. Create common denominators:

   $\frac{1}{2}$ lb $\times \frac{10}{10} = \frac{10}{20}$ lb, $\frac{4}{5}$ lb $\times \frac{4}{4} = \frac{16}{20}$ lb, $\frac{1}{4}$ lb $\times \frac{5}{5} = \frac{5}{20}$ lb, $2 \frac{1}{2}$ lb $= \frac{5}{2}$ lb $\times \frac{10}{10} = \frac{50}{20}$ lb

   Step 2. Add the numerators:

   $\frac{10}{20}$ lb $+ \frac{16}{20}$ lb $+ \frac{5}{20}$ lb $+ \frac{50}{20}$ lb $= \frac{81}{20}$ lb

   Step 3. Simplify:

   $\frac{81}{20}$ lb $= 4 \frac{1}{20}$ lb sugar needed

   Sugar is sold in bags of 2 lb/bag; 2 bags would = 4 lb sugar ($2 \times$ 2lb = 4lb), and we need $\frac{1}{20}$ lb more than that, so 3 bags are needed.

41. 1 bag

   Work: Since we need $4 \frac{1}{20}$ lb sugar (problem 40), one 5 lb bag will provide the sugar needed.

1.3 Problem Set

1. 784.36
2. 0.9
3. 0.2

   Work: $\frac{1}{5} = 1 \div 5 = 0.2$

4. 0.05

   Work: $\frac{1}{20} = 1 \div 20 = 0.05$

5. 4.5

   Work: $4\frac{2}{4} = \frac{18}{4} = 18 \div 4 = 4.5$ or $4\frac{2}{4} = 4\frac{1}{2} = \frac{9}{2} = 4.5$

6. 0.3

   Work: $\frac{30}{100} = 30 \div 100 = 0.3$

7. 0.005

   Work: $\frac{1}{200} = 1 \div 200 = 0.005$

8. 0.002

   Work: $\frac{1}{500} = 1 \div 500 = 0.002$

9. 1.8

   Work: $1\frac{8}{10} = \frac{18}{10} = 18 \div 10 = 1.8$ or $1\frac{8}{10} = 1\frac{4}{5} = \frac{9}{5} = 9 \div 5 = 1.8$

10. 0.04

    Work: $\frac{1}{25} = 1 \div 25 = 0.04$

11. 0.008

    Work: $\frac{1}{125} = 1 \div 125 = 0.008$

12. 4.1
13. 0.6

    Rationale: 0.50 0.56 0.60

14. 2.02

    Rationale: 2.02 2.12 2.10

15. 0.017

    Rationale: 0.160 0.167 0.017

16. 0
17. 6
18. 4
19. hundreds
20. hundredths
21. thousandths
22. ones
23. tenths
24. 1.88
25. 2.729
26. 14.373
27. 3.0983
28. 11.998
29. 467.42
30. 450
31. 1.846
32. 1.333
33. 3.87
34. 0.14
35. 0.08
36. 0.196
37. 0.049
38. 34.9
39. 1.4
40. a. 0.75 mg/dose

    Work: 3 tablets/dose × 0.25 mg/tablet = 0.75 mg/dose

    b. 2.25 mg/day

    Work: 0.75 mg/dose × 3 doses/day = 2.25 mg/day

    c. 126 tablets

    Work: 3 tablets/dose × 3 doses/day × 14 days = 126 tablets

    d. no; the patient will need 26 more tablets

    Work: 126 tablets − 100 tablets = 26 tablets

    e. alprazolam 0.25 mg 100 tablets/$14.95

    Work: $14.95 + $7.59 = $22.54

41. a. 1 mg/dose

    Work: 0.25 mg/tablet × 4 tablets/dose = 1 mg/dose

b. $21.825, rounded to $21.83

   Work: $17.46 × 1.25 = $21.825, rounded to $21.83

c. $11.935, rounded to $11.94

   Work: $23.87 × 0.5 = $11.935, rounded to $11.94

d. 16.7, or 16 full days

   Work: 50 tablets × 1 day/3 tablets = 16.7, or 16 full days

42. a. 8.33 bottles, rounded to 8 bottles

   Work: 1,000 mL × 1 bottle/120 mL = 8.33 bottles, rounded to 8 bottles

   b. 40 mL

   Work: 120 mL/bottle × 8 bottles = 960 mL; 1,000 mL − 960 mL = 40 mL

43. 91.5 mL, rounded to 92 mL

   Work: 8.5 mL/dose × 2 doses/day × 2 days = 34 mL; 5.75 mL/dose × 2 doses/day × 5 days = 57.5 mL; 34 mL + 57.5 mL = 91.5 mL, rounded to 92 mL

44. a. $47   b. $15   c. $4

45. a. $70.08

   b. $111.64

46. a. 0.89

   b. 0.85

   c. 0.92

1.4 Problem Set

1. 68,000 (move decimal point 4 places to the right)

2. 1,870,000 (move decimal point 6 places to the right)

3. 10,300,000 (move decimal point 7 places to the right)

4. 0.00084 (move decimal point 4 places to the left)

5. 0.00768 (move decimal point 3 places to the left)

6. 0.00006239 (move decimal point 5 places to the left)

7. $3.29 × 10^{-9}$

8. $3.9 × 10^{11}$

9. $3.8 × 10^{-3}$

10. $5.2 × 10^{16}$

11. $3.779 × 10^{6}$

12. $2.02 × 10^{-10}$

13. 6

14. 2

15. 2

16. 3

17. 1

18. 4

19. 3

20. 1

21. 8

22. 1

23. 42.8

24. 10.1

25. 0.0427

26. 18.4

27. 0.00392

28. 0.35; 2 significant figures

29. 0.06; 1 significant figure

30. 1.99; 3 significant figures

31. 0.01; 1 significant figure

32. 1.03; 3 significant figures

33. 64

34. 30

35. 163

36. a. 1.784 g, which should be rounded to 1.78 g

   b. 3.2 g

   c. 0.06 g

   Work: 3.2 g + 1.78 g + 2.46 g + 5.87 g = 13.31 g; 13.31 g/0.125 g = 106.48 capsules; 0.48 of a capsule × 0.125 g = 0.06 g

37. a. 21.65 mg × 45 doses = 974.25 mg

   b. 5 significant figures

1.5 Problem Set

1. estimated value: $7; actual value: $6.38

2. estimated value: $12; actual value: $12.25

3. estimated value: $5; actual value: $5.19

4. estimated value: $82; actual value: $81.71

5. estimated value: $50; actual value: $50.58

6. estimated product: 56,000; actual product: 52,060.8

7. estimated product: 1,400; actual product: 1,407.3

8. estimated product: 9; actual product: 8.976

   Work: Round 598.4 to 600 and round 0.015 to 15, ignoring the 3 decimals. Multiply the rounded numbers: 600 × 15 = 9,000. Replace the three decimals. Estimated product: 9; actual product: 8.976

9. estimated product: 500; actual product: 444.1068

   Work: Round 4,569 to 5,000 and round 0.0972 to 1, ignoring the one decimal. Multiply the rounded numbers: 5,000 × 1 = 5,000. Replace the one decimal. Estimated product: 500; actual product: 444.1068

10. estimated product: 120,000; actual product: 111,294

11. estimated product: 9,000; actual product: 11,402.3

12. estimated quotient: 10; actual quotient: 10.28

13. estimated quotient: 300; actual quotient: 321.70

14. estimated quotient: 75; actual quotient: 73

15. estimated quotient: 200; actual quotient: 191.87

16. estimated quotient: 10; actual quotient: 8.79

17. estimated cost: $19; actual cost: $19.10

   Work: (food dye, $2 cost estimate) + (sugar, $8 cost estimate) + (baking soda, $1 cost estimate) + cherry flavoring, $2 cost estimate) + (bleach, $2 cost estimate) + (distilled water, $4 cost estimate) = $19 cost estimate; actual cost: $19.10

18. estimated SWFI 17 mL; 30 mL vial

   Work: 3 mL + 8 mL + 2 mL + 4 mL = 17 mL. Therefore, the 30 mL vial is needed.

19. estimated fluid intake: 2,000 mL

   Work: 1,720 mL IV fluids + 150 mL juice + 130 mL coffee = 2,000 mL

20. estimated parenteral fluid intake: 4,300 mL

   Work: 800 mL + 200 mL + 300 mL + 3,000 mL = 4,300 mL

Chapter 1 Find Solutions

1. 1 tablet

2. estimated number of tablets: 40-45

3. 47 tablets

4. 2,000 mg

   Work: 4 tablets × 500 mg/tablet = 2,000 mg

5. 250 mg

   Work: 0.5 tablet × 500 mg/tablet = 250 mg

6. 2,250 mg

   Work: 2,000 mg + 250 mg = 2,250 mg

7. 3½ tablets

   Work: 4,000 mg – 2,250 mg = 1,750 mg; 1,750 mg × 1 tablet/500 mg = 31/2 tablets

8. The dosing spoon should be filled to ¾ tsp or 3.75 mL.

9. ½ tablet

10. 1 tablet

11. 2.5 mg

   Work: 5 mg/tablet × ½ tablet = 2.5 mg

12. 21 tablets

13. 4 tablets

   Work: 1 tablet/dose × 4 doses/week = 4 tablets

14. 0.500 mg

   Work: 125 mcg/tablet × 4 tablets/week = 500 mcg = 0.500 mg

15. 51 tablets

16. 17 tablets

Chapter 2

2.1 Problem Set

1. $\frac{3}{7}$

2. $\frac{8}{6} = \frac{4}{3} = 1\frac{1}{3}$

3. $\frac{3}{4}$

4. $\frac{4}{6} = \frac{2}{3}$

5. $\frac{1}{7}$

6. 2:3

7. 6:8 = 3:4

8. 5:10 = 1:2

9. 1:9

10. 1:10,000

11. 30 mg:1 capsule or 1 capsule:30 mg

12. 100 mg:1 capsule or 1 capsule:100 mg

13. 250 mg:5 mL or 5 mL:250 mg

14. 90 mg/3 capsules

    Work: x mg/3 capsules = 30 mg/1 capsule;
    x mg = 90 mg

15. 200 mg/2 capsules

    Work: x mg/2 capsules = 100 mg/1 capsule;
    x mg = 200 mg

16. 750 mg/15 mL

    Work: x mg/15 mL = 250 mg/5 mL;
    x mg = 750 mg

17. 10 g; 1,000 mL; 1 g

    Work: x g/100 mL = 10 g/1,000 mL; x = 1 g

18. 1 g, 100 mL, 5 g

    Work: x g/500 mL = 1 g/100 mL; x = 5 g

19. 1 g, 250 mL, 4 g

    Work: x g/1,000 mL = 1 g/250 mL; x = 4 g

20. 1 g; 1,000 mL; 0.05 g

    Work: x g/50 mL = 1 g/1,000 mL; x = 0.05 g

2.2 Problem Set

1. 86%

   Work: $\frac{6}{7}$ = 0.857, rounded to 0.86;
   0.86 $\times$ 100 = 86%

2. 42%

   Work: $\frac{5}{12}$ = 0.416, rounded to 0.42;
   0.42 $\times$ 100 = 42%

3. 25%

   Work: $\frac{1}{4}$ = 0.25; 0.25 $\times$ 100 = 25%

4. 67%

   Work: $\frac{2}{3}$ = 0.666, rounded to 0.67;
   0.67 $\times$ 100 = 67%

5. 5%

   Work: $\frac{0.5}{10}$ = 0.05; 0.05 $\times$ 100 = 5%

6. 66.7%

   Work: $\frac{2}{3}$ = 0.6667, rounded to 0.667;
   0.667 $\times$ 100 = 66.7%

7. 32.3%

   Work: $\frac{1.5}{4.65}$ = 0.3225, rounded to 0.323;
   0.323 $\times$ 100 = 32.3%

8. 0.4%

   Work: $\frac{1}{250}$ = 0.004; 0.004 $\times$ 100 = 0.4%

9. 0.0%

   Work: $\frac{1}{10,000}$ = 0.0001, rounded to 0.000;
   0.000 $\times$ 100 = 0.0%

10. 16.7%

    Work: $\frac{1}{6}$ = 0.1666, rounded to 0.167;
    0.167 $\times$ 100 = 16.7%

11. 50% = $\frac{50}{100}$ = $\frac{5}{10}$ = $\frac{1}{2}$

12. 2% = $\frac{2}{100}$ = $\frac{1}{50}$

13. 6% = $\frac{6}{100}$ = 0.06

14. 12.5% = $\frac{126}{100}$ = 0.125

15. 126% = $\frac{126}{100}$ = 1.26

16. 20 $\times$ 0.05 = 1

17. 60 $\times$ 0.20 = 12

18. 63 $\times$ 0.19 = 11.97

19. 70 $\times$ 1.10 = 77

20. 50 $\times$ 0.002 = 0.1

21. 1:3, 0.33

22. $\frac{1}{40}$, 0.025

23. 50%, 1:2

24. 1%, $\frac{1}{100}$

25. $^9/_{10}$, 9:10

26. $^2/_3$ or $^{67}/_{100}$; 2:3 or 67:100

27. 0.2%, 0.002

28. $^{0.09}/_{20}$ or $^9/_{2,000}$, 0.09:20 or 9:2,000

29. $^1/_{20}$, 0.05

30. 1:5, 0.2

31. 0.01% solution

Work: $^1/_{10,000} = 0.0001 \times 100 = 0.01\%$ solution

32. 5% solution

Work: $^1/_{20} = 0.05 \times 100 = 5\%$ solution

33. 4% solution

Work: $^1/_{25} = 0.04 \times 100 = 4\%$ solution

34. 0.125% solution

Work: $^1/_{800} = 0.00125 \times 100 = 0.125\%$ solution

35. 10% solution

Work: $^1/_{10} = 0.1 \times 100 = 10\%$ solution

2.3 Problem Set

1. 5

2. 0.07843, rounded to 0.08

3. 4.5

4. 0.1

5. 0.16

6. 5.7692, rounded to 5.77

7. 54.4

8. 242.6666, rounded to 242.67

9. 25.9411, rounded to 25.94

10. 16

11. 44.3571, rounded to 44.36

12. 21.3870, rounded to 21.39

13. 78.3333, rounded to 78.33

14. 10.7307, rounded to 10.73

15. 77.3636, rounded to 77.36

16. 28.35%

Work: $x\%/100 = 72\%/254$; $x = 28.3464\%$, rounded to 28.35%

17. 48.89

Work: $x/100\% = 44/90\%$; $x = 48.8888$, rounded to 48.89

18. 227.27

Work: $x/100\% = 100/44\%$; $x = 227.2727$, rounded to 227.27

19. 121.43

Work: $x/100\% = 34/28\%$; $x = 121.4285$, rounded to 121.43

20. 54.44%

Work: $x\%/100 = 24.5\%/45$; $x = 54.4444\%$, rounded to 54.44%

21. 0.1 g

Work: x g/100 mg = 1 g/1,000 mg; $x = 0.1$ g

22. 0.247 g

Work: x g/247 mg = 1 g/1,000 mg; $x = 0.247$ g

23. 1.42 g

Work: x g/1,420 mg = 1 g/1,000 mg; $x = 1.42$ g

24. 0.495 g

Work: x g/495 mg = 1 g/1,000 mg; $x = 0.495$ g

25. 3.781 g

Work: x g/3,781 mg = 1 g/1,000 mg; $x = 3.781$ g

26. 349 mg

Work: x mg/0.349 g = 1,000 mg/1 g; $x = 349$ mg

27. 1,500 mg

Work: x mg/1.5 g = 1,000 mg/1 g; $x = 1,500$ mg

28. 83 mg

Work: x mg/0.083 g = 1,000 mg/1 g; $x = 83$ mg

29. 10 mg

Work: x mg/0.01 g = 1,000 mg/1 g; $x = 10$ mg

30. 2,100 mg

Work: x mg/2.1 g = 1,000 mg/1 g; $x = 2,100$ mg

31. 2.9 kg

Work: x kg/6.3 lb = 1 kg/2.2 lb; x = 2.863 kg, rounded to 2.9 kg

32. 6.8 kg

Work: x kg/15 lb = 1 kg/2.2 lb; x = 6.818 kg, rounded to 6.8 kg

33. 44.1 kg

Work: x kg/97 lb = 1 kg/2.2 lb; x = 44.090 kg, rounded to 44.1 kg

34. 52.3 kg

Work: x kg/115 lb = 1 kg/2.2 lb; x = 52.272 kg, rounded to 52.3 kg

35. 84.5 kg

Work: x kg/186 lb = 1 kg/2.2 lb; x = 84.545 kg, rounded to 84.5 kg

36. 16.5 lb

Work: x lb/7.5 kg = 2.2 lb/1 kg; x = 16.5 lb

37. 7.9 lb

Work: x lb/3.6 kg = 2.2 lb/1 kg; x = 7.92 lb, rounded to 7.9 lb

38. 174.2 lb

Work: x lb/79.2 kg = 2.2 lb/1 kg; x = 174.24 lb, rounded to 174.2 lb

39. 198 lb

Work: x lb/90 kg = 2.2 lb/1 kg; x = 198 lb

40. 1.1 lb

Work: x lb/0.5 kg = 2.2 lb/1 kg; x = 1.1 lb

41. 2 mL

Work: x mL/100 mg = 1 mL/50 mg; x = 2 mL

42. 3 tablets

Work: x tablets/375 mg = 1 tablet/125 mg; x = 3 tablets

43. 15 mL

Work: x mL/300 mg = 1 mL/20 mg; x = 15 mL

44. 2 boxes of 100 folders

Work: x boxes/$15.00 = 1 box/$7.40; x = 2.027 boxes, rounded to 2 boxes of 100 folders

45. 0.6 mL

Work: x mL/10,000 units = 15 mL/250,000 units; x = 0.6 mL

46. 3 mL

Work: x mL/30 mg = 2 mL/20 mg; x = 3 mL

47. 6 mL

Work: x mL/60 mg = 4 mL/40 mg; x = 6 mL

48. 6 mL

Work: x mL/300 mg = 10 mL/500 mg; x = 6 mL

49. 6 mL

Work: x mL/30 mg = 1 mL/5 mg; x = 6 mL

50. 1.5 mL

Work: x mL/30 mg = 1 mL/20 mg; x = 1.5 mL

51. 50 mg

Work: x mg/5 mL = 20 mg/2 mL; x = 50 mg

52. 8 mL

Work: x mL/80 mg = 2 mL/20 mg; x = 8 mL

53. 5 mL

Work: x mL/50 mg = 2 mL/20 mg; x = 5 mL

54. 1.25 mL

Work: x mL/12.5 mg = 2 mL/20 mg; x = 1.25 mL

55. 35 mg

Work: x mg/3.5 mL = 20 mg/2 mL; x = 35 mg

2.4 Problem Set

1. 2.16%

Work: 189 mg − 185 mg = 4 mg; (4 mg/185 mg) × 100 = 2.162%, rounded to 2.16%

2. 4.8%

Work: 500 mg − 476 mg = 24 mg; (24 mg/500 mg) × 100 = 4.8%

3. 25.58%

Work: 1,507 mg − 1,200 mg = 307 mg; (307 mg/1,200 mg) × 100 = 25.583%, rounded to 25.58%

4. 16.67%

   Work: 15 mg − 12.5 mg = 2.5 mg;
   (2.5 mg/15 mg) × 100 = 16.666%,
   rounded to 16.67%

5. 3.75%

   Work: 415 mcg − 400 mcg = 15 mcg;
   (15 mcg/400 mcg) × 100 = 3.75%

6. 26%

   Work: 6.3 mL − 5 mL = 1.3 mL;
   (1.3 mL/5 mL) × 100 = 26%

7. 13.33%

   Work: 15 mL − 13 mL = 2 mL;
   (2 mL/15 mL) × 100 = 13.333%,
   rounded to 13.33%

8. 33.33%

   Work: 20 mL − 15 mL = 5 mL; (5 mL/15 mL)
   × 100 = 33.333%, rounded to 33.33%

9. 3.33%

   Work: 1.5 L − 1.45 L = 0.05 L; (0.05 L/1.5 L)
   × 100 = 3.333%, rounded to 3.33%

10. 3.71%

    Work: 726 mL − 700 mL = 26 mL;
    (26 mL/700 mL) × 100 = 3.714%,
    rounded to 3.71%

11. No. 0.4/3 = 13.3%

12. No. 0.4/12.5 = 3.2%

13. No. 0.3/1.8 = 16.7%

14. Yes. 0.09/3.2 = 2.8%

15. Yes. 1/150 = 0.7%

16. Yes. 8/200 = 4%

17. Yes. 1.5/30 = 5%

18. Yes. 4/454 = 0.9%

19. 199 mL to 201 mL

    Work: 200 mL × 0.005 = 1 mL;
    200 mL − 1 mL = 199 mL;
    200 mL + 1 mL = 201 mL; the acceptable
    range is 199 mL to 201 mL

20. 10.22 mL to 10.38 mL

    Work: 10.3 mL × 0.0075 = 0.07725 mL,
    rounded to 0.08 mL; 10.3 mL − 0.08 mL =

10.22 mL; 10.3 mL + 0.08 mL = 10.38 mL;
the acceptable range is 10.22 mL to 10.38 mL

21. 813.4 mL to 846.6 mL

    Work: 830 mL × 0.02 = 16.6 mL;
    830 mL − 16.6 mL = 813.4 mL;
    830 mL + 16.6 mL = 846.6 mL; the
    acceptable range is 813.4 mL to 846.6 mL

22. 17.97 g to 18.03 g

    Work: 18 g × 0.0015 = 0.027 g, rounded to
    0.03 g; 18 g − 0.03 g = 17.97 g;
    18 g + 0.03 g = 18.03 g; the acceptable
    range is 17.97 g to 18.03 g

23. 747 mg to 753 mg

    Work: 750 mg × 0.004 = 3 mg;
    750 mg − 3 mg = 747 mg; 750 mg + 3 mg
    = 753 mg; the acceptable range is 747 mg
    to 753 mg

24. 80 mg to 120 mg

    Work: 100 mg × 0.2 = 20 mg; so the range
    of accuracy is 80 mg (100 mg − 20 mg) to
    120 mg (100 mg + 20 mg)

25. 440 mg to 560 mg

    Work: 500 mg × 0.12 = 60 mg; so the
    range of vitamin C contained in the tablet
    is 440 mg (500 mg − 60 mg) to 560 mg
    (500 mg + 60 mg)

Chapter 2 Find Solutions

1. The dosing cup is the correct measuring
   device and should be filled to the 20 mL
   graduation mark.

   Work: 50 mg/x mL = 12.5 mg/5 mL;
   50 mg(5 mL) = 12.5 mg(x mL); x = 20 mL

2. 180 mL

   Work: 20 mL/dose(3 doses/day) =
   60 mL/day; 60 mL/day(3 days) = 180 mL

3. 2 bottles

   Work: 180 mL/120 mL/bottle = 1.5 bottles;
   rounded up to 2 whole bottles

4. 4.3 kg

   Work: x kg/9.5 lb = 1 kg/2.2 lb;
   x kg(2.2 lb) = 1 kg(9.5 lb); x = 4.3 kg

5. 1 mL

   Work: 25 mg/x mL = 125 mg/5 mL;
   x mL (125 mg) = 5 mL (25 mg); x = 1 mL

6. 2 mL

   Work: 50 mg/x mL = 25 mg/1 mL; x = 2 mL

7. 20 mL

   Work: 500 mg/x mL = 50 mg/2 mL;
   x = 20 mL

8. 250 mg/10 mL

9. 4%

   Work: error of measurement = 50 mL −
   48 mL = 2 mL; percentage of error =
   (2 mL/50 mL) × 100 = 4%

10. Yes

Chapter 3

3.1 Problem Set

1. The DEA number does not meet standard validity tests. The practice identifier J is not an appropriate initial letter for the DEA number of a medical doctor. Checksum calculation: 2 + 6 + 8 = 16; (1 + 9 + 7) × 2 = 34; 16 + 34 = 50; last digit of checksum matches check digit (0).

2. The DEA number meets standard validity tests. The practice identifier M is appropriate for a mid-level practitioner; the letter G is the first letter of the prescriber's last name. Checksum calculation: 3 + 8 + 6 = 17; (0 + 1 + 5) × 2 = 12; 17 + 12 = 29; last digit of checksum matches check digit (9).

3. The DEA number does not meet standard validity tests. The practice identifier B is an appropriate initial letter for the DEA number of a primary practitioner. The letter H is not the first letter of the prescriber's last name; however, the prescriber's last name may have changed. Checksum calculation: 9 + 9 + 0 = 18; (9 + 8 + 7) × 2 = 48; 18 + 48 = 66; last digit of check sum (6) does not match check digit (0).

4. The DEA number does not meet standard validity tests. The practice identifier A is an appropriate initial letter for the DEA number of a primary practitioner; the

letter L is the first letter of the prescriber's last name. Checksum calculation: 6 + 3 + 6 = 15; (2 + 0 + 1) × 2 = 6; 15 + 6 = 21; last digit of check sum (1) does not match check digit (8).

5. The letter check does not match; however, the DEA checksum matches. The second letter (D) of the DEA number does not match the first letter of the physician's last name (C). This discrepancy could be due to a name change. Checksum calculation: 7 + 3 + 2 = 12; (6 + 8 + 2) × 2 = 32; 12 + 32 = 44; last digit of checksum matches check digit (4).

6. The DEA number meets standard validity tests. The practice identifier B is an appropriate initial letter for the DEA number of a primary practitioner; the letter N is the first letter of the prescriber's last name. Checksum calculation: 4 + 1 + 2 = 7; (4 + 2 + 0) × 2 = 12; 7 + 12 = 19; last digit of checksum matches check digit (9).

7. The DEA number meets standard validity tests. The practice identifier A is an appropriate initial letter for the DEA number of a primary practitioner; the letter K is the first letter of the prescriber's last name. Checksum calculation: 3 + 5 + 4 = 12; (0 + 1 + 9) × 2 = 20; 12 + 20 = 32; last digit of checksum matches check digit (2).

8. The DEA number meets standard validity tests. The practice identifier M is an appropriate initial letter for the DEA number of a mid-level practitioner; the letter S is the first letter of the prescriber's last name. Checksum calculation: 2 + 6 + 2 = 10; (8 + 4 + 2) × 2 = 28; 10 + 28 = 38; last digit of checksum matches check digit (8).

9. The DEA number meets standard validity tests. The practice identifier B is an appropriate initial letter for the DEA number of a primary practitioner; the letter K is the first letter of the prescriber's last name. Checksum calculation: 1 + 7 + 8 = 16; (1 + 9 + 7) × 2 = 34; 16 + 34 = 50; last digit of checksum matches the check digit (0).

10. The DEA number meets standard validity tests. The practice identifier A is an

appropriate initial letter for the DEA number of a primary practitioner; the letter *A* is the first letter of the prescriber's last name. Checksum calculation: $2 + 7 + 7 = 16$; $(1 + 0 + 5) \times 2 = 12$; $16 + 12 = 28$; last digit of checksum matches check digit (8).

11. Brand name: Macrobid

    Generic name: nitrofurantoin monohydrate/ macrocrystals

    Dosage form: capsules

    Strength: 100 mg

    Total quantity: 100 capsules

    Storage requirements: Store between 20° and 25° C (68° to 77° F); excursions permitted to 15° to 50° C (59° to 86° F).

    Manufacturer: Paradigm Drug Therapies

    NDC number: 0000-0000-000

12. Brand name: Prozac

    Generic name: fluoxetine

    Dosage form: capsules

    Strength: 20 mg

    Total quantity: 100 capsules

    Storage requirement(s): Keep tightly closed. Store between 20° and 25° C (68° to 77° F); excursions permitted to 15° to 50° C (59° to 86° F).

    Manufacturer: Paradigm Drug Therapies

    NDC number: 0000-0000-000

13. Brand name: Strattera

    Generic name: atomoxetine HCl

    Dosage form: capsules

    Strength: 18 mg

    Total quantity: 30 capsules

    Storage requirements: Keep tightly closed. Store at controlled room temperature 20° to 25° C (68° to 77° F); excursions permitted to 15° to 50° C (59° to 86° F).

    Manufacturer: Paradigm Drug Therapies

    NDC number: 0000-0000-000

14. Brand name: none provided on label

    Generic name: spironolactone

    Dosage form: tablets

    Strength: 50 mg

    Total quantity: 100 tablets

    Storage requirements: Store at controlled room temperature 20° to 25° C (68° to 77° F); excursions permitted to 15° to 50° C (59° to 86° F) in a light-resistant container.

    Manufacturer: Paradigm Drug Therapies

    NDC number: 0000-0000-000

15. Brand name: Vistaril

    Generic name: hydroxyzine pamoate

    Dosage form: capsules

    Strength: 50 mg

    Total quantity: 100 capsules

    Storage requirements: Store between 20° and 25° C (68° to 77° F); excursions permitted to 15° to 50° C (59° to 86° F).

    Manufacturer: Paradigm Drug Therapies

    NDC number: 0000-0000-000

16. Brand name: Restoril

    Generic name: temazepam

    Dosage form: capsule

    Strength: 7.5 mg

    Total quantity: 100 capsules

    Storage requirement(s): Store between 20° and 25° C (68° to 77° F); excursions permitted to 15° to 50° C (59° to 86° F).

    Manufacturer: Paradigm Drug Therapies

    NDC number: 0000-0000-000

17. 20 tablets; XX is Roman numeral for 20

18. 30 capsules.

    Work: 3 capsules/day × 10 days = 30 capsules

19. 48 tablets.

    Work: Determine number of tablets needed for each part of the prescription: 4 tablets/

dose × 2 doses/day × 2 days = 16 tablets;
3 tablets/dose × 2 doses/day × 2 days =
12 tablets; 4 tablets/dose × 1 dose/day ×
2 days = 8 tablets; 3 tablets/dose ×
1 dose/day × 2 days = 6 tablets;
2 tablets/dose × 1 dose/day × 2 days =
4 tablets; 1 tablet/dose × 1 dose/day
× 2 days = 2 tablets. Add the subtotals to
determine the total number to dispense:
16 tablets + 12 tablets + 8 tablets + 6
tablets + 4 tablets + 2 tablets = 48 tablets.

20. 7 oz

    Work: 1 oz/day × 7 days/week = 7 oz for a
    1-week supply

21. 150 capsules; #CL = Roman numeral C
    (100) plus Roman numeral L (50)

22. 14 days

    Work: 28 capsules/2 daily = 14 days

23. 90 days

    Work: 90 tablets/1 daily = 90 days

24. 30 days

    Work: 120 capsules/4 daily = 30 days

25. 60 days

    Work: 120 doses/2 daily = 60 days

3.2 Problem Set

1. g

2. c

3. b

4. a

5. d

6. e

7. f

8. 0730

9. 1628

10. 0045

11. 2120

12. 0224

13. 2258

14. 2350

15. 0120

16. 0003

17. 1220

18. 5:30 p.m.

19. 11:49 p.m.

20. 3:22 p.m.

21. 12:34 a.m.

22. 12:04 p.m.

23. 3:55 a.m.

24. 10:45 p.m.

25. 5:19 p.m.

26. 1:00 p.m.

27. 1:45 a.m.

28. 0815; 1315; 1900

29. 0500

30. 10:00 p.m.

31. Between 6:00 and 7:00 p.m.

32. 1500; 1505; 1510

3.3 Problem Set

1. bid = twice a day

2. DAW = dispense as written

3. IM = intramuscular

4. IV = intravenous

5. mL = milliliter

6. NKA = no known allergy

7. npo = nothing by mouth

8. q3h = every 3 hours

9. qid = four times a day

10. tid = three times a day

11. Take two capsules by mouth four times a
    day as needed for itching.

12. Apply one patch every night at bedtime and
    remove every morning.

13. Apply one-half inch (7.5 mg) of ointment twice a day every morning and six hours after first (dose) application.

14. Take two tablets by mouth three times a day before meals.

15. Take one-half tablet by mouth twice a day.

3.4 Problem Set

1. This type of prescription is a written prescription.

2. Beth Arnold

3. Duane Yamaguchi

4. MY4756687

5. The DEA number meets standard validity tests. The letter *M* is an appropriate initial letter for the DEA number of a midlevel practitioner; the letter *Y* is the first letter of the prescriber's last name. Checksum calculation: $4 + 5 + 6 = 15$; $(7 + 6 + 8) \times 2 = 42$; $15 + 42 = 57$; last digit of the checksum matches the last digit (7).

6. glipizide 10 mg tablets

7. The product pictured in the second label (glipizide 10 mg) should be used.

8. glipizide one tablet by mouth three times daily before meals

9. The days' supply of the prescription is 30, and 90 tablets should be dispensed for a 30 days' supply.

10. 5 refills

11. This medication order is an admission order.

12. Caycie Pasqual.

13. The patient has no known allergies.

14. The patient's weight is 132 pounds, and the patient's height is 5'3".

15. Greg Galangal, MD

16. The prescriber is an MD, or medical doctor.

17. 11/16/25

18. The medication order was written at 1430 (2:30 p.m.).

19. warfarin 10 mg PO tonight for one dose; docusate 100 mg by mouth every 12 hours, hold for loose stool; Benadryl 50 mg by mouth every night at bedtime as needed for insomnia

20. 2000 or 8:00 p.m.

Chapter 3 Find Solutions

1. The DEA number provided is not valid.

   Work: Checksum calculation: $4 + 2 + 9 = 15$; $4 + 3 + 2 = 9$; $2 \times 9 = 18$; $15 + 18 = 33$. The last digit of the checksum is 3, but the DEA number has a 1 as the check digit (in the last place).

2. Take three tablets four times daily or as needed.

3. NORCO is the brand name, and hydrocodone/acetaminophen is the generic name. Prescribers typically do not write both brand names and generic names on a prescription.

4. Take one tablet by mouth every day in the morning for edema.

5. Take one tablet by mouth twice a day for GERD.

6. Take one tablet by mouth four times a day for five days for shingles.

7. Take one tablet by mouth three times a day for angina.

8. Take one tablet by mouth at bedtime for sleep.

9. Students should have selected the oral syringe. The 1 tsp oral syringe should be filled to the ½ tsp graduation mark.

10. Students should have selected the medicine cup. The 2 tbsp medicine cup should be filled to the 2 tsp graduation mark.

11. The DEA number could be valid.

    Work: Checksum calculation $3 + 5 + 7 = 15$; $4 + 6 + 8 = 18$; $2 \times 18 = 36$; $15 + 36 = 51$. The last digit of the checksum is 1, and the DEA number has a 1 as the check digit (in the last place).

12. 1 tab PO qam

13. 30 days

14. 90 tablets

15. five refills

16. Take 2 tablets by mouth immediately for 1 dose.

17. You would include "before meals" in the translation.

Chapter 4

4.1 Problem Set

1. mcg

2. mg

3. L

4. g

5. kg

6. m

7. cm

8. mL

9. mcL

10. dL

11. 0.6 g

12. 50 kg

13. 0.4 mg

14. 0.04 L

15. 4.2 g

16. 0.005 g

17. 0.06 g

18. 2.6 L

19. 0.03 L

20. 0.02 mL

4.2 Problem Set

1. 1.964 mg

   Work: x mg/1,964 mcg = 1 mg/1,000 mcg; x = 1.964 mg

2. 0.418 g

   Work: x g/418 mg = 1 g/1,000 mg; x = 0.418 g

3. 651,000 mcg

   Work: x mcg/651 mg = 1,000 mcg/1 mg; x = 651,000 mcg

4. 840 mcg

   Work: x mcg/0.84 mg = 1,000 mcg/1 mg; x = 840 mcg

5. 12,000 mcg

   Work: x mcg/0.012 g = 1,000,000 mcg/1 g; x = 12,000 mcg

6. 9.213406

   Work: x g/9,213,406 mcg = 1 g/1,000,000 mcg; x = 9.213406 g

7. 0.284 g

   Work: x g/284 mg = 1 g/1,000 mg; x = 0.284 g

8. 9.3825 mg

   Work: x mg/9,382.5 mcg = 1 mg/1,000 mcg; x = 9.3825 mg

9. 0.012321 g

   Work: x g/12,321 mcg = 1 g/1,000,000 mcg; x = 0.012321 g

10. 0.184 kg

    Work: x kg/184 g = 1 kg/1,000 g; x = 0.184 kg

11. 0.052 L

    Work: 52 mL × 1 L/1,000 mL = 0.052 L

12. 2,060 mg

    Work: 2.06 g × 1,000 mg/1 g = 2,060 mg

13. 16,000 mcg

    Work: 16 mg × 1,000 mcg/1 mg = 16,000 mcg

14. 0.256 g

    Work: 256 mg × 1 g/1,000 mg = 0.256 g

15. 2.703 g

    Work: 2,703,000 mcg × 1 g/1,000,000 mcg = 2.703 g

16. 6,900 mL

Work: 6.9 L $\times$ 1,000 mL/1 L = 6,900 mL

17. 0.0625 g

Work: 62.5 mg $\times$ 1 g/1,000 mg = 0.0625 g

18. 15,000 g

Work: 15 kg $\times$ 1,000 g/1 kg = 15,000 g

19. 2.785 g

Work: 2,785,000 mcg $\times$ 1 mg/1,000 mcg $\times$ 1 g/1,000 mg = 2.785 g

20. 8.234 mcg

Work: 8.234 mg $\times$ 1,000 mcg/1 mg = 8,234 mcg

21. 2,000,000 mg

Work: 2 kg $\times$ 1,000,000 mg/1 kg = 2,000,000 mg; or x mg/2 kg = 1,000 g/1 kg; x = 2,000 g; x mg/2,000 g = 1,000 mg/1 g; x = 2,000,000 mg, x = 2,000,000 mg

22. 21,000 mL

Work: 21 L $\times$ 1,000 mL/1 L = 21,000 mL; or x mL/21 L = 1,000 mL/1 L, x = 21,000 mL

23. 0.576 L

Work: 576 mL $\times$ 1 L/1,000 mL = 0.576 L; or x L/576 mL = 1 L/1,000 mL; x = 0.576 L

24. 823,000,000 mg

Work: 823 kg $\times$ 1,000 g/1 kg $\times$ 1,000 mg/1 g = 823,000,000 or x g/823 kg = 1,000 g mg/1 kg$x$ = 823,000 g; x mg/823,000 g = 1,000 mg/1 g; x = 823,000,000; x = 823,000,000 mg

25. 0.027 mg

Work: 27 mcg $\times$ 1 mg/1,000 mcg = 0.027 mg; or x mg/27 mcg = 1 mg/1,000 mcg; x = 0.027 mg

26. 5 mg

Work: 5,000 mcg $\times$ 1 mg/1,000 mcg = 5 mg; or x mg/5,000 mcg = 1 mg/1,000 mcg; x = 5 mg

27. 0.02 mg

Work: 20 mcg $\times$ 1 mg/1,000 mcg = 0.02 mg; or x mg/20 mcg = 1 mg/1,000 mcg; x = 0.02 mg

28. 4,624 mcg

Work: 4.624 mg $\times$ 1,000 mcg/1 mg = 4,624 mcg; or x mcg/4.624 mg = 1,000 mcg/1 mg; x = 4,624 mcg

29. 3,190 mg

Work: 3.19 g $\times$ 1,000 mg/1 g = 3,190 mg; or x mg/3.19 g = 1,000 mg/1 g; x = 3,190 mg

30. 8.736 mg

Work: 8,736 mcg $\times$ 1 mg/1,000 mcg = 8.736 mg; or x mg/8,736 mcg = 1 mg/1,000 mcg; x = 8.736 mg

31. 0.83 L

Work: 830 mL $\times$ 1 L/1,000 mL = 0.83 L; or x L/830 mL = 1 L/1,000 mL; x = 0.83 L

32. 940 mL

Work: 0.94 L $\times$ 1,000 mL/1 L = 940 mL; or x mL/0.94 L = 1,000 mL/1 L; x = 940 mL

33. 1,840 mg

Work: 1.84 g $\times$ 1,000 mg/1 g = 1,840 mg; or x mg/1.84 g = 1,000 mg/1 g; x = 1,840 mg

34. 0.56 g

Work: 560 mg $\times$ 1 g/1,000 mg = 0.56 g; or x g/560 mg = 1 g/1,000 mg; x = 0.56 g

35. 1.2 mg

Work: 1,200 mcg $\times$ 1 mg/1,000 mcg = 1.2 mg; or x mg/1,200 mcg = 1 mg/1,000 mcg; x = 1.2 mg

36. 0.125 mg

Work: 125 mcg $\times$ 1 mg/1,000 mcg = 0.125 mg; or x mg/125 mcg = 1 mg/1,000 mcg; x = 0.125 mg

37. 275 mcg

Work: 0.275 mg $\times$ 1,000 mcg/1 mg = 275 mcg; or x mcg/0.275 mg = 1,000 mcg/1 mg; x = 275 mcg

38. 0.48 L

Work: 480 mL $\times$ 1 L/1,000 mL = 0.48 L; or x L/480 mL = 1 L/1,000 mL; x = 0.48 L

39. 0.239 g

   Work: 239 mg × 1 g/1,000 mg = 0.239 g
   or x g/239 mg = 1 g/1,000 mg; x = 0.239 g

40. 1.5 g

   Work: 1,500 mg × 1 g/1,000 mg = 1.5 g;
   or x g/1,500 mg = 1 g/1,000 mg; x = 1.5 g

41. a. 20 mL/day

   Work: a. 2 tsp/dose × 5 mL/tsp ×
   2 doses/day = 20 mL/day

   b. 140 mL/course of treatment

   Work: 20 mL/day × 7 days/course of
   treatment = 140 mL/course of treatment

   c. 0.5 g

   Work: 20 mL/day × 125 mg/5 mL × 1 g/
   1,000 mg = 0.5 g

   d. Because each bottle contains 100 mL, two
   bottles will be needed (200 mL − 140 mL
   = 60 mL to be discarded).

42. 6 capsules

   Work: (1) Convert 1.5 g to
   milligrams: x mg/1.5 g = 1,000 mg/1 g;
   x = 1,500 mg.

   (2) Determine number of capsules:
   1,500 mg × 1 capsule/250 mg = 6 capsules

43. a. Convert the prescribed dose to grams,
   1,000 mg = 1 g. Because one vial contains
   10 g, there are ten 1 g doses in one vial.

   b. 5 days

   Work: x days/10 doses = 1 day/
   2 doses; x = 5 days; 10 doses × 1 day/
   2 doses = 5 days

4.3 Problem Set

1. tsp

2. lb

3. tbsp

4. fl oz

5. pt

6. qt

7. gal

8. 1

9. 8

10. 16

11. 1

12. 2

13. 2

14. 2 tbsp

15. 6 tbsp

4.4 Problem Set

1. 4 pt

   Work: 8 cups × 1 pt/2 cups = 4 pt

2. 48 fl oz

   Work: 3 pt × 2 cups/1 pt × 8 fl oz/1 cup =
   48 fl oz or x cups/3 pt = 2 cups/1 pt;
   x = 6 cups; × fl oz/6 cups = 8 fl oz/1 cup;
   x = 48 fl oz

3. 16 fl oz

   Work: 1 pt × 2 cups/1 pt × 8 fl oz/
   1 cup × 2 tbsp/1 fl oz = 32 tbsp, or 16 fl oz
   or 1 pt = 2 cups; x fl oz/2 cups = 8 fl oz/
   1 cup; x = 16 fl oz

4. 96 fl oz

   Work: 3 qt × 2 pt/1 qt × 2 cups/1 pt ×
   8 fl oz/1 cup = 96 fl oz or x pt/3 qt = 2 pt/
   1 qt ; x = 6 pt; x cups/6 pt = 2 cups/
   1 pt; x = 12 cups; x fl oz/12 cups = 8 fl oz/
   1 cup ; x = 96 fl oz

5. 4.67 fl oz or 4 2/3 fl oz

   Work: 28 tsp × 1 tbsp/3 tsp = 9.333 tbsp,
   rounded to 9.33 tbsp; 9.33 tbsp × 1 fl oz/
   2 tbsp = 4.665 fl oz, rounded to 4.67 fl oz
   or 4 2/3 fl oz

6. 0.5 qt or ½ qt

   Work: 1 pt × 1 qt/2 pt = 0.5 qt or ½ qt

7. 288 tsp

   Work: 6 cups × 8 fl oz/1 cup × 2 tbsp/
   1 fl oz × 3 tsp/1 tbsp = 288 tsp or x fl oz/
   6 cups = 8 fl oz/1 cup; x = 48 fl oz; x tbsp/

48 fl oz = 3 tbsp/1 fl oz; x = 96 tbsp; x tsp/96 tbsp = 3 tsp/1 tbsp; x = 288 tsp

8. 228 tsp

   Work: 2 pt = 2 pt × 2 cups/1 pt × 8 fl oz/ 1 cup × 2 tbsp/1 fl oz × 3 tsp/1 tbsp = 192 tsp and 6 fl oz = 6 fl oz × 2 tbsp/ 1 fl oz × 3 tsp/1 tbsp = 36 tsp; 192 tsp + 36 tsp = 228 tsp

9. 72 doses

   Work: 3 cups × 8 fl oz/1 cup × 2 tbsp/ 1 fl oz × 3 tsp/1 tbsp × 1 dose/2 tsp = 72 doses

10. 384 doses

    Work: 12 bottles × 16 fl oz/1 bottle × 3 tbsp/1 fl oz × 1 dose/1 tbsp = 384 doses

4.5 Problem Set

1. 45 mL

   Work: 3 tbsp × 15 mL/1 tbsp = 45 mL

2. 30 mL

   Work: 1 fl oz × 30 mL/1 fl oz = 30 mL

3. 60 mL

   Work: 2 fl oz × 30 mL/1 fl oz = 60 mL

4. 90 mL

   Work: 3 fl oz × 30 mL/1 fl oz = 90 mL

5. 120 mL

   Work: 4 fl oz × 30 mL/1 fl oz = 120 mL

6. 150 mL

   Work: 5 fl oz × 30 mL/1 fl oz = 150 mL

7. 180 mL

   Work: 6 fl oz × 30 mL/1 fl oz = 180 mL

8. 210 mL

   Work: 7 fl oz × 30 mL/1 fl oz = 210 mL

9. 240 mL

   Work: 8 fl oz × 30 mL/1 fl oz = 240 mL

10. 360 mL

    Work: 12 fl oz × 30 mL/1 fl oz = 360 mL

11. 480 mL

    Work: 16 fl oz × 30 mL/1 fl oz = 480 mL

12. 5.3 tbsp

    Work: 80 mL × 1 fl oz/30 mL × 2 tbsp/ 1 fl oz = $^{160}/_{30}$ tbsp = $^{16}/_3$ tbsp = $5\frac{1}{3}$ tbsp = 5.3 tbsp

13. 180 mL

    Work: 6 fl oz × 30 mL/1 fl oz = 180 mL

14. 3 fl oz

    Work: 90 mL × 1 fl oz/30 mL = 3 fl oz

15. 1.7 pt

    Work: 800 mL × 1 oz/30 mL × 1 pt/ 16 oz = $^5/_3$ pt = $1\frac{2}{3}$ pt = 1.67 = 1.7 pt

16. 10.6 tsp

    Work: 53 mL × 1 tsp/5 mL = $10\,^3/_5$ tsp = 10.6 tsp

17. 7 tsp

    Work: 35 mL × 1 tsp/5 mL = 7 tsp

18. 2.6 gal

    Work: 10 L = 10,000 mL; 10,000 mL × 1 gal/3,840 mL = 2.604 gal, rounded to 2.6 gal

19. 60 mL

    Work: 4 tbsp × 1 fl oz/2 tbsp × 30 mL/ 1 fl oz = 60 mL

20. 3 tsp

    Work: 15 mL × 1 tsp/5 mL = 3 tsp

21. 1.5 pt, or 1 ½ pt

    Work: 720 mL × 1 pt/480 mL = 1.5 pt, or 1 ½ pt

22. 150 mL

    Work: 30 tsp × 5 mL/1 tsp = 150 mL

23. 4 fl oz

    Work: 120 mL × 1 fl oz/30 mL = 4 fl oz

24. 1,920 mL

Work: ½ gal = 0.5 gal × 3,840 mL/
1 gal = 1,920 mL

25. 4.2 pt

Work: 2 L = 2,000 mL; 2,000 mL × 1 pt/
480 mL = 4.166 pt, rounded to 4.2 pt

26. 1.6 kg

Work: 3.5 lb × 1 kg/2.2 lb = 1.59 kg,
rounded to 1.6 kg

27. 6.4 kg

Work: 14 lb × 1 kg/2.2 lb = 6.364 kg,
rounded to 6.4 kg

28. 19.1 kg

Work: 42 lb × 1 kg/2.2 lb = 19.09 kg,
rounded to 19.1 kg

29. 44.1 kg

Work: 97 lb × 1 kg/2.2 lb = 44.09 kg,
rounded to 44.1 kg

30. 50.9 kg

Work: 112 lb × 1 kg/2.2 lb = 50.909 kg,
rounded to 50.9 kg

31. 75 kg

Work: 165 lb × 1 kg/2.2 lb = 75 kg

32. 80.9 kg

Work: 178 lb × 1 kg/2.2 lb = 80.909 kg,
rounded to 80.9 kg

33. 112.3 kg

Work: 247 lb × 1 kg/2.2 lb = 112.27 kg,
rounded to 112.3 kg

34. 60 g

Work: 2 oz × 30 g/1 oz = 60 g

35. 45 g

Work: 1.5 oz × 30 g/1 oz = 45 g

36. 240 g

Work: 8 oz × 30 g/1 oz = 240 g

37. 2 lb

Work: 906 g × 1 lb/454 g = 1.995 lb,
rounded to 2 lb

38. 0.1 lb

Work: 30 g × 1 lb/454 g = 0.0660 lb,
rounded to 0.1 lb

39. 24 g

Work: 0.8 oz × 30 g/1 oz = 24 g

40. 30 doses

Work: 5 fl oz = 150 mL; 150 mL × 1 dose/
5 mL = 30 doses

41. 32 doses

Work: 1 pt = 480 mL; 480 mL × 1 dose/
15 mL = 32 doses

42. 135 mL/day

Work: 1.5 fl oz = 45 mL; 45 mL ×
3 times/day = 135 mL/day

43. 32 doses

Work: 8 fl oz = 240 mL; 240 mL ×
1 dose/7.5 mL = 32 doses

44. 25 mg

Work: ½ tsp × 5 mL/1 tsp × 10 mg/
1 mL = 25 mg

45. 60 days

Work: 4 fl oz × 30 mL/1 fl oz × 10 mg/
mL × 1 day/20 mg = 60 days

46. 0.5 tsp

Work: 2.5 mL × 1 tsp/5 mL = 0.5 tsp

47. 21 full days

Work: 320 mL × 1 day/3 tsp × 1 tsp/
5 mL = 21.3 days or 21 full days

48. 25 doses

Work: (conversions) 180 lb × 1 kg/
2.2 lb = 81.8181 kg, rounded to 81.8 kg;
2 tsp × 5 mL/1 tsp = 10 mL; 81.8 kg ×
10 mL/68 kg = 12.029411 mL, rounded to
12 mL; 300 mL × 1 dose/12 mL = 25 doses

49. 20 doses

Work: (conversions) 52 lb × 1 kg/
2.2 lb = 23.636 kg, rounded to 23.6 kg;
1 tsp/20 kg × 23.6 kg = 1.18 tsp;
4 fl oz × 30 mL/1 fl oz × 1 tsp/5 mL ×
1 dose/1.18 tsp = 20.3 doses, rounded to
20 doses

50. 7 full doses

Work: (conversions) 172 lb × 1 kg/ 2.2 lb = 78.181 kg, rounded to 78.2 kg; 2 tbsp × 15 mL/1 tbsp = 30 mL; 12 fl oz × 30 mL/1 fl oz = 360 mL; 78.2 kg × 30 mL/50 kg = 46.92 mL, rounded to 46.9 mL; 360 mL × 1 dose/ 46.9 mL = 7.6759 doses, or 7 full doses

4.6 Problem Set

1. −17.8° C

Work: (0° − 32°) ÷ 1.8 = −17.777° C, rounded to −17.8° C

2. −5° C

Work: (23° − 32°) ÷ 1.8 = −5° C

3. 2.2° C

Work: (36° − 32°) ÷ 1.8 = 2.222° C, rounded to 2.2° C

4. 4.4° C

Work: (40° − 32°) ÷ 1.8 = 4.444° C, rounded to 4.4° C

5. 17.8° C

Work: (64° − 32°) ÷ 1.8 = 17.777° C, rounded to 17.8° C

6. 22.2° C

Work: (72° − 32°) ÷ 1.8 = 22.222° C, rounded to 22.2° C

7. 37° C

Work: (98.6° − 32°) ÷ 1.8 = 37° C

8. 38.1° C

Work: (100.5° − 32°) ÷ 1.8 = 38.055° C, rounded to 38.1° C

9. 39.3° C

Work: (102.8° − 32°) ÷ 1.8 = 39.333° C, rounded to 39.3° C

10. 40.6° C

Work: (105° − 32°) ÷ 1.8 = 40.555° C, rounded to 40.6° C

11. 5° F

Work: (1.8 × −15°) + 32 = 5° F

12. 64.4° F

Work: (1.8 × 18°) + 32 = 64.4° F

13. 80.6° F

Work: (1.8 × 27°) + 32 = 80.6° F

14. 87.8° F

Work: (1.8 × 31°) + 32 = 87.8° F

15. 100.4° F

Work: (1.8 × 38°) + 32 = 100.4° F

16. 104° F

Work: (1.8 × 40°) + 32 = 104° F

17. 120.2° F

Work: (1.8 × 49°) + 32 = 120.2° F

18. 145.4° F

Work: (1.8 × 63°) + 32 = 145.4° F

19. 211.6° F

Work: (1.8 × 99.8°) + 32 = 211.64° F, rounded to 211.6° F

20. 214.5° F

Work: (1.8 × 101.4°) + 32 = 214.52° F, rounded to 214.5° F

21. 266° F

Work: (1.8 × 130°) + 32 = 266° F

22. a. −4° F

Work: (1.8 × −20°) + 32 = −4° F

b. August 1, 2025

Work: 2/1/2025 + 6 months = August 1, 2025

23. 148.9° C

Work: (300° − 32°) ÷ 1.8 = 148.888° C, rounded to 148.9° C

24. a. 2.3° C

    b. 3.2° C

    c. 3.9° C

    d. 2.1° C

    e. 2.7° C

f. 1.6° C; too cold

g. 2.4° C

h. 2.7° C

i. 1.9° C; too cold

j. 3.8° C

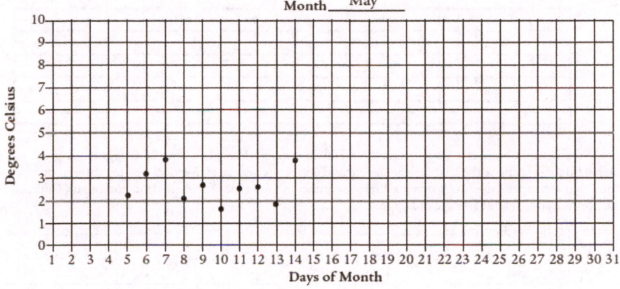

Month ___May___

Graph refrigerator temperature on chart once daily. If temperature is less than **2 degrees** or greater than **5 degrees,** check the thermostat setting and correct as necessary. Recheck temperature in one hour, and if temperature is out of stand range, contact maintenance for evaluation and repair. Contact the appropriate area for storage of supplies.

Documentation of Repairs: _____

_____

_____

_____

Documentation of Cleaning: _____

_____

_____

_____

25. a. 35.2° F; too cold

    b. 37.6° F

    c. 37° F

    d. 37.4° F

    e. 40.1° F

f. 37.8° F

g. 39° F

h. 36.5° F

i. 39.4° F

j. 40.5° F

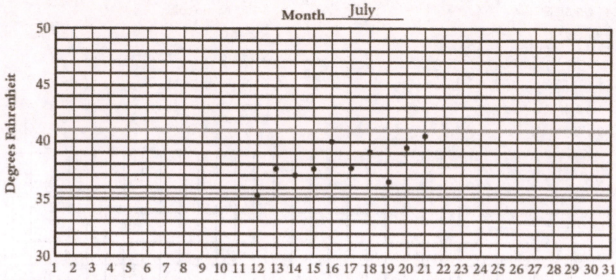

Month ___July___

Graph refrigerator temperature on chart once daily. If temperature is less than **35.6 degrees** or greater than **41 degrees,** check the thermostat setting and correct as necessary. Recheck temperature in one hour, and if temperature is out of stated range, contact maintenance for evaluation and repair. Contact the appropriate area for storage of supplies.

Documentation of Repairs: _____   Documentation of Cleaning: _____

_____   _____

_____   _____

_____   _____

Chapter 4 Find Solutions

1. Yes. One way to check is to see if the means equal the extremes.

    Work: 2.5 mg/mL = 12.5 mg/5 mL;
    2.5 mg:1 mL :: 12.5 mg:5 mL;
    $1 \times 12.5 = 2.5 \times 5$; 12.5 = 12.5

2. 5 mL

    Work: 5 mL/tsp $\times$ 1 tsp = 5 mL

3. 15 mL

    Work: 5 mL/dose $\times$ 3 doses/day =
    15 mL/day

4. 1 tbsp

    Work: 1 tbsp/15 mL $\times$ 15 mL = 1 tbsp

5. 480 mL

6. 960 mL

    Work: 480 mL $\times$ 2 = 960 mL

7. 20 mL

    Work: x mL/1,000 mg = 5 mL/250 mg;
    x = 20 mL; the medicine cup should be
    filled to 20 mL

8. 4 tsp

    Work: x tsp/20 mL = 1 tsp/5 mL; x = 4 tsp

9. 800 mL

    Work: 20 mL $\times$ 4 doses/day = 80 mL;
    80 mL $\times$ 10 days = 800 mL

10. 102.2° F

    Work: ° F = (1.8 $\times$ 39) + 32°

5.1 Problem Set

1. 4 tablets

    Work: x tablets/30 mg =
    1 tablet/7.5 mg; x = 4 tablets

2. 1.6 mL

    Work: x mL/20 mg = 2 mL/25 mg;
    x = 1.6 mL

3. 6.3 mL

Work: x mL/125 mg = 5 mL/100 mg; x = 6.25 mL, rounded to 6.3 mL

4. 0.8 mL

Work: x mL/4 mg = 1 mL/5 mg; x = 0.8 mL

5. 7 capsules

Work: x capsules/1,750 mg = 1 capsule/250 mg; x = 7 capsules

6. 2 mL

Work: x mL/40 mg = 5 mL/100 mg; x = 2 mL

7. 10 mL

Work: x mL/400 mg = 5 mL/200 mg; x = 10 mL

8. a.   20 mL

Work: x mL/1,000 mg = 5 mL/250 mg; x = 20 mL

b. 13.3 mL

Work: x mL/800 mg = 5 mL/300 mg; x = 13.3 mL

c. 2 tablets/day

Work: x tablets/500 mg = 1 tablet/1,000 mg; x = 0.5 tablet; 0.5 tablet/dose × 4 doses/day = 2 tablets/day

9. 250 mL

Work: Convert 10 mg to 10,000 mcg; x mL/10,000 mcg = 1 mL/40 mcg; x = 250 mL

10. 20 mg

Work: x mg/2 mL = 20 mg/2 mL; x = 20 mg

11. 2.5 mL

Work: 1 mg/1 × 1000 mcg/1 mg × mL/400 mcg = 2.5 mL; x = 2.5 mL

12. 480 mcg

Work: x mcg/1.2 mL = 400 mcg/1 mL; x = 480 mcg

13. 3,360 mcg

Work: Convert 80 mg to 80,000 mcg; x mcg/0.63 mL = 80,000 mcg/15 mL; x = 3,360 mcg

14. 30,000 capsules

Work: 1.05 kg = 1,050 g = 1,050,000 mg; x capsules/1,050,000 mg = 1 capsule/35 mg; x = 30,000 capsules

15. 22 doses

Work: x doses/880 mg = 2 doses/80 mg; x = 22 doses

16. 11,429 mcg

Work: Convert 1,600 mg to 1,600,000 mcg; x mcg/4 mL = 1,600,000 mcg/560 mL; x = 11,428.571 mcg, rounded to 11,429 mcg

17. 250 mL

Work: Convert 10 mg to 10,000 mcg; x mL/10,000 mcg = 1 mL/40 mcg; x = 250 mL

18. 2 mL

Work: x mL/2,000 units = 1 mL/1,000 units; x = 2 mL

19. 6 mL

Work: x mL/900 mg = 1 mL/150 mg; x = 6 mL

20. 600 mg

Work: x mg/4 mL = 150 mg/1 mL; x = 600 mg

21. 125 mg

Work: x mg/12.5 mL = 50 mg/5 mL; x = 125 mg

22. 10 mL

Work: x mL/100 mg = 5 mL/50 mg; x = 10 mL

23. 5 mg

Work: x mg/0.5 mL = 10 mg/mL; x = 5 mg

24. 8 mg

Work: x mg/0.8 mL = 10 mg/1 mL; x = 8 mg

25. 7.5 mL

Work: x mL/150 mg = 5 mL/100 mg; x = 7.5 mL

26. 25 mL

Work: Convert 0.5 g to 500 mg; x mL/500 mg = 5 mL/100 mg; x = 25 mL

27. 10 mL

Work: x mL/50 mg = 1 mL/5 mg; x = 10 mL

28. 4 mg

Work: x mg/0.8 mL = 5 mg/1 mL; x = 4 mg

29. 4 mL

Work: x mL/100 mg = 5 mL/125 mg; x = 4 mL

30. 187.5 mg

Work: x mg/7.5 mL = 125 mg/5 mL; x = 187.5 mg

31. 8 mL

Work: x mL/20 mg = 5 mL/12.5 mg; x = 8 mL

32. 20 mL

Work: x mL/50 mg = 5 mL/12.5 mg; x = 20 mL

33. a. 75 mg capsules

Work: Because 150 mg × 1 capsule/25 mg = 6 capsules, 150 mg × 1 capsule/50 mg = 3 capsules, and 150 mg × 1 capsule/75 mg = 2 capsules, then the 75 mg/capsule product will result in the fewest capsules taken per day, which is 2 capsules.

b. 14 capsules

Work: 2 capsules/day × 7 days/week = 14 capsules/week

34. a. 40 mL

Work: 500 mg/dose × 4 doses/day = 2,000 mg/day; 2,000 mg × 5 mL/250 mg = 40 mL

b. 2 tablets

Work: 50 mg × 1 tablet/25 mg = 2 tablets

c. 19.2 mL

Work: 480 mg × 5 mL/125 mg = 19.2 mL

d. 30 mL

Work: 200 mg/dose × 3 doses/day = 600 mg/day; 600 mg × 5 mL/100 mg = 30 mL

5.2 Problem Set

1. 90 tablets

Work: 3 tablets/day × 30 days = 90 tablets

2. 15 tablets

Work: (4 tablets × 2/day) + (3 tablets × 2/day) + 1 tablet × 1/day) = 15 tablets

3. 26.7 mg

Work: 5 mL × 80 mg/15 mL = 26.7 mg

4. ½ tsp

Work: 60 mg × 5 mL/120 mg = 2.5 mL or ½ tsp

5. 1.152 g

Work: 240 mL × 24 mg/5 mL = 1,152 mg or 1.152 g

6. 520 mg

Work: 120 mL × 65 mg/15 mL = 520 mg

7. 417 mg

Work: 10 mL × 2,500 mg/60 mL = 416.67 mg, rounded to 417 mg

8. 6.5 mg

Work: 15 mL × 260 mg/600 mL = 6.5 mg

9. 3 g

Work: 600 mL × 25 mg/5 mL = 3,000 mg or 3 g

10. 90 mg

Work: 30 mg/5 mL = x mg/15 mL; x = 90 mg

11. 19.2 g

Work: 480 mL × 40 mg/1 mL = 19,200 mg or 19.2 g

12. a. 13.3 days

Work: 150 mL × 1 dose/3.75 mL = 40 doses; 40 doses × 1 day/3 doses = 13.3 days

b. 37.5 mL

Work: 3.75 mL/dose × 3 doses/day = 11.25 mL/day × 10 days = 112.5 mL; 150 mL − 112.5 mL = 37.5 mL

13. a. 150 mL bottle

Work: 1 tsp = 5 mL; 10 mL/day ×
14 days = 140 mL; 150 mL bottle selected

   b. 10 mL

Work: 150 mL − 140 mL = 10 mL

14. 8 days

Work: 1 tbsp = 15 mL and 12 fl oz/bottle
= 360 mL/bottle; 15 mL/dose ×
3 doses/day = 45 mL/day; 360 mL/bottle ×
1 day/45 mL = 8 days/bottle

15. 24 days

Work: 2 tsp = 10 mL and 1 tbsp = 15 mL,
so 25 mL is being taken every 2 days;
300 mL/25 mL every 2 days = 24 days

16. 1 g

Work: 600 mL × 25 mg/15 mL = 1,000 mg
or 1 g

17. 5 bottles

Work: 12 fl oz/bottle = 360 mL/bottle and
1 fl oz × 4 doses/day = 30 mL × 4 doses/
day = 120 mL/day; 120 mL/day × 14 days/
treatment = 1,680 mL/treatment; 1,680 mL/
treatment × 1 bottle/360 mL = 4.666 bottles,
or a total of 5 bottles to be purchased

18. 30 tablets

Work: (4 tablets × 4 days) + (3 tablets ×
3 days) + (2 tablets × 2 days) + (1 tablet
× 1 day) = 16 + 9 + 4 + 1 = 30 tablets

19. 160 mL

Work: 24 hr/day × 1 dose/3 hr = 8 doses/day;
8 doses/day × 10 days = 80 doses;
80 doses × (1 mL/dose × 2 cheeks) = 160 mL

20. 1,800 mg

Work: 12 fl oz/bottle = 360 mL/bottle,
1 tsp/dose = 5 mL/dose; 360 mL/bottle ×
25 mg/5 mL = 1,800 mg/bottle

21. 15 fl oz

Work: 2 tsp/dose = 10 mL/dose;
3 doses/day × 10 mL/dose = 30 mL/day;
30 mL/day × 15 days/treatment = 450 mL/
treatment; 450 mL/treatment × 1 fl oz/
30 mL = 15 fl oz/treatment

22. 1,800 mL

Work: 2 tbsp/dose = 30 mL/dose; 3 doses/
day × 30 mL/dose = 90 mL/day; 20 days/
treatment × 90 mL/day = 1,800 mL/
treatment

23. 2 bottles

Work: 1 tsp = 5 mL; Child 1: 5 mL/dose ×
3 doses/day = 15 mL/day; 15 mL/day ×
4 days = 60 mL; Child 2: 10 mL/dose ×
3 doses/day = 30 mL/day; 30 mL/day ×
4 days = 120 mL; 60 mL + 120 mL =
180 mL. Because 1 bottle = 4 fl oz, 4 fl oz/
bottle × 30 mL/1 fl oz = 120 mL/bottle.
The mother will need 2 bottles, or 240 mL.

24. Child 1: 25 mg; Child 2: 50 mg

Work: Child 1: 5 mL × 25 mg/5 mL;
x = 25 mg; Child 2: 10 mL × 25 mg/5 mL;
x = 50 mg

25. 140.25 mg

Work: ¾ tsp = 0.75 tsp; 0.75 tsp × 5 mL/
tsp = 3.75 mL; 3.75 mL × 187 mg/
5 mL = 140.25 mg

26. 280.5 mg

Work: 1½ tsp = 1.5 tsp;
1.5 tsp × 5 mL/tsp = 7.5 mL;
7.5 mL × 187 mg/5 mL = 280.5 mg

27. 3.34 mL

Work: 125 mg × 5 mL/187 mg =
3.3422 mL, rounded to 3.34 mL

28. 13.37 mL

Work: 500 mg × 5 mL/187 mg =
13.3689 mL, rounded to 13.37 mL

29. 6 syringes

Work: 12 fl oz bottle × 30 mL/1 fl oz =
360 mL; 360 mL × 1 syringe/60 mL =
6 syringes

30. 243 mg

31. 324 mg

32. 405 mg

33. 648 mg

34. 27.3 mcg to 40.9 mcg

Work: 6 lb/(2.2 kg/lb) = 2.727;
2.727 × 10 = 27.27 mcg;

$2.727 \times 15 = 40.905$ mcg; rounded dosage: 27.3 mcg to 40.9 mcg

35. 35.2 mcg to 52.9 mcg

    Work: 12 oz/x lb = 16 oz/1 lb; x = 0.75; 7 lb 12 oz = 7.75 lb; 7.75 lb/(2.2 kg/lb) = 3.523; $3.523 \times 10 = 35.23$; $3.523 \times 15 = 52.845$; rounded dosage: 35.2 mcg to 52.9 mcg

36. 62.7 mcg to 83.6 mcg

    Work: 23 lb/(2.2 kg/lb) = 10.454; $10.454 \times 6 = 62.724$; $10.454 \times 8 = 83.632$; rounded dosage: 62.7 mcg to 83.6 mcg

37. 40.9 mcg to 49.1 mcg

    Work: 18 lb/(2.2 kg/lb) = 10.454; $8.182 \times 5 = 40.91$; $8.182 \times 6 = 49.092$; rounded dosage: 40.9 mcg to 49.1 mcg

5.3 Problem Set

1. 28 mg

   Work: 56 kg $\times$ 0.5 mg/kg = 28 mg

2. 1,812.5 mg

   Work: 87 kg $\times$ 125 mg/kg = 10,875 mg per day; for each dose, 10,875 mg/6 doses = 1,812.5 mg

3. 5.6 mL

   Work: 1.4 kg $\times$ 4 mL/kg = 5.6 mL

4. a. 50 mg

      Work: 80 kg $\times$ 0.625 mg/kg = 50 mg

   b. 16.67 mg

      Work: 50 mg/3 doses = 16.6666 mg/dose, rounded to 16.67 mg/dose

5. 15 mg

   Work: 6 kg $\times$ 5 mg/kg/day = 30 mg/day; 30 mg/2 doses = 15 mg/dose

6. 8,580 mg

   Work: 68.64 kg $\times$ 125 mg/kg/day = 8,580 mg/day

7. 50 mg

   Work: 10 kg $\times$ 10 mg/kg/day = 100 mg/day; 1 day = 24 hr; 100 mg/day = 100 mg/24 hr;

100 mg/2 = 50 mg; 24 hr/2 = 12 hr; 50 mg/12 hr

8. 13.75 mg

   Work: 1.1 m² $\times$ 25 mg/m² = 27.5 mg; 27.5 mg/2 doses = 13.75 mg/dose

9. 0.50 mg

   Work: 0.67 m² $\times$ 0.75 mg/m² = 0.5025 mg, rounded to 0.50 mg

10. 85 mg

    Work: 0.85 m² $\times$ 100 mg/m² = 85 mg

11. 177.5 mg

    Work: 0.71 m² $\times$ 250 mg/m² = 177.5 mg

12. 2.7 mg

    Work: 0.83 m² $\times$ 3.3 mg/m² = 2.739 mg, rounded to 2.7 mg

13. The physician has ordered a dose higher than the recommended dose.

    Work: 0.7 m² $\times$ 2 mg/m² = 1.4 mg. 1.9 mg is greater than 1.4 mg.

14. The physician has ordered a dose higher than the recommended dose.

    Work: 0.48 m² $\times$ 3.3 mg/m² = 1.584 mg, rounded to 1.6 mg. 2.5 mg is greater than 1.6 mg.

15. The physician has ordered a dose higher than the recommended dose.

    Work: 0.47 m² $\times$ 250 mg/m² = 117.5 mg. 200 mg is greater than 117.5 mg.

16. The physician's dose is under the recommended dose.

    Work: 40.9 kg $\times$ 50 mg/kg/day = 2,045 mg/day (recommended dose); order is 300 mg $\times$ 3 doses/day = 900 mg/day, which is under the recommended dose per day.

17. a. 1,820 mg

       Work: 36.4 kg $\times$ 50 mg/kg = 1,820 mg

    b. 3,640 mg

       Work: 36.4 kg $\times$ 100 mg/kg = 3,640 mg

    c. The physician's dose is under the minimum recommended dose.

Work: 250 mg × 3 doses/day =
750 mg/day, which is under the
minimum recommended dose

   d. 25 mL

Work: 250 mg/dose × 50 mL/
500 mg = 25 mL/dose

18. a. 109 mg

Work: 5.45 kg × 20 mg/kg = 109 mg

   b. 218 mg

Work: 5.45 kg × 40 mg/kg = 218 mg

   c. The physician's dose is higher than the
maximum recommended dose.

Work: 125 mg × 3 doses/day = 375 mg,
which is higher than the maximum
recommended dose

   d. 5 mL

Work: 125 mg/dose × 5 mL/125 mg =
5 mL/dose

19. a. 5.9 mg

Work: 11.8 kg × 0.5 mg/kg = 5.9 mg

   b. 11.8 mg

Work: 11.8 kg × 1 mg/kg = 11.8 mg

   c. 24 mg

Work: 10 mL × 12 mg/5 mL = 24 mg

   d. No, it is not a safe dose. It is higher than
11.8 mg, the maximum recommended
dose.

20. a. 139.8 mg/day

Work: 9.32 kg × 5 mg/kg = 46.6 mg;
24 hr/day × 1 dose/8 hr = 3 doses/day;
46.6 mg × 3 doses/day = 139.8 mg/day

   b. 372.8 mg/day

Work: 9.32 kg × 10 mg/kg = 93.2 mg;
24 hr/day × 1 dose/6 hr = 4 doses/day;
93.2 mg × 4 doses/day = 372.8 mg/day

   c. The physician's dose is higher than the
maximum recommended dose.

Work: 125 mg/dose × 3 doses/day
= 375 mg/day, which is higher than the
maximum recommended dose

   d. 6.25 mL

Work: 125 mg × 5 mL/100 mg =
6.25 mL

21. a. 1,250 mg

Work: 50 kg × 25 mg/kg = 1,250 mg

   b. 2,500 mg

Work: 50 kg × 50 mg/kg = 2,500 mg

   c. The physician's dose is under the
minimum recommended dose.

Work: 500 mg × 2 doses/day
= 1,000 mg/day, which is under the
minimum recommended dose

   d. 10 mL

Work: 500 mg × 5 mL/250 mg = 10 mL

22. a. 286 mg

Work: 28.6 kg × 10 mg/kg = 286 mg

   b. 429 mg

Work: 28.6 kg × 15 mg/kg = 429 mg

   c. It is within the recommended range.

   d. 10.1 mL

Work: 325 mg × 5 mL/160 mg =
10.156 mL, rounded down to 10.1 mL
(pediatric dose)

Chapter 5 Find Solutions

1. 10 kg

Work: 22 lb × 1 kg/2.2 lb = 10 kg

2. 10 mg

Work: 10 kg × 1 mg/kg = 10 mg

3. 5 mg

Work: 10 mg/2 doses = 5 mg

4. The 5 mL oral syringe should be filled to
0.62 mL

Work: x mL/5 mg × 5 mL/40 mg; x =
0.625 mL, rounded down to 0.62; the 5 mL
oral syringe should be filled to 0.62 mL.

5. less than 1 teaspoonful

6. An oral syringe provides a more exact measurement of the dose than a teaspoonful.

7. 21 capsules

    Work: 7 days × 3 capsules/day = 21 capsules

8. 30 capsules

    Work: 10 days × 3 capsules/day = 30 capsules

9. 5 days

    Work: 15 capsules × day/3 capsules = 5 days

10. 14 days

    Work: 42 capsules × day/3 capsules = 14 days

6.1 Problem Set

1. 5 mL syringe filled to 5 mL

    Work: x mL/50 mg = 1 mL/10 mg; x = 5 mL (5 mL syringe filled to 5 mL)

2. 10 mL syringe filled to 6 mL

    Work: x mL/60 mg = 4 mL/40 mg; x = 6 mL (10 mL syringe filled to 6 mL)

3. 10 mL syringe filled to 8 mL

    Work: x mL/80 mg = 10 mL/100 mg; x = 8 mL (10 mL syringe filled to 8 mL)

4. 1 mL syringe filled to 0.75 mL

    Work: x mL/0.75 mg = 1 mL/1 mg; x = 0.75 mL (1 mL syringe filled to 0.75 mL)

5. 3 mL syringe filled to 2 mL

    Work: x mL/100 mg = 1 mL/50 mg; x = 2 mL (3 mL syringe filled to 2 mL)

6. 3 mL syringe filled to 3 mL

    Work: x mL/30 mg = 2 mL/20 mg; x = 3 mL (3 mL syringe filled to 3 mL)

7. 5 mL syringe filled to 4 mL

    Work: x mL/40 mg = 2 mL/20 mg; x = 4 mL (5 mL syringe filled to 4 mL)

8. 3 mL syringe filled to 2.5 mL

    Work: Reconstitute to 100 mg/mL; x mL/250 mg = 1 mL/100 mg; x = 2.5 mL (3 mL syringe filled to 2.5 mL)

9. 5 mL syringe filled to 4 mL

    Work: Reconstitute to 100 mg/mL; x mL/400 mg = 1 mL/100 mg; x = 4 mL (5 mL syringe filled to 4 mL)

10. 60 mL syringe filled to 50 mL

    Work: x mL/50 mg = 100 mL/100 mg; x = 50 mL (60 mL syringe filled to 50 mL)

11. 7.5 mg

    Work: x mg/0.5 mL = 15 mg/1 mL; x = 7.5 mg

12. 52.5 mg

    Work: x mg/1.75 mL = 60 mg/2 mL; x = 52.5 mg

13. 75 mg

    Work: x mg/3.75 mL = 20 mg/1 mL; x = 75 mg

14. 1.3 mg

    Work: x mg/1.3 mL = 2 mg/2 mL; x = 1.3 mg

15. 25 mg

    Work: x mg/5 mL = 50 mg/10 mL; x = 25 mg

16. 25 mg

    Work: x mg/5 mL = 25 mg/5 mL; x = 25 mg

17. 5 mg

    Work: x mg/5 mL = 10 mg/10 mL; x = 5 mg

18. 32 mg

    Work: x mg/8 mL = 4 mg/1 mL; x = 32 mg

19. 3 mg

    Work: x mg/1.5 mL = 4 mg/2 mL; x = 3 mg

20. 125 mg

    Work: x mg/2.5 mL = 50 mg/1 mL; x = 125 mg

21. 2 mg

    Work: x g/2 mL = 1 g/1,000 mL; x = 0.002 g = 2 mg

22. 200 mcg

    Work: x g/1 mL = 1 g/5,000 mL; x = 0.0002 g = 0.2 mg = 200 mcg

23. 150 mcg

Work: x g/1.5 mL = 1 g/10,000 mL;
x = 0.00015 g = 0.15 mg = 150 mcg

24. 700 mcg

Work: x g/1.4 mL = 1 g/2,000 mL;
x = 0.0007 g = 0.7 mg = 700 mcg

25. 250 mcg

Work: x mg/2.5 mL = 1 g/10,000 mL;
x = 0.00025 g = 0.25 mg = 250 mcg

26. 500 mL

Work: Convert 500 mg to 0.5 g; x mL/
0.5 g = 1,000 mL/1 g; x = 500 mL

27. 500 mL

Work: Convert 50 mg to 0.05 g; x mL/
0.05 g = 10,000 mL/1 g; x = 500 mL

28. 180 mL

Work: Convert 600 mg to 0.6 g; x mL/
0.6 g = 300 mL/1 g; x = 180 mL

29. 125 mL

Work: Convert 250 mg to 0.25 g; x mL/
0.25 g = 500 mL/1 g; x = 125 mL

30. 7.5 mL

Work: x mL/0.01 g = 750 mL/1 g;
x = 7.5 mL

6.2 Problem Set

1. 0.7 mL

Work: Convert 375 mg to 0.375 g; x mL/
1.5 g = 1 mL/0.375 g; x = 4 mL; 4 mL final
volume – 3.3 mL diluent volume = 0.7 mL
powder volume

2. 91.4 mL

Work: Convert 250 mg to 0.25 g and note
that 1 tsp = 5 mL; x mL/5 g = 5 mL/0.25 g;
x = 100 mL final volume; 100 mL final
volume – 8.6 mL powder volume = 91.4 mL
diluent volume

3. 1.6 mL

Work: Convert 1 g to
1,000 mg; x mL/1,000 mg = 2 mL/125 mg;

x = 16 mL final volume; 16 mL final volume
– 14.4 mL diluent volume = 1.6 mL powder
volume

4. 1.2 mL

Work: Convert 250 mg to 0.25 g; x mL/
2 g = 1 mL/0.25 g; x = 8 mL final volume;
8 mL final volume – 6.8 mL diluent
volume = 1.2 mL powder volume

5. 14.8 mL

Work: Convert 125 mg to 0.125 g; x mL/
2 g = 1 mL/0.125 g; x = 16 mL final
volume; Using the powder volume calculated
in #4, 16 mL final volume – 1.2 mL powder
volume = 14.8 mL diluent volume

6. 4.3 mL

Work: Convert 250 mg to 0.25 g; x mL/
4 g = 1 mL/0.25 g; x = 16 mL final volume;
16 mL final volume – 11.7 mL diluent
volume = 4.3 mL powder volume

7. 1,200 mg/mL

Work: x mL/6 g = 2.5 mL/1 g; x = 15 mL
final volume; 15 mL final volume – 12.5 mL
diluent volume = 2.5 mL powder volume;
2.5 mL powder volume + 2.5 mL diluent
volume = 5 mL final volume; 6 g/
5 mL = 1.2 g/mL = 1,200 mg/mL

8. 0.7 mL

Work: 4 mL final volume – 3.3 mL diluent
volume = 0.7 mL powder volume

9. 0.4 mL

Work: Using the information from #8, 1 g/4
mL, convert 1 g to 1,000 mg; x mL/100 mg =
4 mL/1,000 mg; x = 0.4 mL

10. 1.2 mL

Work: x mL/2 g = 1 mL/0.2 g; x = 10 mL
final volume; 10 mL final volume – 8.8 mL
diluent volume = 1.2 mL powder volume

11. 200 mg

Work: Convert 10 g to 10,000 mg; 45 mL
diluent volume + 5 mL powder volume =
50 mL final volume; x mg/1 mL =
10,000 mg/50 mL; x = 200 mg
(or 200 mg/mL)

12. 200 mg

Work: Convert 8 g to 8,000 mg and note that 1 tsp = 5 mL; x mg/5 mL = 8,000 mg/200 mL; x = 200 mg (or 200 mg/tsp)

13. 46 mL

Work: x mL/20 g = 6 mL/1 g; x = 20 mL final volume; 120 mL final volume − 106 mL diluent volume = 14 mL powder volume; x mL/20 g = 3 mL/1 g; x = 60 mL final volume; 60 mL final volume − 14 mL powder volume = 46 mL diluent volume

14. 1.8 mL

Work: Convert 2 g to 2,000 mg; x mL/2,000 mg = 1 mL/375 mg; x = 5.3 mL final volume; 5.3 mL final volume − 3.5 mL diluent volume = 1.8 mL powder volume

15. 32.1 mL

Work: Convert 2.5 g to 2,500 mg; x mL/2,500 mg = 5 mL/300 mg; x = 41.7 mL final volume; 41.7 mL final volume − 9.6 mL powder volume = 32.1 mL diluent volume

16. 11.4 mL

Work: Convert 5 g to 5,000 mg; x mL/5,000 mg = 1 mL/250 mg; x = 20 mL final volume; 20 mL final volume − 8.6 mL diluent volume = 11.4 mL powder volume

17. 250 mg/mL

Work: x mg/10 g = 2.5 mL/1 g; x = 5 mL final volume; 25 mL final volume − 20 mL diluent volume = 5 mL powder volume; 5 mL powder volume + 35 mL new diluent volume = 40 mL final volume; 10 g/40 mL = 0.25 g/mL or 250 mg/mL

18. 0.7 mL

Work: 5 mL final volume − 4.3 mL diluent volume = 0.7 mL powder volume

19. 167 mg

Work: 25 mL diluent volume + 5 mL powder volume = 30 mL final volume; Convert 5 g to 5,000 mg; x mg/1 mL =5,000 mg/30 mL; x = 167 mg (or 167 mg/mL)

20. 200 mg

Work: 90 mL diluent volume + 10 mL powder volume = 100 mL final volume; Convert 20 g to 20,000 mg; x mg/1 mL = 20,000 mg/100 mL; x = 200 mg (or 200 mg/mL)

21. 120 mg

Work: 20 mL diluent volume + 5 mL powder volume = 25 mL final volume; Convert 3 g to 3,000 mg; x mg/1 mL = 3,000 mg/25 mL; x = 120 mg (or 120 mg/mL)

22. 33 mL

Work: 100 mL final volume − 67 mL diluent volume = 33 mL powder volume

23. 350 mg/mL

Work: Convert 35 g to 35,000 mg; x mg/1 mL = 35,000 mg/100 mL; x = 350 mg (or 350 mg/mL)

6.3 Problem Set

1. 10 mL syringe filled to 6.8 mL graduation mark

   Work: x mL/30 mEq = 1 mL/4.4 mEq; x = 6.81818 mL, rounded to 6.8 mL (10 mL syringe filled to 6.8 mL graduation mark)

2. 10 mL syringe filled to 10 mL graduation mark

   Work: x mL/44 mEq = 1 mL/4.4 mEq; x = 10 mL (10 mL syringe filled to 10 mL graduation mark)

3. 4 tablets

   Work : x tablets/32 mEq = 1 tablet/8 mEq; x = 4 tablets

4. 10 mL syringe filled to 5.6 mL graduation mark

   Work: x mL/30 mEq = 15 mL/40 mEq; x = 11.25 mL; 11.25 mL/2 doses = 5.625 mL, rounded to 5.6 mL (10 mL syringe filled to 5.6 mL graduation mark)

5. 30 mEq

   Work : x mEq/15 mL = 20 mEq/10 mL;
   x = 30 mEq

6. 30 mL syringe filled to 27 mL graduation
   mark

   Work: x mL/36 mEq = 15 mL/20 mEq;
   x = 27 mL (30 mL syringe filled to 27 mL
   graduation mark)

7. 10 mL syringe filled to 7 mL graduation
   mark

   Work: Select the 20 mEq vial; x mL/
   14 mEq = 1 mL/2 mEq; x = 7 mL (10 mL
   syringe filled to 7 mL graduation mark)

8. 10 mL syringe filled to 10 mL graduation
   mark

   Work: Select the 20 mEq vial; x mL/
   20 mEq = 1 mL/2 mEq; x = 10 mL (10 mL
   syringe filled to 10 mL graduation mark)

9. 13.5 mL

   Work: Select the 40 mEq vial; x mL/
   27 mEq = 1 mL/2 mEq; x = 13.5 mL

10. 25 mL

    Work: Select the 40 mEq plus the 10 mEq
    vial; x mL/50 mEq = 1 mL/2 mEq;
    x = 25 mL

11. 16 mEq

    Work: x mEq/8 mL = 60 mEq/30 mL;
    x = 16 mEq; or x mEq/8 mL = 2 mEq/
    1 mL; x = 16 mEq

12. 30 mEq

    Work: x mEq/15 mL = 40 mEq/20 mL;
    x = 30 mEq; or x mEq/15 mL = 2 mEq/
    1 mL; x = 30 mEq

13. 60 mL syringe filled to 33 mL graduation
    mark

    Work: x mL/132 mEq = 1 mL/4 mEq;
    x = 33 mL (60 mL syringe filled to 33 mL
    graduation mark)

14. 30 mL syringe filled to 30 mL graduation
    mark

    Work: x mL/120 mEq = 1 mL/4 mEq;
    x = 30 mL (30 mL syringe filled to 30 mL
    graduation mark)

15. 0.4 mL

    Work: x mL/4 units = 1 mL/10 units;
    x = 0.4 mL

16. 3 mL syringe filled to 2.8 mL graduation
    mark

    Work: x units/2.8 mL = 10 units/1 mL;
    x = 28 units (3 mL syringe filled to 2.8 mL
    graduation mark)

17. 3.5 mL

    Work: x mL/3,500 units = 1 mL/1,000 units;
    x = 3.5 mL

18. 10,750 units

    Work: x units/0.43 mL = 20,000 units/
    0.8 mL; x = 10,750 units

19. 0.7 mL

    Work: x mL/7,000 units = 1 mL/
    10,000 units; x = 0.7 mL

20. 2.4 mL

    Work: x mL/24,000 units = 1 mL/
    10,000 units; x = 2.4 mL

21. 0.3 mL

    Work: x mL/30 mg = 0.8 mL/80 mg;
    x = 0.3 mL

22. 0.35 mL

    Work: x mL/175,000 units = 1 mL/
    500,000 units; x = 0.35 mL

23. 2 mL

    Work: x mL/1,200,000 units = 1 mL/
    600,000 units; x = 2 mL

24. 7.7 mL

    Work: x mL/385,000 units = 1 mL/
    50,000 units; x = 7.7 mL

25. 0.45 mL

    Work: x mL/45 units = 1 mL/100 units;
    x = 0.45 mL

26. 35 days

    Work: Calculate morning dose: x mL/
    18 units = 1 mL/100 units; x = 0.18 mL;
    Calculate evening dose: x mL/10 units =
    1 mL/100 units; x = 0.1 mL; Add morning
    and evening doses: 0.18 mL/morning +

0.1 mL/evening = 0.28 mL/day; Because the vial shown on the label contains 10 mL, calculate time for 10 mL vial to last: x days/10 mL vial = 1 day/0.28 mL; x = 35.714 days, rounded to 35 days

27. a. 38 units

    Work: Add morning and evening units: 20 units + 18 units = 38 units/day

    b. 2 vials

    Work: x mL/38 units = 1 mL/100 units; x = 0.38 mL. Calculate the number of days of therapy in a 10 mL vial: 10 mL/0.38 mL = 26.3 days, rounded down to 26 days for 1 vial. Therefore, 2 vials will be needed for 30 days of therapy.

28. Humulin R: 1 vial; Humulin 70/30: 1 vial

    Work: Humulin R: 10 units/dose × 1 dose/day × 30 days = 300 units for month; 300 units × 1 mL/100 units = 3 mL; 1 vial will be needed; Humulin 70/30: 15 units/dose × 2 doses/day × 30 days = 900 units for month; 900 units × 1 mL/100 units = 9 mL; 1 vial will be needed

29. 50 units

    Work: x units/0.5 mL = 100 units/1 mL; x = 50 units

30. 50 days

    Work: 20 units/dose × 2 doses/day = 40 units/day; x mL/40 units = 1 mL/100 units; x = 0.4 mL (used daily); x days/20 mL = 1 day/0.4 mL; x = 50 days

Chapter 6 Find Solutions

1. 0.5 mL

   Work: 5,000 units × mL/10,000 units = 0.5 mL

2. 0.25 mL

   Work: 5,000 units × mL/20,000 units = 0.25 mL

3. 33.3 mL

   Work: 2,000,000 units × mL/60,000 units = 33.3 mL

4. 133.3 mL

   Work: 2,000,000 units/dose × 4 doses/day × mL/60,000 = 133.3 mL

5. 100 mL

   Work: 2,000,000 units × mL/20,000 units = 100 mL

6. 400 mL

   Work: 2,000,000 units/dose × 4 doses/day × mL/20,000 units = 400 mL

7. 20 mL

   Work: 40 mEq/dose × 10 mL/20 mEq = 20 mL

8. 100 mL

   Work: 40 mEq/dose × 50 mL/20 mEq = 100 mL

9. 30 mL

   Work: 40 mEq/dose × 15 mL/20 mEq = 30 mL

10. 30 mEq

    Work: 15 mL × 10 mEq/5 mL = 30 mEq

Chapter 7

7.1 Problem Set

1. You will need 1 g of coal tar, 0.25 g of salicylic acid, 3.75 g of triamcinolone 0.1%, and 25 g of hydrophilic petrolatum base ointment.

   Work: Because 30 g/120 g = 30/120 = ¼ ratio you would divide each number by 4 (or multiply by ¼).

   Coal tar: 4 g/4 = 1 g

   salicylic acid 1: 1 g/4 = 0.25 g

   triamcinolone 0.1%: 15 g/4 = 3.75 g

   hydrophilic petrolatum base ointment: 100 g/4 = 25 g

2. You will need 12 g of progesterone, 150 g of polyethylene glycol 3350, and 450 g of polyethylene glycol 1000.

Work: Because 150/30 = 5/1 ratio, you would multiply each number by 5.

progesterone: 2.4 g × 5 = 12 g

polyethylene glycol 3350: 30 g × 5 = 150 g

polyethylene glycol 1000: 90 g × 5 = 450 g

3. You will need 30 mL of podophyllum resin 25% and QSAD 120 mL of benzoin tincture.

Work: Because 120/20 = 6/1 ratio you will multiply by 6.

podophyllum resin 5 mL × 6 = 30 mL

5 mL × 6 = 30 mL

benzoin tincture QSAD 20 mL × 6 = 120 mL

Note: You could also solve this problem by multiplying 120 × 0.25 = 30 mL; 120−30 = 90 mL.

4. You will need 8 capsules of tetracycline 500 mg, 7.5 mL of hydrocortisone suspension, 10 mL of lidocaine oral suspension, and QSAD 120 mL of Mylanta suspension.

Work: 8 oz = 240 mL

120/240 = ½ ratio

tetracycline 500 mg capsules: 16/2 = 8 capsules

hydrocortisone suspension 15 mL: 15/2 = 7.5 mL

lidocaine oral suspension 30 mL: 30/2 = 15 mL

Mylanta suspension: QSAD 240 mL; 240/2 = QSAD 120 mL

5. You will need 3.6 g of antipyrine, 1 g of benzocaine, and QSAD to 60 mL of glycerin.

Work: 4 × 15 = 60 mL

60/30 = 2/1 ratio

antipyrine: 1.8 g × 2 = 3.6 g

benzocaine: 0.5 g × 2 = 1 g

glycerin: QSAD 30 mL × 2 = QSAD 60 mL

7.2 Problem Set

1. 100 mL of $D_{10}W$ and 100 mL of D_5W

10		2.5 parts of 10%
	7.5	
5		2.5 parts of 5%

2.5 + 2.5 = 5 (total number of parts)

2.5/5 = x/200 = 100; x = 100 mL of $D_{10}W$

2.5/5 = x/200 = 100; x = 100 mL of 5% D_5W

2. 80 mL of $D_{20}W$ and 320 mL of D_5W

20		3 parts of 20%
	8	
5		12 parts of 5%

3 + 12 = 15 (total number of parts)

3/15 = x/400 = 80; x = 80 mL of $D_{20}W$

12/15 = x/400 = 320; x = 320 mL of D_5W

3. 58 mL of $D_{70}W$ and 442 mL of D_5W

70		7.5 parts of 70%
	12.5	
5		57.5 parts of 5%

7.5 + 57.5 = 65 (total number of parts)

7.5/65 = x/500 = 57.69; x = 57.69, rounded to 58 mL of $D_{70}W$

57.5/65 = x/500 = 442.31; x = 442.31, rounded to 442 mL of D_5W

4. 200 mL of D_5W and 50 mL of $D_{10}W$

10		1 part of 10%
	6	
5		4 parts of 5%

4 + 1 = 5 (total number of parts)

4/5 = x/250 = 200; x = 200 mL of D_5W

1/5 = x/250 = 50; x = 50 mL of $D_{10}W$

5. 28 mL of $D_{50}W$ and 472 mL of D_5W

50		2.5 parts of 50%
	7.5	
5		42.5 parts of 5%

2.5 + 42.5 = 45 (total number of parts)

2.5/45 = x/500 = 27.78; x = 27.78, rounded to 28 mL of $D_{50}W$

42.5/45 = x/500 = 472.22; x = 472.22, rounded to 472 mL of D_5W

6. 50 mL of $D_{20}W$ and 200 mL of D_5W

20		3 parts of 20%
	8	
5		12 parts of 5%

3 + 12 = 15 (total number of parts)

3/15 = x/250 = 50; x = 50 mL of 20%

12/15 = x/250 = 200; x = 200 mL of 5%

7. 50 mL of $D_{20}W$ and 250 mL of D_5W

20		2.5 parts of 20%
	7.5	
5		12.5 parts of 5%

2.5 + 12.5 = 15 (total number of parts)

2.5/15 = x/300 = 50; x = 50 mL of $D_{20}W$

12.5/15 = x/300 = 250; x = 250 mLof D_5W

8. 125 mL of $D_{20}W$ and 375 mL of $D_{10}W$

20		2.5 parts of 20%
	12.5	
10		7.5 parts of 10%

2.5 + 7.5 = 10 parts total

2.5/10 = x/500 = 125; x = 125 mL of $D_{20}W$

7.5/10 = x/500 = 375; x = 375 mL of $D_{10}W$

9. 75 mL of $D_{10}W$ and 75 mL of D_5W

10		2.5 parts of 10%
	7.5	
5		2.5 parts of 5%

2.5 + 2.5 = 5 (total number of parts)

2.5/5 = x/150 = 75; x = 75 mL of $D_{10}W$

2.5/5 = x/150 = 75; x = 75 mL of D_5W

10. 63 mL of $D_{20}W$ and 188 mL of $D_{10}W$

20		2.5 parts of 20%
	12.5	
10		7.5 parts of 10%

2.5 + 7.5 = 10 (total number of parts)

2.5/10 = x/250 = 62.5; x = 62.5, rounded to 63 mL of $D_{20}W$

7.5/10 = x/250 = 187.5; x = 187.5, rounded to 188 mL of $D_{10}W$

11. 13 g of 10% cream and 47 g of 1% cream

10		2 parts of 10%
	3	
1		7 parts of 1%

2 + 7 = 9 (total number of parts)

2/9 = x/60 = 13.33; x = 13.33, rounded to 13 g of 10% cream

7/9 = x/60 = 46.66; x = 46.66, rounded to 47 g of 1% cream

12. 8 g of 15% cream and 23 g of 5% cream

15		2.5 parts of 15%
	7.5	
5		7.5 parts of 5%

7.5 + 2.5 = 10 (total number of parts)

2.5/10 = x/30 = 7.5; x = 7.5, rounded to 8 g of 15% cream

7.5/10 = x/30 = 22.5; x = 22.5, rounded to 23 g of 5% cream

13. 60 g of 5% cream and 60 g of 1% cream

$4 \times 30 = 120$ g

5		2 parts of 5%
	3	
1		2 parts of 1%

2 + 2 = 4 (total number of parts)

$2/4 = x/120 = 60; x = 60$ g of 5% cream

$2/4 = x/120 = 60; x = 60$ g of 1% cream

14. 15 g of 20% zinc oxide ointment and 30 g of 5% zinc oxide ointment

20		5 parts of 20%
	10	
5		10 parts of 5%

10 + 5 = 15 (total number of parts)

$5/15 = x/45 = 15; x = 15$ g of 20%

$10/15 = x/45 = 30; x = 30$ g of 5%

15. 60 g of 10% cream and 40 g of 5% cream

10		3 parts of 10%
	8	
5		2 parts of 5%

3 + 2 = 5 (total number of parts)

$3/5 = x/100 = 60; x = 60$ g of 10% cream

$2/5 = x/100 = 40; x = 40$ g of 5% cream

7.3 Problem Set

1. 1.5 g

Work: $2\% = 2$ g/100 g; 2 g/100 g = x g/75 g;

$x = 1.5$ g

Therefore, there are 1.5 g of hydrocortisone in 75 g of the cream.

2. 1.8%

Work: 8 g/454 g = x g/100 g;

$x = 1.8$ g

Therefore, the percentage strength of the compound is 1.8%.

3. 2.5 g

Work: $2.5\% = 2.5$ g/100 g

Therefore, 2.5 g of acyclovir will be needed for this preparation.

4. 16.7%

Work: 10 g + 50 g = 60 g; 10 g/60 g = x g/100 g;

10 × 100 = 1,000; 1,000/60 = 16.66 g;

$x = 16.7$ g

Therefore, the percentage strength of the compound is 16.7%.

5. 0.6 g

Work: $2\% = 2$ g/100 g; 2 g/100 g = x g/30 g;

2 × 30 = 60; 60/100 = 0.6; $x = 0.6$ g

Therefore, 0.6 g of triamcinolone will be needed for this prescription.

6. 0.0075 g

Work: $0.05\% = 0.05$ g/100 g; 0.05 g/100 g = x g/15 g;

0.05 × 15 = 0.75; 0.75/100 = 0.0075 g

Therefore, 0.0075 g of mometasone fumarate will be needed to prepare the prescription.

7. a. 20 g

Work: 200 mg/sup × 100 sup/1 × 1 g/1,000 mg = 20 g

b. 20%

Work: 200 mg/sup × 1 g/1,000 mg = 0.2 g; x g/100 g = 0.2 g/1 g; $x = 20$

Therefore, the percentage strength is 20%.

8. 0.23 g

Work: $0.75\% = 0.75$ g/100 g; 0.75 g/100 g = x g/30 g; 0.75 × 30 = 22.5; 22.5/100 = 0.225 g (rounded to 0.23 g) of metronidazole needed for this prescription

9. 0.02 g

Work: $0.05\% = 0.05$ g/100 g

0.05 g/100 g = x g/30 g

0.05 × 30 = 1.5/100 = 0.02 g, rounded to 0.02 g

Therefore, 0.015 g of clindamycin is needed to prepare this prescription.

10. a. 5 g

Work: 10% = 10 g/100 g; 10 g/100 g = x g/50 g; 10 × 50 = 500; 500/100 = 5 g

Therefore, 5 g of acyclovir are needed to prepare this prescription.

b. 50 doses

Work: 1 dose = 1 g; 1 g/1 dose = 50 g/x doses; 50 × 1 = 50; 50/1 = 50 doses

Therefore, there are 50 doses.

Chapter 7 Find Solutions

1. 0.1 g

2. 0.03 g

Work: 0.1 g/100 g × 30 g = 0.03 g

3. 0.015 g

Work: 0.1 g/100 g × 15 g = 0.015 g

4. 2.5%

Work: 2.5 g/100 g = x g/100 g; x = 2.5%

5. 6.7%

Work: 3 g/45 g = x g/100 g; x = 6.7%

6. 16 oz

Work: 480 mL × 1 oz/30 mL = 16 oz

7. 1.3 oz

Work: 80 mL/2 = 40 mL; 40 mL × 1 oz/30 mL = 1.3 oz

8. 100 mg

Work: 12.5 mg/5 mL × 40 mL = 100 mg

9. 120 mg

Work: 15 mg/5 mL × 40 mL = 120 mg

10. Swish, gargle, and spit 5–10 mL every six hours as needed for irritation.

A (higher %) 10		D (parts of higher %; the difference of B − C) 2
	B (desired %) 3	
C (lower %) 1		E (parts of lower %; the difference of A − B) 7

2 + 7 = 9 parts total

$$\frac{x}{454 \text{ g}} = \frac{2}{9}$$

x = 100.9 g of zinc oxide cream 10%

$$\frac{x}{454 \text{ g}} = \frac{7}{9}$$

x = 353.1 g of zinc oxide cream 1%

11. 3

12. 2

13. 7

14. 9

15. 100.9 g of zinc oxide cream 10% and 353.1 g of zinc oxide cream 1%

Chapter 8

8.1 Problem Set

1. one quarter

2. $10 bill

3. one $10 bill, four $1 bills, and one quarter

4. one penny

5. $1 bill

6. one penny, two quarters, one $1 bill, and two $20 bills

8.2 Problem Set

1. 1 bottle of 500

2. 2 bottles of 100

3. 1 bottle of 500

4. no purchase necessary

5. 1 bottle of 100

6. no purchase necessary

7. 1 bottle of 50

8. no purchase necessary

9. no purchase necessary

10. 3 of the 15 g; 4 of the 80 g

11. 1 of the 15 g; 1 of the 60 g; 2 of the 80 g

12. 1 of the 60 mL

13. 1 of the 15 g; 1 of the 60 g

14. 3 of the 60 g

15. 1 of the 15 g; 1 of the 60 g; 0 of the 4 oz

16. 2 of the 15 g; 1 of the 60 g

17. 0 of the 15 g; 0 of the 45 g

18. 0 of the 15 g; 1 of the 30 g; 0 of the 60 g; 1 of the 120 g

19. 0 of the 15 g; 0 of the 30 g; 1 of the 60 g

20. 0 of the 15 g; 0 of the 30 g; 1 of the 60 g; 0 of the 120 g

21. 1 of the 20 mL; 1 of the 60 mL

22. 1 bottle of 100

23. 1 bottle of 100

24. 1 bottle of 100

25. 2 bottle of 60

26. 1 bottle of 100

27. 1 bottle of 1,000

28. 0 (or 1) bottles of 100

29. 1 bottle of 1,000

30. 1 bottle of 100

31. 1 bottle of 300

32. 1 bottle of 100

33. 0 (or 1) bottles of 100

34. 1 bottle of 1,000

35. 1 bottle of 100

36. 0 bottles of 100

37. a. 7 jars

    b. 2 bottles of 1,000

    c. 20 bottles

    d. 11 bottles

    e. 3 bottles

38. a. 34 inventory days' supply

    Work: \$183,445.00/
    (38,207.00/7) = 33.61, rounded to 34

    b. \$32,748.84, which makes the pharmacy six days over its goal

    Work: \$5458.14 $\times$ 6 = \$32,748.84

39. a. 33 inventory days' supply

    Work: \$123,490.00/
    (\$26,504.00/7) = 32.62, rounded to 33

    b. \$26,504.00, which makes the pharmacy seven days over its goal

    Work: (\$26,504.00/7) $\times$ 7 = \$26504.00

40. \$42,936.25

    Work: \$147,210.00/24 = \$6133.75;
    the approximate cost of goods sold in one day was \$6133.75; \$6133.75 $\times$ 7 days = \$42936.25; the cost of products sold last week is \$42936.25

41. The pharmacy's daily sales average must be \$8,040.00.

    Work: \$51,280.00 + \$5,000.00 = \$56,280.00; \$56,280.00/7 = \$8,040.00

42. The turnover rate was 12.13.

    Work: \$1,612,000.00/\$132,936.00 = 12.126, rounded to 12.13

43. The turnover rate was 11.32.

    Work: \$1,768,000.00/\$156,200.00 = 11.31, rounded to 11.32

44. The turnover rate is 40.

    Work: \$20,800.00/\$520.00 = 40

45. The turnover rate is 32.36.

    Work: $5,760.00/$178.00 = 32.36

46. The turnover rate is 20.04.

    Work: $7,213.00/$360.00 = 20.04

47. The turnover rate is 15.81.

    Work: $5,060.00/$320.00 = 15.81

48. The turnover rate is 15.58.

    Work: $6,000.00/$385.00 = 15.58

49. The turnover rate is 10.5.

    Work: $52,500.00/$5,000.00 5 10.5

50. The annual depreciation is $1,026.00.

    Work: $8,294.00 − $2,138.00 = $6,156.00;

    $6,156.00/6 = $1,026.00

51. The annual depreciation amount for both cabinets is $2,797.17.

    Work: $18,350.00 × 2 = $36,700.00;
    $1,567.00 × 2 = $3,134.00;
    $36,700.00 − $3,134.00 = $33,566.00;
    $33,566.00/12 = $2,797.17

52. 500 tablets/bottle, $35.30

    Work: ($35.30/500=$0.07/tablet)

53. 1,480

8.3 Problem Set

1. The pharmacy's desired income goal for 18% profit is $1,156,400.00.

    Work: $135,000.00 + $52,000.00 +
    $23,000.00 + $6,000.00 + $4,000.00
    + $2,000.00 + $4,000.00 + $4,000.00
    + $750,000.00 = $980,000.00;
    $980,000.00 × 0.18 = $176,400.00;
    $980,000.00 + $176,400.00 = $1,156,400.00

2. The pharmacy's percentage of profit is 30%.

    Work: $1,401,489.00 − $980,000.00 =
    $421,489.00;

    $421,480.00/$1,401,490.00 = 0.30 = 30%

3. The pharmacy's percentage of profit is 18%.

    Work: $1,191,692.00 − $980,000.00 =
    $211,692.00;

$211,692.00/$1,191,692.00 = 0.178 = 17.8%, rounded to 18%

4. The desired income goal for 20% profit is $244,200.00.

    Work: $72,000.00 + $52,000.00 +
    $13,000.00 + $5,500.00 + $2,000.00
    + $1,500.00 + $4,000.00 + $3,500.00
    + $50,000.00 + $203,500.00;
    $203,500.00 × 0.2 = $40,700.00;
    $203,500.00 + $40,700.00 = $244,200.00;

5. The pharmacy's percentage of profit is 79%.

    Work: $991,982.00 − $203,500.00 =
    $788,482.00;

    $788,482.00/$991,982.00 = 0.79 = 79%

6. The pharmacy's percentage of profit is 84%.

    Work: $1,248,301.00 − $203,500.00 =
    $1,044,801.00;
    $1,044,801.00/$1,248,301.00 =
    0.837 = 83.7%, rounded to 84%;

7. The pharmacy's overhead for the week is $50,916.70.

    Work: $54,617.53 − $3,700.83= $50,916.70

8. For this pharmacy to make a 22% profit, its weekly sales must be $15,900.33.

    Work: $13,033.06 × 0.22 = $2,867.27;
    $2,867.27 + $13,033.06 = $15,900.33

9. The net profit for this prescription drug item is $2.36.

    Work: $3.96/100 × 50 = $1.98; $8.59 −
    $1.98 − $4.25 = $2.36

10. The net profit for this prescription drug item is $10.04.

    Work: $8.50/500 × 30 = $0.51; $14.80 −
    $0.51 − $4.25 = $10.04 net profit

11. The net profit for this prescription drug item is $5.70.

    Work: $118.50/100 tablets × 30 = $35.55;
    $45.50 − $35.55 − $4.25 = $5.70 net profit

12. The net profit for this prescription drug item is $2.21.

    Work: $83.50/500 tablets × 100 = $16.70;
    $23.16 − $16.70 − $4.25 = $2.21 net profit

13. The net profit for this prescription drug item is $0.37.

    Work: $41.20/100 tablets × 90 = $37.08; $41.70 − $37.08 − $4.25 = $0.37 net profit

14. The markup amount is $7.84; the markup rate is 44.8%.

    Work: $25.34 − $17.50 = $7.84 markup amount; $7.84/$17.50 × 100 = 44.8% markup rate

15. The markup amount is $5.60; the markup rate is 45.5%.

    Work: $17.90 − $12.30 = $5.60 markup amount; $5.60/$12.30 × 100 = 45.5%

16. The discounted selling price is $4.71.

    Work: $5.89 × 0.2 = $1.18; $5.89 − $1.18 = $4.71

17. The discounted selling price is $1.01.

    Work: $1.19 × 0.15 = $0.18; $1.19 − $0.18 = $1.01

18. The discounted selling price is $5.10.

    Work: $7.29 × 0.30 = $2.19; $7.29 − $2.19 = $5.10

19. The discounted selling price is $4.84.

    Work: $5.69 × 0.15 = $0.85; $5.69 − $0.85 = $4.84

20. The discounted selling price is $2.92.

    Work: $3.89 × 0.25 = $0.97; $3.89 − $0.97 = $2.92

21. The discounted selling price is $2.98.

    Work: $4.26 × 0.30 = $1.28; $4.26 − $1.28 = $2.98

22. The discounted selling price is $4.35.

    Work: $8.70 × 0.5 = $4.35; $8.70 − $4.35 = $4.35

23. The discounted selling price is $1.79.

    Work: $2.99 × 0.40 = $1.20; $2.99 − $1.20 = $1.79

24. The total selling price of a box of 12 tubes is $195.00.

    Work: $12.50 × 0.3 = $3.75; $12.50 + $3.75 = $16.25; $16.25 × 12 tubes = $195.00

25. The selling price is $4.85 per bottle.

    Work: $111.60/36 = $3.10 (purchase price per bottle); $3.10 + $1.75 = $4.85

26. The markup amount is $3.90; the selling price is $19.50.

    Work: $15.60 × 0.25 = $3.9; is $3.90 (markup amount); $15.60 + $3.90 = $19.50 (selling price)

27. The markup rate is 24.0%.

    Work: $30.75 − $24.80 = $5.95; $5.95/$24.80 × 100; $5.95/$24.80 = 0.2399; 0.2399 × 100 = 23.99, rounded to 24.0%

28. The gross profit is $130.00.

    Work: $650.00 − $520.00 = $130.00

29. The net profit for selling one tablet is $0.11. C

    Work: $130/1,000 tablets = $0.13/tablet; $2.05/100 tablets = $0.02/tablet; $0.13/tablet − $0.02/tablet = $0.11/tablet

30. The pharmacy's markup amount is $30.13; the pharmacy's selling price is $150.63.

    Work: $120.50 × 0.25 = $30.13 (markup amount); $120.50 + $30.13 = $150.63 (selling price)

31. The pharmacy's markup amount is $3.60; the pharmacy's selling price is $27.60.

    Work: $24.00 × 0.15 = $3.60 (markup amount); $24.00 + $3.60 = $27.60 (selling price)

32. The pharmacy's markup amount is $54.00; the pharmacy's selling price is $254.00.

    Work: $200.00 × 0.27 = $54.00 (markup amount); $200.00 + $54.00 = $254.00 (selling price)

33. The pharmacy's markup amount is $5.78; the pharmacy's selling price is $33.28.

    Work: $27.50 × 0.21 = $5.78 (markup amount); $27.50 + $5.78 = $33.28 (selling price)

34. The pharmacy's markup amount is $12.15; the pharmacy's selling price is $79.65.

   Work: $67.50 × 0.18 = $12.15 (markup amount); $67.50 + $12.15 = $79.65 (selling price)

35. The pharmacy's markup amount is $268.80; the pharmacy's selling price is $1,108.80.

   Work: $840.00 × 0.32 = $268.80 (markup amount); $840.00 + $268.80 = $1,108.80 (selling price)

36. The pharmacy's markup amount is $165.00; the pharmacy's selling price is $715.00.

   Work: $550.00 × 0.30 = $165.00 (markup amount); $550.00 + $165.00 = $715.00 (selling price)

37. The total amount the pharmacy spent on this shipment was $1,829.50; the amount the pharmacy made upon selling the items was $539.46; the overall markup rate for the entire shipment was 29%.

   Work: $120.50 + $24.00 + $200.00 + $27.50 + $67.50 + $840.00 + $550.00 = $1,829.50 (total amount spent on shipment); $150.63 + $27.60 + $254.00 + $33.28 + $79.65 + 1,108.80 + $715.00 = $2,368.96; $2,368.96 − $1,829.50 = $539.46 (total amount for selling all items); $539.46/$1,829.50 × 100; $539.46/$1,829.50=0.2948;0.2948×100=29.49 rounded to 29 or 29% (overall markup rate for entire shipment)

8.4 Problem Set

1. The reimbursement for this prescription based on AWP less than 13% is $14.18.

   Work: $48.90 × 0.13 = $6.36; $48.90 − $6.36 = $42.54; $42.54/60 tablets = $x/20 tablets; x = $14.18

2. The reimbursement for this prescription based on AWP less than 13% is $21.94.

   Work: $84.07 × 0.13 = $10.93; $84.07 − $10.93 = $73.14; $73.14/100 tablets = $x/30 tablets; x = $21.94

3. The reimbursement for this prescription based on AWP less than 13% is $2.63.

   Work: $30.25 × 0.13 = $3.93; $30.25 − $3.93 = $26.32; $26.32/1,000 tablets = $x/100 tablets; x = $2.63

4. The reimbursement for this prescription based on AWP plus 4% is $13.78.

   Work: $120.68 × 0.04 = $4.83; $120.68 + $4.83 = $125.51; $125.51/500 = $x/30 tablets; x = $7.53; $7.53 + $6.25 = $13.78

5. The reimbursement for this prescription based on AWP plus 4% is $31.07.

   Work: $39.78 × 0.04 = $1.59; $39.78 + $1.59 = $41.37; $41.37/100 tablets = $x/60 tablets; x = $24.82; $24.82 + $6.25 = $31.07

6. The reimbursement for this prescription based on AWP plus 4% is $226.38.

   Work: $317.50 × 0.04 = $12.70; $317.50 + $12.70 = $330.20; $330.20/30 tablets = $x/20 tablets; x = $220.13; $220.13 + $6.25 = $226.38

7. a. The pharmacy's medication cost is $35.68.

   Work: $71.35/100 = $x/50; x = $35.68

   b. The reimbursement for this prescription is $41.43.

   Work: $35.68 + ($35.68 × 0.035) + $4.50 = $41.43

   c. The gross profit for this prescription is $5.75.

   Work: $41.43 − $35.68 = $5.75

8. a. The pharmacy's medication cost is $70.52.

   Work: $36.35 × 0.03 = $1.09; $36.35 − $1.09 = $35.26; $35.26 × 2 5 $70.52

   b. The reimbursement for this prescription is $76.34.

   Work: $72.70 + ($72.70 × 0.05) = $76.34

   c. The gross profit for this prescription is $5.82.

   Work: $76.34 − $70.52 = $5.82

9. a. The pharmacy's medication cost is $100.78.

   Work: $302.35/30 = x/10; x = $100.78

   b. The reimbursement for this prescription is $104.76.

   Work: $100.78 − ($100.78 × 0.03) + $7.00 = $104.76

   c. The gross profit for this prescription is $3.98.

   Work: $104.76 − $100.78 = $3.98

10. a. The pharmacy's cost of the prescription is $70.41.

   Work: $117.35/50 = x/30; x = $70.41

   b. The pharmacy will submit $76.52 to the insurance company for this prescription.

   Work: $70.41 + ($70.41 ×.03) + $4.00 = $76.52

   c. The pharmacy's profit for this prescription is $6.11.

   Work: $76.52 − $70.41 = $6.11

11. a. The pharmacy's cost of the prescription is $16.00.

   Work: $85.35/80 = x/15; x = $16.00

   b. The pharmacy will submit $16.72 to the insurance company for this prescription.

   Work: $16.00 + ($16.00 × 0.04) 5 = $16.72

   c. The pharmacy's profit for this prescription is $0.72.

   Work: $16.72 − $16.00 = $0.72

12. a. The total amount the HMO reimbursed for capitation fees is $1,860.00.

   Work: $310.00 × 6 = $1,860.00

   b. The pharmacy's purchase price for all prescriptions on this plan is $1,698.80.

   Work: $15.75 + $106.50 + $27.80 + $210.00 + $47.50 + $105.25 + $160.00 + $52.00 + $150.00 + $210.00 + $76.00 + $10.50 + $28.00 + $62.50 + $210.00 + $210.00 + $17.00 = $1,698.80

   c. The pharmacy made a profit.

d. The pharmacy's profit is $161.20.

   Work: $1,860.00 − $1,698.80 = $161.20

13. a. The pharmacy's purchase price for all prescriptions on the plan is $1,698.80.

   Work: $15.75 + $106.50 + $27.80 + 210.00 + 47.50 + 105.25 + 160.00 + $52.00 + $150.00 + $210.00 + $76.00 + $10.50 + $28.00 + $62.50 + $210.00 + $210.00 + $17.00 = $1,698.80

   b. The pharmacy will submit $1,783.76 for insurance reimbursement on this plan.

   Work: $1,698.80 + ($1,698.80 × 0.03) + ($2.00 × 17) = $1,783.76

   c. The pharmacy made a profit.

   d. The gross profit for this prescription is $84.96.

   Work: $1,783.76 − $1,698.80 = $84.96

   e. The pharmacy made a profit of $76.24 under Mountain HMO's capitation plan.

   Work: $161.20 − $84.96 = $76.24

14. a. The total amount of capitation fees reimbursed from the HMO to the pharmacy is $2,750.00.

   Work: $275.00 × 10 = $2,750.00

   b. The pharmacy's medication cost for all prescriptions on this plan is $800.87.

   Work: $89.63 + $126.54 + $420.45 + $117.50 + $46.75 = $800.87

   c. The pharmacy made a profit.

   d. The amount of the pharmacy's profit is $1,949.13.

   Work: $2,750.00 − $800.87 = $1,949.13

15. a. The total amount of capitation fees reimbursed from the HMO to the pharmacy is $3,300.00.

   Work: a. $275.00 × 12 = $3,300.00

   b. The pharmacy's medication cost for all prescriptions on this plan is $538.55.

   Work: $78.26 + $75.23 + $25.48 + $128.46 + $21.86 + $61.89 + $41.20 + $16.59 + $5.80 + $3.87 + $21.67 + $58.24 = $538.55

c. The pharmacy made a profit.

d. The pharmacy's profit is $2,761.45.

Work: $3,300.00 − $538.55 = $2,761.45

16. a. The total amount reimbursed from the HMO to the pharmacy in August was $9,060.00.

Work: $225.00 × 40 = $9,000.00; $9,000.00 + $60.00 = $9,060.00

b. The pharmacy made a profit.

c. The pharmacy's profit was $7,192.50.

Work: $9,060.00 − $1,867.50 = $7,192.50

17. a. The total amount reimbursed from the insurance company to the pharmacy in September was $9,049.50.

Work: $210.00 × 42 = $8,820.00; $4.25 × 54 = $229.50; $8,820.00 + $229.50 = $9,049.50

b. The pharmacy lost money

c. The pharmacy's loss was −$585.23.

Work: $9049.50 − $9,634.73 = − $585.23

Chapter 8 Find Solutions

1. 250-count bottle at $4.65 per bottle = $0.02 per capsule

2. one bottle

3. $4.65

4. The amount the HMO reimbursed the pharmacy was $19,105.00.

Work: $149.00 × 127 = $18,923.00; $3.50 × 52 = $182.00; $18,923.00 + $182.00 = $19,105.00.

5. $6,283.24

6. The pharmacy made a profit.

7. The pharmacy made a profit of $12,821.76.

Work: $19,105.00 − $6,283.24 = $12,821.76

8. $1,190,000

9. $1,404,200

Work: $1,190,000 × 0.18 = $214,200; $1,190,000 + $214,200 = $1,404,200

10. $1,582,700

Work: $1,190,000 × 0.33 = $392,700; $1,190,000 + $392,700 = $1,582,700

11. 3

Work: $750,000/$238,000 = 3.15, round to 3

12. 25.7%

Work: $1,601,489 − $1,190,000 = $411,489; $411,489/$1,601,489 = 25.7%

13. 37.1%

Work: $1,891,692 − $1,190,000 = $701,692; $701,692/$1,891,692= 37.1%

14. $18.80

Work: ($200 − $12)/10 = $18.80

15. $5

Work: ($50 − $15)/7 = $5.00

Chapter 9

9.1 Problem Set

1. w/v = 10 g/100 mL

2. w/v = 0.45 g/100 mL

3. 50 g

Work: 10% = 10 g/100 mL; 10 g/100 mL = x g/500 mL; x = 50 g

4. 26 mg

Work: 2% = 2 g/100 mL = x g/1.3 mL; x = 0.026 g = 26 mg

5. 4%

Work: 20 g/500 mL × 100 = 4%

6. 15%

Work: 0.15 g/1 mL × 100 = 15%

7. 3%

Work: 0.03 g/1 mL × 100 = 3%

8. 0.5%

Work: 0.005 g/1 mL × 100 = 0.5%

9. 0.2%

Work: 0.002 g/1 mL × 100 = 0.2%

10. 1%

   Work: 0.01 g/1 mL $\times$ 100 = 1%

11. 2%

   Work: 0.02 g/1 mL $\times$ 100 = 2%

12. 87.5 g

   Work: 3.5% = 3.5 g/100 mL = x g/2,500 mL;
   x = 87.5 g

13. 100 g

   Work: 10% = 10 g/100 mL = x g/1,000 mL;
   x = 100 g

14. 0.9 g

   Work: 0.9% = 0.9 g per 100 mL; 0.9 g

15. 20 g

   Work: 4% = 4 g/100 mL = x g/500 mL;
   x = 20 g

16. 4.5 g

   Work: 0.45% = 0.45 g/100 mL = x g/
   1,000 mL; x = 4.5 g

17. 50 g

   Work: 5% = 5 g/100 mL = x g/1,000 mL;
   x = 50 g

18. 2 g

   Work: 0.4% = 0.4 g/100 mL = x g/500 mL;
   x = 2 g

19. 20 g

   Work: 4% = 4 g/100 mL = x g/500 mL;
   x = 20 g

20. 5 g

   Work: 2% = 2 g/100 mL = x g/250 mL;
   x = 5 g

21. 375 mg

   Work: 7.5% = 7.5 g/100 mL = x g/5 mL;
   x = 0.375 g; x mg/0.375 g = 1,000 mg/1 g;
   x = 375 mg

22. 250 mg

   Work: 0.5% = 0.5 g/100 mL = x g/50 mL;
   x = 0.25 g; x mg/0.25 g = 1,000 mg/1g;
   x = 250 mg

23. 5 mg

   Work: 1% = 1 g/100 mL = x g/0.5 mL;
   x = 0.005 g; x mg/0.005 g = 1,000 mg/1 g;
   x = 5 mg

24. 1 mg

   Work: 0.1% = 0.1 g/100 mL = x g/1 mL;
   x = 0.001 g; x mg/0.001 g = 1,000 mg/1g;
   x = 1 mg

25. 10 mg

   Work: 0.2% = 0.2 g/100 mL = x g/5 mL;
   x = 0.01 g; x mg/0.01 g = 1,000 mg/1g;
   x = 10 mg

26. 2.25 g

   Work: 0.9 g/100 mL = x g/250 mL;
   x = 2.25 g

27. 4.5 g

   Work: 0.9 g/100 mL = x g/500 mL; x = 4.5 g

28. 9 g

   Work: 0.9 g/100 mL = x g/1,000 mL; x = 9 g

29. 20.03 g

   Work: 0.9 g/100 mL = x g/2,225 mL;
   x = 20.03 g

30. 0.56 g

   Work: 0.45 g/100 mL = x g/125 mL;
   x = 0.563, rounded to 0.56 g

31. 1.13 g

   Work: 0.45 g/100 mL = x g/250 mL;
   x = 1.125, rounded to 1.13 g

32. 3.38 g

   Work: 0.45 g/100 mL = x g/750 mL;
   x = 3.375, rounded to 3.38 g

33. 8.1 g

   Work: 0.45 g/100 mL = x g/1,800 mL;
   x = 8.1 g

34. 11.7 g

   Work: 0.45 g/100 mL = x g/2,600 mL;
   x = 11.7 g

35. 3.75 g

   Work: 5 g/100 mL = x g/75 mL; x = 3.75 g

36. 19.25 g

   Work: 5 g/100 mL = x g/385 mL; x = 19.25 g

37. 26.25 g

   Work: 5 g/100 mL = x g/525 mL; x = 26.25 g

38. 67.5 g

   Work: 5 g/100 mL = x g/1,350 mL; x = 67.5 g

39. 10 g

   Work: 10 g/100 mL = x g/100 mL; x = 10 g

40. 32.5 g

   Work: 10 g/100 mL = x g/325 mL; x = 32.5 g

41. 45 g

   Work: 10 g/100 mL = x g/450 mL; x = 45 g

42. 87.5 g

   Work: 10 g/100 mL = x g/875 mL; x = 87.5 g

9.2 Problem Set

1. v/v = 0.25 mL/100 mL

2. v/v = 2 mL/100 mL

3. v/v = 70 mL/100 mL

4. v/v = 99 mL/100 mL

5. 200 mL

   Work: 2 L × 1,000 mL/L × 10 mL/
   100 mL = 200 mL

6. 10 mL

   Work: 500 mL × 2 mL/100 mL = 10 mL

7. 3.75 mL

   Work: 50 mL × 7.5 mL/100 mL = 3.75 mL

8. 3.75 mL

   Work: 1,500 mL × 0.25 mL/100 mL = 3.75 mL

9. 860.86 mL

   Work: 946 mL × 91 mL/100 mL = 860.86 mL

10. 682.5 mL

   Work: 750 mL × 91 mL/100 mL = 682.5 mL

11. 91 mL

   Work: 100 mL × 91 mL/100 mL = 91 mL

12. 68.25 mL

   Work: 75 mL × 91 mL/100 mL = 68.25 mL

13. 2.5 mL

   Work: 1,000 mL × 0.25 mL/100 mL = 2.5 mL

14. 0.94 mL

   Work: 375 mL × 0.25 mL/100 mL = 0.94 mL

15. 2.5 mL

   Work: 500 mL × 0.5 mL/100 mL = 2.5 mL

16. 3.75 mL

   Work: 750 mL × 0.5 mL/100 mL = 3.75 mL

17. 7.5%

   Work: 75 mL/1,000 mL × 100 = 7.5%

18. 15%

   Work: 75 mL/500 mL × 100 = 15%

19. 18%

   Work: 90 mL/500 mL × 100 = 18%

20. 6%

   Work: 90 mL/1,500 mL × 100 = 6%

9.3 Problem Set

1. 20 hr

   Work: 1,000 mL/50 mL/hr = 20 hr

2. 5 a.m.

   Work: 1,000 mL/100 mL/hr = 10 hr;
   10 hr from 7 p.m. is 5 a.m.

3. 16.67 hr

   Work: 500 mL/30 mL/hr = 16.666 rounded
   to 16.67 hr; or approximately 16 hr and
   40 min

4. 100 mL/hr

   Work: 75 mL/45 min = x mL/60 min;
   x = 100 mL/hr

5. 133 mL/hr

   Work: 100 mL/45 min = x mL/60 min;
   x = 133 mL/hr

6. 50 mL/hr

   Work: 250 mL/5 hr = 50 mL/hr

7. 300 mg/hr

Work: 1,500 mg/5 hr = 300 mg/hr

8. Rate is 50 mL over 60 min or 50 mL/hr

9. Dosage is 500 mg over 60 min or 500 mg/hr

10. 100 mL/hr

11. 10 hr

Work: 1,000 mL/100 mL/hr= 10 hr

12. 3 IV bags

Work: 1 bag = 10 hr; 24/10 = 2.4;
2.4, rounded up to 3 IV bags

13. 2 mEq/hr

Work: 20 mEq/10 hr = 2 mEq/hr

14. 2 IV bags

Work: 1,000 mL/50 mL/hr = 20 hr;
24/20 = 1.2, rounded up to 2 IV bags

15. 2 IV bags

Work: 1,000/75 mL/hr = 13.33 hr;
24/13.33 = 1.8, rounded up to 2 IV bags

16. 3 IV bags

Work: 1,000 mL/100 mL/hr= 10 hr;
24/10 = 2.4, rounded up to 3 IV bags

17. 3 IV bags

Work: 1,000 mL/120 mL/hr = 8.33 hr;
24/8.33 = 2.88, rounded up to 3 IV bags

18. 3 IV bags

Work: 1,000 mL/125 mL/hr = 8 hr;
24/8 = 3 IV bags

19. 4 IV bags

Work: 1,000 mL/130 mL/hr = 7.69 hr;
24/7.69 = 3.12, rounded up to 4 IV bags

20. 4 IV bags

Work: 1,000 mL/150 mL/hr = 6.67 hr;
24/6.67 = 3.6, rounded up to 4 IV bags

21. 5 IV bags

Work: 1,000 mL/175 mL/hr = 5.71 hr;
24/5.71 = 4.2, rounded up to 5 IV bags

22. 5 IV bags

Work: 1,000 mL/200 mL/hr = 5 hr;
24/5 = 4.8, rounded up to 5 IV bags

23. 6 IV bags

Work: 1,000 mL/225 mL/hr = 4.44 hr;
24/4.44 = 5.41, rounded up to 6 IV bags

24. a. 62.5 mL/hr

Work: 250 mL/4 hr = 62.5 mL/hr

b. 62.5 mg/hr

Work: 250 mg/4 hr = 62.5 mg/hr

25. a. 41.67 mL/hr

Work: 500 mL/12 hr = 41.666, rounded
to 41.67 mL/hr

b. 1,000,000 units/hr

Work: 12,000,000 units/
12 hr = 1,000,000 units/hr

26. a. 20 mL/hr

Work: 4% = 4 g/100 mL = x g/500 mL;
x = 20 g; 20 g = 20,000 mg;
20,000/500 = 40; 40 mg/
1 mL = 800 mg/x mL; x = 20 mL/hr

b. 25 hr

Work: 500 mL/20 mL/hr = 25 hr

27. a. 40 mL/hr

Work: 250 mg/500 mL = 20 mg/x mL;
x = 40 mL/hr

b. 12.5 hr

Work: 20 mg/1 hr = 250 mg/x hr;
x = 12.5 hr

28. a. 75 mL/hr

Work: 500 mL/1600 mcg ×
4 mcg/min × 60 min/1 hr = 75 mL/hr

b. 240 mcg/hr

Work: 4 mcg/1 min = x mcg/60 min;
x = 240; 240 mcg/hr

29. a. 20 mL

Work: 200 mg/5 mL = 800 mg/x mL;
x = 20 mL

b. 1.56 mL/hr

Work: 5 mg/hr × 250 mL/800 mg =
1.56 mL/hr

30. a. 2 mg/kg × 176 lb/1 × 1 kg/2.2 lb × mL/40 mg = 4 mL

 b. 100 mL/hr

9.4 Problem Set

1. 1 gtt/min

 Work: 10 mL/60 min × 10 gtts/mL = 1.67, rounded down to 1 gtt/min

2. 35 gtts/min

 Work: 35 mL/60 min × 60 gtts/mL = 35 gtts/min

3. 16 gtts/min

 Work: 100 mL/60 min × 10 gtts/mL = 16.66, rounded down to 16 gtts/min

4. 100 gtts/min

 Work: 60 gtts/mL × 50 mL/30 min = 100 gtts/min

5. 5 gtts/min

 Work: 15 gtts/mL × 500 mL/24 hr × 1 hr/60 min = 5.21, rounded down to 5 gtts/min

6. 62 gtts/min

 Work: 250 mL/60 min × 15 gtts/mL = 62.5, rounded down to 62 gtts/min

7. 12 gtts/min

 Work: 50 mL/60 min × 15 gtts/mL = 12.5, rounded down to 12 gtts/min

8. 31 gtts/min

 Work: 95 mL/60 min × 20 gtts/mL = 31.67, rounded down to 31 gtts/min

9. 0.04 mEq/gtt

 Work: 1 mL/10 gtts × 40 mEq/100 mL = 0.04 mEq/gtt

10. 6 gtts/min

 Work: 25 mL/60 min × 15 gtts/mL = 6.25, rounded down to 6 gtts/min

11. 50 gtts/min

 Work: 50 mL/60 min × 60 gtts/mL = 50 gtts/min

12. 3 gtts/min

 Work: 10 mL/60 min × 20 gtts/mL = 3.33, rounded to 3 gtts/min

13. 0.03 mg/gtt

 Work: mg/gtt = 450 mg/250 mL × 1 mL/60 gtts = 0.03 mg/gtt

14. 0.0032 mg/gtt

 Work: mg/gtt = 8 mg/250 mL × 1 mL/10 gtts = 0.0032 mg/gtt

15. 4 gtts/min

 Work: 25 mL/60 min × 10 gtts/mL = 4.17, rounded down to 4 gtts/min

16. 0.00033 mgEq/gtt

 Work: mEq/gtt = 10 mEq/500 mL × 1 mL/60 gtts = 0.00033 mgEq/gtt

9.5 Problem Set

1. a. 100 mg

  Work: 10 mg/1 mL = x mg/10 mL; x = 100 mg

 b. 1 mL

  Work: 100 mg/mL = 1 mL

 c. 9 mL

  Work: 10 mL − 1 mL = 9 mL

2. a. 50 mg

  Work: 10 mg/1 mL = x mg/5 mL; x = 50 mg

 b. 1.25 mL

  Work: 40 mg/1 mL = 50 mg/x mL; x = 1.25 mL

 c. 3.75 mL

  Work: 5 mL − 1.25 mL = 3.75 mL

3. a. 100 mg

  Work: 10 mg/1 mL = x mg/10 mL; x = 100 mg

 b. 1 mL

  Work: 500 mg/5 mL = 100 mg/x mL; x = 1 mL

c. 9 mL

Work: 10 mL − 1 mL = 9 mL

4. a. 5 mg

Work: 1 mg/1 mL = x mg/5 mL;
x = 5 mg

b. 1.25 mL

Work: 4 mg/1 mL = 5 mg/x mL;
1 × 5 = 5; 5/4 = 1.25; x = 1.25 mL

c. 3.75 mL

Work: 5 mL − 1.25 mL = 3.75 mL

5. a. 10 mg

Work: 1 mg/1 mL = x mg/10 mL;
x = 10 mg

b. 1 mL

Work: 20 mg/2 mL = 10 mg/x mL;
x = 1 mL

c. 9 mL

Work: 10 mL − 1 mL = 9 mL

6. a. 107 mL of 70% dextrose

Work: 500 mL/70% × 15% = 107.14 mL,
rounded to 107 mL of 70% dextrose

b. 393 mL of SWFI 500 − 107 = 393 mL of
SWFI

7. a. 400 mL of 50% dextrose

Work: 2,000 mL/50% × 10% 400 mL of
50% dextrose

b. 1,600 mL of SWFI

Work: 2,000 mL − 400 mL = 1,600 mL
of SWFI

8. a. 200 mL of 50% dextrose

Work: 1,000 mL/50% × 10% 200 mL of
50% dextrose

b. 800 mL of SWFI

Work: 1,000 mL − 200 mL = 800 mL of
SWFI

9. a. 120 mL of 50% dextrose

Work: 750 mL/50% × 8% = 120 mL of
50% dextrose

b. 630 mL of SWFI

Work: 750 mL − 120 mL = 630 mL
of SWFI

10. a. 27 mL of 70% dextrose

Work: 250 mL/70% × 7.5% = 26.79 mL,
rounded to 27 mL of 70% dextrose

b. 223 mL of SWFI

Work: 250 mL − 27 mL = 223 mL
of SWFI

11. a. 364.29 mL of $D_{70}W$

Work: 1,500 mL/70% × 17% =
364.29 mL of $D_{70}W$

b. 450.00 mL of Aminosyn 10%

Work: 1,500 mL/10% × 3% = 450.00 mL
of Aminosyn 10%

c. 187.50 mL of Liposyn 20%

Work: 1,500 mL/20% × 2.5% =
187.50 mL of Liposyn 20%

d. 7.50 mL of sodium chloride

Work: 20 mEq/L × 1.5 L = 30 mEq;
30 mEq/4 mEq/mL = 7.50 mL of sodium
chloride

e. 11.25 mL of potassium chloride

Work: 15 mEq/L × 1.5 L = 22.5 mEq;
22.5 mEq/2 mEq/mL = 11.25 mL of
potassium chloride

f. 5.00 mL of potassium phosphate

Work: 10 mM/L × 1.5 L = 15 mM;
15 mM/3 mM/mL = 5.00 mL of
potassium phosphate

g. 1.50 mL of sodium phosphate

Work: 3 mM/L × 1.5 L = 4.5 mM;
4.5 mM/3 mM/mL = 1.50 mL of sodium
phosphate

h. 3.69 mL of magnesium sulfate

Work: 10 mEq/L × 1.5 L = 15 mEq;
15 mEq/4.06 mEq/mL = mEq/mL 3.6946
rounded to 3.69 mL of magnesium sulfate

i. 10.00 mL of MVI

j. 459.27 mL of SWFI

Work: SWFI QSAD to 1,500 mL; 364.29 + 450 + 187.5 + 7.5 + 11.25 + 5 + 1.5 + 3.69 + 10 = 1040.74

1,500 − 1040.73 = 459.27 mL of SWFI

k. 1,500.00 mL

12. a. 321.43 mL of $D_{70}W$

Work: 1500 mL/70% × 15% = 321.43 mL of $D_{70}W$

b. 600.00 mL of Amniosyn 10%

Work: 1500 mL/10% × 4% = 600.00 mL of Aminosyn 10%

c. 225.00 mL of Liposyn 20%

Work: 1500 mL/20% × 3% = 225.00 mL of Liposyn 20%

d. 9.38 mL of sodium chloride

Work: 25 mEq/L × 1 L/1,000 mL × 1,500 mL × 1 mL/4 mEq = 9.38 mL of sodium chloride

e. 9.38 mL of potassium chloride

Work: 12.5 mEq/L × 1 L/1,000 mL × 1,500 mL × 1 mL/2 mEq = 9.38 mL of potassium chloride

f. 5.00 mL of potassium phosphate

Work: 10 mM/L × 1 L/1,000 mL × 1,500 mL × 1 mL/3 mM = 5.00 mL of potassium phosphate

g. 1.00 mL of sodium phosphate

Work: 2 mM/L × 1 L/1,000 mL × 1,500 mL × 1 mL/3 mM = 1.00 mL of sodium phosphate

h. 3.69 mL of magnesium sulfate

Work: 10 mEq/L × 1 L/1,000 mL × 1,500 mL × 1 mL/4.06 mEq = 3.69 mL of magnesium sulfate

i. 10.00 mL of MVI

j. 315.12 mL SWFI

Work: SWFI QSAD to 1,500 mL; 1,500 mL − (321.43 mL + 600.00 mL + 225.00 mL 1 9.38 mL + 9.38 mL + 5.00 mL + 1.00 mL + 3.69 mL + 10.00 mL) = 315.12 mL sterile water

k. 1500.00 mL

Chapter 9 Find Solutions

1. 60 mEq of potassium chloride

Work: 125 mL/hr × 24 hr/1 × 1 L/1,000 mL= 3 L; 20 mEq/L × 3 L = 60 mEq

2. 150 g of dextrose

Work: 5 g/100 mL × 125 mL/hr × 24 hr/1 = 150 g

3. 27 g of sodium chloride in 24 hr

Work: 0.9 g/100 mL × 125 mL/hr × 24 hr/1= 27 g

4. 24 g of dextrose

Work: 5 g/100 mL × 20 mL/hr × 24 hr/1 = 24 g

5. 960 mg of aminophylline

Work: 1,000 mg/500 mL × 20 mL/hr × 24 hr/1 = 960 mg

6. 480 mL

Work: 20 mL/1 hr × 24 hr/1 = 480 mL

7. 3 vials

Work: 1,500 mg/x vials = 500 mg/1 vial; x = 3 vials

8. 0.3% w/v

Work: 100 mL/x g = 500 mL/1.5 g; x = 0.3 g; 0.3% w/v

9. This concentration is appropriate.

Work: Concentration is 1,500 mg/500 mL = 3 mg/mL; this concentration is appropriate since it is less than 5 mg/mL.

10. 90 mins, or 1.5 hrs

Work: 1,500 mg/x mins = 500 mg/30 mins; x = 90 mins

11. 16.7 mL/hr

Work: 0.5 mg/min × 250 mL/450 mg × 60 min/hr = 16.7 mL/hr

12. 4 gtts/min

Work: 16.7 mL/hr × 15 gtts/mL × 1 hr/60 mins = 4.18 gtts/min

13. 2 bags will be needed.

Work: 16.7 mL/hr × 18 hr/1 × 1 bag/250 mL = 1.2 bags, rounded up to 2 bags

14. 0900 the next morning

    Work: 250 mL/bag $\times$ 1 hr/16.7 mL = 14.97, rounded to 15 hr; so IV bag will need to be replaced after 15 hours, or at 0900 the next morning.

15. 3,600.0 mL will be needed for 24 hours.

    Work: 150 mL/1 hr = x mL/24 hr; x = 3,600.0 mL will be needed for 24 hours.

16. 771.4 mL of $D_{70}W$

    Work: 3,600 mL/70% $\times$ 15% = 771.4 mL of $D_{70}W$

17. 1,800.0 mL of Aminosyn 10%

    Work: 3,600 mL/10% $\times$ 5% = 1,800.0 mL of Aminosyn

18. 900.0 mL of Liposyn 10%

    Work: 3,600 mL/10% $\times$ 2.5% = 900.0 mL of Liposyn

19. 9.0 mL of NaCl

    Work: 3,600 mL $\times$ 1 L/1,000 mL = 3.6 L; 10 mEq/L $\times$ 3.6 L = 36 mEq; 36 mEq/ 4 mEq/mL = 9.0 mL of NaCl

20. 18.0 mL of KCl

    Work: 10 mEq/L $\times$ 3.6 L = 36 mEq; 36 mEq/2 mEq/mL = 18.0 mL of KCl

21. 2.2 mL of MgSO4

    Work: 2.5 mEq/L $\times$ 3.6 L = 9 mEq; 9 mEq/4.06 mEq/mL = 2.2 mL of MgSO4

22. 0.7 mL of insulin

    Work: 20 units/L $\times$ 3.6 L = 72 units; 72 units/100 units/mL = 0.72 mL, rounded to 0.7 mL of insulin.

23. 10.0 mL of MVIs

24. 88.6 mL of SWFI

    Work: 771.4 + 1,800.00 + 900.00 + 9.00 + 18.00 + 2.2 + 0.7 + 10.00 = 3,511.3; 3,600 − 3,511.3 = 88.7 mL of SWFI

B

Common Pharmacy Abbreviations and Acronyms

The abbreviations with lines through them are ones that are still in use but are discouraged by Institute for Safe Medication Practices (ISMP). The ISMP recommends the use of the correct words instead. Many of these discouraged abbreviations are also on the Joint Commission's Official "Do Not Use" List of Abbreviations.

Abbreviation	Meaning
A-B-C	
aaa	apply to affected area
~~ac; a.c.; AC~~	before meals
ACE	angiotensin-converting enzyme inhibitors
ad; a.d.; AD	right ear
ADR	adverse drug reaction
AM; a.m.	morning
APAP	acetaminophen; Tylenol
ARBs	angiotensin receptor blockers
~~as; a.s.; AS~~	left ear
ASA	aspirin
~~au; a.u.; AU~~	both ears; each ear
b.i.d.; BID	twice daily
BMI	Body Mass Index
BP	blood pressure
BUD	beyond-use date
°C	degrees centigrade; temperature in degrees centigrade
Ca^{++}	calcium
Cap, cap	capsule
CSP	compounded sterile preparation
CV	cardiovascular
D-E-F	
D$_5$; D$_5$W; D5W	dextrose 5% in water
D$_5$ ¼; D5 1/4	dextrose 5% in ¼ normal saline; dextrose 5% in 0.225% sodium chloride
D$_5$ ⅓; D5 1/3	dextrose 5% in ⅓ normal saline; dextrose 5% in 0.33% sodium chloride

Abbreviation	Meaning
D$_5$ ½; D5 1/2	dextrose 5% in ½ normal saline; dextrose 5% in 0.45% sodium chloride
D$_5$LR; D5LR	dextrose 5% in lactated Ringer's solution
D$_5$NS; D5NS	dextrose 5% in normal saline; dextrose 5% in 0.9% sodium chloride
DAW	dispense as written
DC; d/c	discontinue
D/C	discharge
DCA	direct compounding area
disp	dispense
EC	enteric-coated
Elix	elixir
eMAR	electronic medication administration record
EPO	epoetin alfa; erythropoietin
ER; XR; XL	extended-release
°F	degrees Fahrenheit; temperature in degrees Fahrenheit
FeSO$_4$	ferrous sulfate; iron
G-H-I	
g, G	gram
gr	grain
gtt; gtts	drop; drops
h; hr	hour
h.s.; HS	bedtime (comes from Latin hora somni <italic hora somni> meaning "hour of sleep")
IBU	ibuprofen; Motrin
IM	intramuscular
Inj	injection
IPA	isopropyl alcohol
ISMP	Institute for Safe Medication Practices
IV	intravenous
IVF	intravenous fluid
IVP	intravenous push
IVPB	intravenous piggyback
J-K-L	
K; K+	potassium
KCl	potassium chloride
kg	kilogram
L	liter
LAFW	laminar airflow workbench; hood
lb	pound
LD	loading dose
LVP	large-volume parenteral

Abbreviation	Meaning
JCAHO	Joint Commission on the Accreditation of Healthcare Organizations
M-N-O	
Mag; Mg; MAG	magnesium
mcg	microgram
MDI	metered-dose inhaler
MDV	multiple-dose vial
mEq	milliequivalent
mg	milligram
$MgSO_4$	magnesium sulfate; magnesium
mL	milliliter
mL/hr	milliliters per hour
mL/min	milliliters per minute
MMR	measles, mumps, and rubella vaccine
MRSA	methiciliin-resistant S. aureaus
MOM; M.O.M.	milk of magnesia
M.S.	morphine sulfate (save MS for multiple sclerosis)
MU; mu	million units
MVI; MVI-12	multiple vitamin injection; multivitamins for parenteral administration
Na^+	sodium
NaCl	sodium chloride; salt
NDC	National Drug Code
NF; non-form	nonformulary
NKA	no known allergies
NKDA	no known drug allergies
NPO, npo	nothing by mouth
NR; d.n.r.	no refills; do not repeat
NS	normal saline; 0.9% sodium chloride
½ NS	one-half normal saline; 0.45% sodium chloride
¼ NS	one-quarter normal saline; 0.225% sodium chloride
NSAID	nonsteroidal anti-inflammatory drug
NTG	nitroglycerin
OC	oral contraceptive
od; o.d.; OD	right eye
ODT	orally disintegrating tablet
OPTH; OPHTH; Opth	ophthalmic
os; o.s.; OS	left eye

Abbreviation	Meaning
OTC	over the counter; no prescription required
ou; o.u.; OU	both eyes; each eye
oz	ounce
P-Q-R	
p.c.; PC	after meals
PM; p.m.	afternoon; evening
PN	paternal nutrition
PO; po	orally; by mouth
PPE	personal protective equipment
PR	per rectum; rectally
PRN; p.r.n.	as needed; as occasion requires
PV	per vagina; vaginally
PVC	polyvinyl chloride
q	every
q.h.; qhour	every hour
q2h	every 2 hours
q4h	every 4 hours
q6h	every 6 hours
q8h	every 8 hours
q12h	every 12 hours
q24h	every 24 hours
q48h	every 48 hours
QA	quality assurance
QAM; qam	every morning
qDay; QD	every day
q.i.d.; QID	four times daily
QOD; Q other day; Q.O. Day	every other day
QPM; qpm	every evening
qs; qsad	quantity sufficient; a sufficient quantity to make
QTY; qty	quantity
qwk; qweek	every week
Rx	prescription; pharmacy; medication; drug; recipe; take
S-T	
sig	write on label; signa; directions
SL; sub-L	sublingual
SR	sustained-release

Abbreviation	Meaning
SS; ss	one-half
STAT, Stat	immediately; now
Sub-Q; SC; SQ; sq, subcut, SUBCUT	subcutaneous
SUPP; Supp	suppository
susp	suspension
SVP	small-volume parenteral
SW	sterile water
SWFI	sterile water for injection
Tab; tab	tablet
TB	tuberculosis
TBSP; tbsp	tablespoon; tablespoonful; 15 mL
TDS	transdermal delivery system
t.i.d.; TID	three times daily
t.i.w.; TIW	three times a week
TKO; TKVO; KO; KVO	to keep open; to keep vein open; keep open; keep vein open (a slow IV flow rate)
TNA	Total Nutrition Admixture
TPN	total parenteral nutrition
TSP; tsp	teaspoon; teaspoonful; 5 mL
U-V-W	
U or u	unit
u.d., UD, ut dictum utd	as directed
ung	ointment
USP	U.S. Pharmacopoeial Convention
USP-NF	*U.S. Pharmacopeia-National Forumulary*
UV	ultraviolet light
VAG; vag	vagina; vaginally
VO; V.O.; V/O	verbal order
w/o	without
X-Y-Z	
Zn	zinc

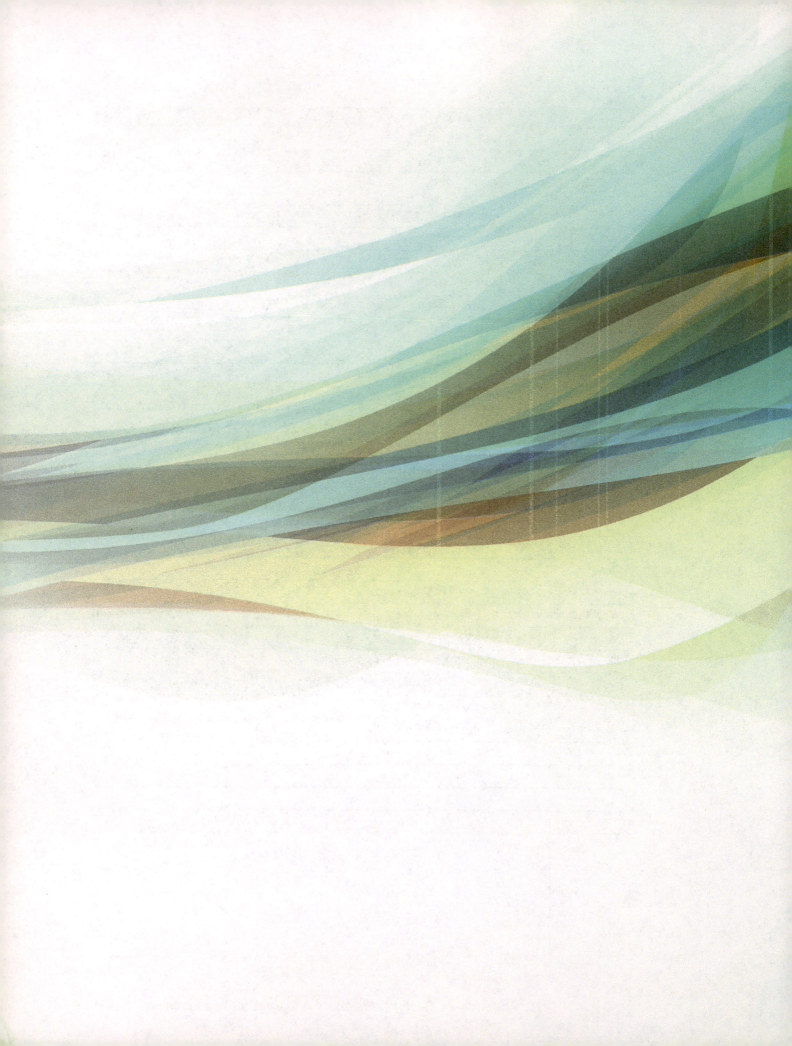

Measures and Conversions

Metric	*Volume*		
	1 L = 1,000 mL		
	1 mL = 1 cc		
	Weight		
	1 g = 1,000 mg		
	1 mg = 1,000 mcg		
Household	*Volume*	*Weight*	
	1 gal = 4 qt	1 lb = 16 oz	
	1 qt = 2 pt	*Length*	
	1 pt = 2 cups = 16 fl oz	1 yd = 3 ft	
	1 fl oz = 2 tbsp = 6 tsp	1 ft = 12 in	

CONVERSIONS

	Household	Apothecary	Metric
Volume	1 qt 5 32 fl oz		0.96 L
	1 pint 5 16 fl oz		480 mL*
	1 cup 5 8 fl oz		240 mL
	2 tbsp 5 1 fl oz	6 f ʒ 1 f ℥	30 mL*
	1 tbsp	3 f ʒ	15 mL
	1 tsp	1 f ʒ	5 mL†
		1 ℳ	0.0625 mL
Weight	2.2 lb		1 kg
	1 lb		454 g
	1 oz	8 ʒ	30 g
Length	1 in		2.5 cm

*There are actually 29.57 mL in 1 fl oz, but 30 mL is usually used. When packaging a pint, companies will typically include 473 mL, rather than the full 480 mL, thus saving money over time.

†There are actually 3.75 mL in an apothecary f. However, convention dictates that 1 f ʒ 5 mL 5 1 tsp.

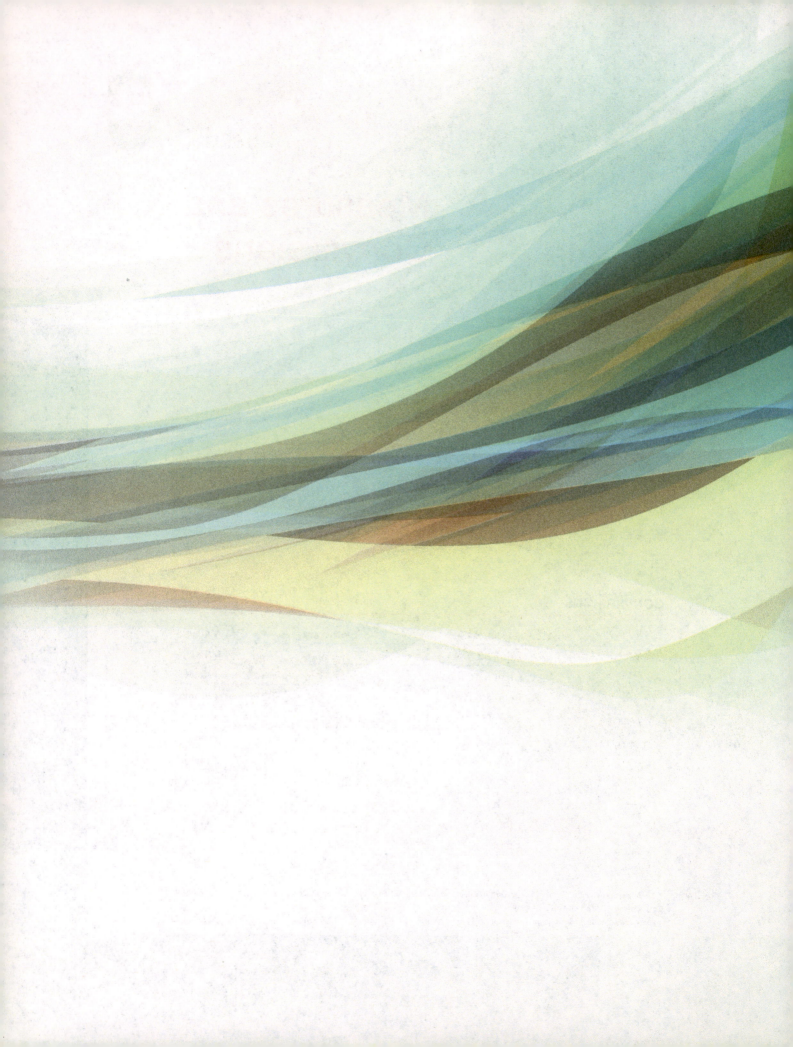

ASHP/ACPE Accreditation Standards

The following identifies the *ASHP/ACPE Accreditation Standards* addressed in each chapter of Paradigm's *Pharmacy Calculations for Technicians*, Seventh Edition. This appendix identifies the *ASHP/ACPE Standards* associated with the chapter content. This list is meant for guidance purposes only and was compiled by the authors and editor. Neither ASHP nor ACPE has participated in or had any role in creating the list of standards or any other content that is included in this book.

Unit 1: Fundamentals of Pharmacy Calculations

Chapter 1: Understanding Number Systems and Operations

> 1.4, 1.8, 1.10, 2.6

Chapter 2: Performing Ratio, Percent, and Proportion Calculations

> 1.8, 1.10, 2.6, 4.2

Chapter 3: Developing Prescription and Medication Order Literacy Skills

> 1.4, 1.8, 2.6, 3.2, 4.2

Unit 2: Common Pharmacy Calculations

Chapter 4: Understanding Measurement Systems and Conversions

> 1.4, 1.8, 1.10, 2.6, 4.2

Chapter 5: Calculating Doses for Oral Medications

> 1.8, 1.10, 2.6, 3.2, 4.2

Chapter 6: Calculating Doses for Injectable Medications

> 1.8, 1.10, 2.6, 3.2, 3.15, 4.2

Unit 3: Specialized and Advanced Pharmacy Calculations

Chapter 7: Performing Calculations for Compounding

> 1.4, 1.8, 1.10, 2.6, 3.15, 4.2

Chapter 8: Conducting Business Operations

> 1.4, 1.8, 1.10, 2.6, 3.19

Chapter 9: Performing Calculations for Sterile Parenteral Solutions

> 1.4, 1.8, 1.10, 2.6, 3.15, 4.2

Index

When the letter *t* or *f* follows a page number, the reference relates to either a *table* or a *figure*.

Photo Credits

Chapter 6 pg. 206 © magicoven/Shutterstock.com, pg. 207 George Brainard/© Paradigm Education Solutions, pg. 208 © Paradigm Education Solutions, pg. 209 © Paradigm Education Solutions, pg. 210 © Paradigm Education Solutions, pg. 211 © Paradigm Education Solutions, pg. 217 © Paradigm Education Solutions, pg. 218 © Paradigm Education Solutions, pg. 219 © Paradigm Education Solutions, pg. 220 © Looka/Shutterstock.com, pg. 229 © Paradigm Education Solutions, pg. 230 © Paradigm Education Solutions, pg. 231 © Paradigm Education Solutions, pg. 233 Image used with permission from Fresenius Kabi USA, LLC., © Paradigm Education Solutions, pg. 234 © Paradigm Education Solutions, pg. 235 © Paradigm Education Solutions, pg. 236 © Orawan Pattarawimonchai/Shutterstock.com, pg. 237 © Paradigm Education Solutions, pg. 239 © Paradigm Education Solutions, pg. 240 © Paradigm Education Solutions, pg. 241 © Paradigm Education Solutions, pg. 242 © Paradigm Education Solutions, pg. 243 © Paradigm Education Solutions, pg. 244 © Paradigm Education Solutions, pg. 245 © Paradigm Education Solutions, pg. 246 © Paradigm Education Solutions

Unit 3 pg. 251 © hedgehog94/Shutterstock.com

Chapter 7 pg. 255 © semyon lorbeg/ Shutterstock.com, pg. 269 George Brainard/ © Paradigm Education Solutions, pg. 271 © Paradigm Education Solutions, pg. 272 © Paradigm Education Solutions, pg. 276 © Paradigm Education Solutions

Chapter 8 pg. 280 © Natali55522/Shutterstock .com, pg. 283 © Dragna Gordic/Shutterstock .com, pg. 285 © Paradigm Education Solutions

Chapter 9 pg. 330 © Paradigm Education Solutions, pg. 331 © Paradigm Education Solutions, pg. 334 © Paradigm Education Solutions, pg. 335 © Paradigm Education Solutions, pg. 336 © Paradigm Education Solutions, pg. 337 © Paradigm Education Solutions, pg. 338 © Paradigm Education Solutions, pg. 340 © Paradigm Education Solutions, pg. 353 © Paradigm Education Solutions, pg. 357 © Paradigm Education Solutions, pg. 358 © Paradigm Education Solutions, pg. 368 © Paradigm Education Solutions, pg. 369 © Paradigm Education Solutions, pg. 375 © Paradigm Education Solutions, pg. 376 © Paradigm Education Solutions

Appendix A pg. 387 © Paradigm Education Solutions, pg. 398 © Paradigm Education Solutions